CHALLENGES IN PARKINSON'S DISEASE

Edited by **Jolanta Dorszewska**
and **Wojciech Kozubski**

Challenges in Parkinson's Disease
http://dx.doi.org/10.5772/61880
Edited by Jolanta Dorszewska and Wojciech Kozubski

Contributors
Patrick Flood, Monika Sharma, Naik Arbabzada, Michelle Hyczy De Siqueira Tosin, Beatriz Oliveira, Massimo Piacentino, Giacomo Beggio, Lorenzo Volpin, Sarat Chandra Yenisetti, Priyanka Modi, Ayajuddin Mohamad, Limamanen Phom, Zevelou Koza, Abhik Das, Rahul Chaurasia, Saikat Samadder, Bovito Achumi, Rajesh Singh Pukhrambam, Muralidhara, Davide Vito Moretti, Anahí Chavarría, Perla Ugalde-MUñiz, Jesús Pérez-H, Satoshi Goto, David Eidelberg, Hideo Mure, Chi-Meng Tzeng, Zhiming Li, Maria Satue, Vicente Polo, Sofia Otin, Jose M. Larrosa, Luis E. Pablo, Elena Garcia-Martin, Javier Obis, Sebastiano Cavallaro, Valentina La Cognata, Francesca Cavalcanti, Velia D'Agata, Iván Galtier, Antonieta Nieto, José Barroso, Fabin Han, Javier Blesa, Ines Trigo-Damas, Ana Quiroga-Varela, Natalia Lopez-Gonzalez Del Rey, Jose A. Obeso, Jasna Saponjic, Jelena Petrovic, Katarina Lazic, Jelena Ciric, Unax Lertxundi, Rafael Hernández, Saioa Domingo-Echaburu, Javier Peral-Aguirregoitia, Juan Medrano, Jolanta Dorszewska, Wojciech Kozubski, Samuel Sw Tay, Meenalochani Sivasubramanian, Thameem Dheen, Keun-A Chang, Seonghan Kim, Susanne Schmid, Andrea R. DiSebastiano, Michael D Staudt, Matthew O. Hebb, Hu Xu, Simon Benoit

Published by InTech
Janeza Trdine 9, 51000 Rijeka, Croatia

Publishing Process Manager Ana Simcic
Technical Editor SPi Global
Cover InTech Design team

First published August, 2016
Printed in Croatia

Additional hard copies can be obtained from orders@intechopen.com

Challenges in Parkinson's Disease, Edited by Jolanta Dorszewska and Wojciech Kozubski
p. cm.
Print ISBN 978-953-51-2463-4
Online ISBN 978-953-51-2464-1

For EU product safety concerns:
IN TECH d.o.o., Prolaz Marije Krucifikse Kozulić 3, 51000 Rijeka, Croatia,
info@intechopen.com or visit our website at intechopen.com.

Meet the editors

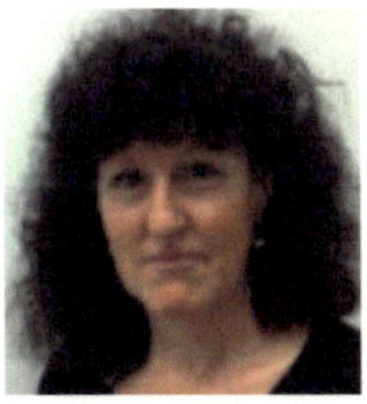

Associate Professor Jolanta Dorszewska is Chief of Laboratory of Neurobiology, Department of Neurology, Poznan University of Medical Sciences (PUMS), Poznan, Poland. She graduated from PUMS (M.Sc. Pharmacy, 1987), obtained PhD degree at PUMS (1996) and D.Sc. in Medical Sciences at PUMS (2004). Between the years 1999 and 2000, she worked as a Research Scientist at the Institute for Basic Research in Developmental Disabilities, New York, USA. Associate Professor Dorszewska has authored and co-authored about 100 papers mainly concerning the pathophysiology of Parkinson's and Alzheimer's diseases as well as epilepsy and migraine. She is a co-author and co-editor of books on genetic and biochemical factors in neurological diseases. She is a guest editor of two theme issue in Current Genomics (2014, 2013) and a member of editorial board in Advanced Alzheimer's Disease and Austin Alzheimer's and Parkinson's Disease (USA).

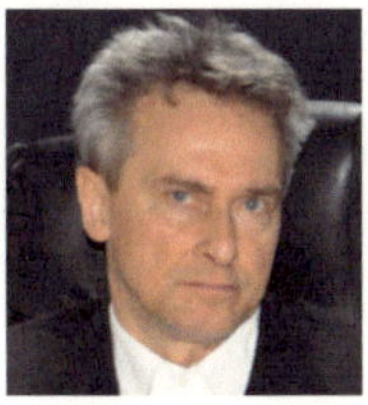

Prof. Wojciech Kozubski is Head of Chair & Department of Neurology, University of Medical Sciences in Poznan, Poland. Prof. Wojciech Kozubski graduated in Medical School in Lodz, Poland, in 1980. During the years 1980–1983, he was a PhD student in the Department of Neurology, Medical School in Lodz, and next—after his PhD degree—an assistant, adjunct scientific worker and assistant professor in this department. He was scholarshiped in Academic Unit of Neuroscience of Charing Cross & Westminster Medical School, University of London (1987–1988); Department of Neurology in Sackler School of Medicine, University of Tel-Aviv (1990) and in Department of Neurology in University of Trondheim, Norway (1990–1991). Prof. Kozubski is an author and co-author of over 290 papers (102 of them are original) concerning mainly the pathophysiology of migraine and related headaches, pathophysiology of stroke, dementia, treatment of headaches and stroke. He is a co-author and co-editor of the Handbook of Clinical Neurology for neurologists, on brain tumors, affective diseases of nervous system, therapy in neurology. He is an editor of the Handbook of Treatment in Neurology and co-author and co-editor of the Handbooks of Clinical Neurology for medical students. He is a co-author of the monograph on stroke aphasia. During the years 2011–2014, he was the President of Polish Neurological Society; in the years 1999–2001, President of Polish Headache Society.

Contents

Preface

Despite being discovered almost 200 years ago, Parkinson's disease is still not fully understood. Current state of knowledge concerning Parkinson's disease and other movement disorders is growing rapidly. This development is related to numerous discoveries in the field of genetics and significant improvement in neuroimaging techniques and surgical protocols, especially deep brain stimulation treatment. There is also a continuing search for markers of early diagnosis and the establishment of effective pharmacotherapy.

This publication is a sum up of knowledge on the genetic factors and neuronal death mechanisms induced by excitotoxic and inflammatory agents. We summarize the pathophysiology observed both in patients with Parkinson's disease and in experimental models. The book also contains the latest views on drug therapy used in the treatment of parkinsonism and other therapeutic approaches for Parkinson's disease.

We hope that this book may help in understanding the complex mechanisms behind Parkinson's disease pathogenesis and guide clinicians to right diagnosis and therapy.

Associate Professor Jolanta Dorszewska, MDs, PhD
Laboratory of Neurobiology,
Department of Neurology,
Poznan University of Medical Sciences,
Poland

Professor Wojciech Kozubski, MD, PhD
Chair and Department of Neurology,
Poznan University of Medical Sciences,
Poland

Chapter 1

Introductory Chapter - Genetic and Biochemical Factors in Parkinson's Disease

Jolanta Dorszewska and Wojciech Kozubski

Additional information is available at the end of the chapter

http://dx.doi.org/10.5772/64216

1. Introduction

Worldwide increased life expectancy, which was seen in the second half of the twentieth century, has contributed to an increased number of cases of diseases typical of old age, including Parkinson's disease (PD). At present, PD is one of the most common degenerative diseases of the central nervous system (CNS) and affects nearly 2% of the population over the age of 65 and 5% over the age of 85. Moreover, the estimates show that in the face of population aging, the number of patients with this neurodegenerative disease will maintain an upward trend.

Although PD was first described nearly 200 years ago, it is still an incurable disease and its cause is not fully understood. It is known that disturbances in the structure of two pathological proteins of PD, alpha-synuclein (ASN) and Parkin, may lead to the formation of Lewy bodies (LB), which lead to damage of dopaminergic neurons and decreased levels of dopamine (DA). The disturbances in the structure of ASN and Parkin are due to both genetic and environmental factors. Despite numerous reports in the literature concerning the molecular basis of this disease, little is known about the interactions occurring between the individual genes responsible for encoding these proteins and the pathological manifestation of PD [1–8].

As a result of the lack of knowledge of PD pathomechanism, it is also not possible to have early, potentially intravital, diagnosis of this disease. Currently, the diagnosis of PD is based on clinical criteria, supported with neuroimaging, and is only a probable diagnosis of this disease. Reliable detection of PD is only possible after testing for the presence of neuropathological changes in the brain that is typical for this disease and is carried out *postmortem*. It is known that lack of early and definite diagnosis of PD may make it difficult to provide effective therapy to slow down the progression of the disease and can decrease the quality of life of patients [9].

PD belongs to the disorders of the extrapyramidal system (EPS), in which we observe symptoms in a number of nonmotor (NMS) symptoms, such as dementia, hallucinations, depression, and orthostatic hypotension, in addition to motor disorders [9–12].

Many studies are currently being conducted on the pathogenesis of PD in many research centers around the world, and knowledge of this disease is growing rapidly. In the last two decades, new genes associated with PD (PARK1-PARK18) were discovered, and there was a remarkable progress of surgical treatment techniques using deep brain stimulation (DBS) of selected brain structures [6].

2. Genes important for pathogenesis of Parkinson's disease

The causes of PD are both genetic and environmental. To date, a number of genes associated with the presence of PD have been described within distinct patient families (familial PD, FPD) and/or corresponding locations of genes identified as PARK (PARK1-PARK16) as described in [5]. It is believed that genetic factors include mutations of the *SNCA* gene (PARK1, PARK4), encoding the ASN protein, may also be responsible for increased susceptibility in sporadic PD (SPD) [6,7].

It has been shown that approximately 5–10% of all known PD patients are people with FPD, a monogenic condition that is classically inherited in a recessive or dominant manner. The molecular mechanisms responsible for RPD also play an important role in the pathogenesis of SPD.

Moreover, SPD occurs due to the influence of various factors, including signal transduction, vesicular transport, the process of autophagy, and mitochondrial dysfunction. It is also suggested that the clinical heterogeneity of PD, including SPD, may involve interactions not only in genetic and environmental factors, as well as in the reactions between genes, such as *SNCA, PRKN, LRRK2, PINK1*, and their protein products: ASN, Parkin, LRRK2, and PINK1, respectively [1–8].

3. Oxidative damage and hyperhomocysteinemia and biogenic amines in Parkinson's disease

It is known that the degenerative process in PD occurs for many years before the manifestation of clinical symptoms. There are several hypotheses to explain the pathological processes in PD. One of them indicates the participation of oxidative stress in the damage that occurs to dopaminergic neurons [13–15]. In oxidative neuron damage, it is possible that impaired metabolism of homocysteine (Hcy) and other biothiols, such as methionine (Met), cysteine (Cys), and glutathione (GSH), may be involved. Moreover, Hcy, or its oxidative product homocysteine acid, may increase prooxidative activity, most probably through its direct interaction with NMDA receptors (as agonist of NMDA receptor). Many of the literature reports indicate that pathogenesis of PD is associated with increased apoptosis [13,15–18].

Homocysteine in physiological condition is converted to Met and Cys, depending on the activity of enzymes MTHFR, MTR, MTHFD1, and CBS, encoded by genes *MTHFR, MTR, MTHFD1,* and *CBS,* respectively [13]. Activity of these enzymes depends on the genotype of the gene encoding a given enzyme. As also shown in [13], the following genotypes are included in the pathogenesis of PD, for Hcy metabolites, Met [MTR, AA (A2756G)], Cys [MTR, AG (A2756G)], and Met/Hcy [MTHFR: CC, CT (C677T), and AA (A1298C), and GG (G1793A); MTHFD1 AA (G1958A); MTR AA (A2756G)] and Hcy [MTHFR: CT (C677T) and GG (G1793A); MTR, AG (A2756G)].

Biogenic amines are also involved in the generation of oxidative stress in the course of PD and include catecholamines such as norepinephrine (NE), epinephrine (E), DA and serotonin (5-HT). Catecholamines are subject to nonenzymatic autoxidation and form highly reactive derivatives. Increased endogenous neurotoxin levels may lead to the formation of ubiquitin and ASN-positive cytoplasmic inclusions (LB) [10–12]. Regulation of plasma biogenic amine levels in PD affects both coding by genes the enzymes responsible for metabolism (*COMT, MAO-A* and *MAO-B*), and the amines' transport and reuptake (*NET, DAT, SERT*). Polymorphisms in genes related to trading of biogenic amines may influence the manifestation of this disease, especially *NET* GA (c.1287G>A) and *NET* AA (c.1287G>A) [12].

4. L-Dopa therapy effects in Parkinson's disease

The strategy of therapy of patients with movement disorders, particularly PD, is based essentially on the strengthening of dopaminergic transmission with exogenous L-dihydroxy-phenylalanine (L-dopa) and DA agonists [9]. It has been shown that long-term treatment of PD patients with L-dopa improves their motor functions by increasing the level of central DA.

At the same time, it has been shown that increasing dopaminergic neuronal damage in PD may reduce the effectiveness of L-dopa and DA agonist therapy. Moreover, in patients with PD, due to the loss of dopaminergic neurons in the *striatum,* L-dopa may penetrate other dopaminergic neurons, especially the mesolimbic, and lead to emotional and neuropsychiatric disorders in these patients.

L-Dopa therapy in PD may also induce cardiovascular disease and stroke by increasing the plasma levels of risk factors for vascular diseases, such as asymmetric dimethylarginine (ADMA) and Hcy. Moreover, L-dopa leads to increased levels of 8-oxo-2'-deoxyguanosine (8-oxo2dG), a parameter of oxidative stress, and changes levels of biogenic amines and proteins involved in apoptosis [9,15,19–21].

5. Summary

Although PD has been known and studied since the early nineteenth century, the cause of death of dopaminergic neurons remains unknown and the treatment of this disease focuses on treating symptoms.

In PD, as in other neurodegenerative diseases, research seeks to determine biomarkers to enable early definite diagnosis of this disease and the development of effective neuroprotective or modulatory disease drugs. PD patients who do not respond to conventional drug treatment are currently treated using one of the new surgical techniques, including DBS.

Currently, research in PD is looking for a therapy that can ensure effective antiparkinsonian treatment, eliminate dyskinesia, and slow or stop the progression of this disease.

Author details

Jolanta Dorszewska[1*] and Wojciech Kozubski[2]

*Address all correspondence to: dorszewskaj@yahoo.com

1 Laboratory of Neurobiology, Department of Neurology, Poznan University of Medical Sciences, Poznan, Poland

2 Chair and Department of Neurology, Poznan University of Medical Sciences, Poznan, Poland

References

[1] Polrolniczak A, Dorszewska J, Florczak J, Owecki M, Rozycka A, Rubis B, Jagodziński PP, Kozubski W. Analysis of *SNCA* and *PARK2* mutations in sporadic Parkinson's disease. In: 10th International Conference on Alzheimer's and Parkinson's Diseases; 9–13 March 2011; Barcelona, Spain. Neurodegenerative Diseases. 2011; 8(Supp. 1):P1.

[2] Dorszewska J. Genetic factors in Parkinson's disease. Current Genomics. 2013;14:485. doi: 10.2174/1389202914081402061138l0

[3] Oczkowska A, Kozubski W, Lianeri M, Dorszewska J. Mutations in *PRKN* and SNCA genes important for the progress of Parkinson's disease. Current Genomics. 2013;14:502–517. doi: 10.2174/13892029146661312l0205839

[4] Oczkowska A, Lianeri M, Kozubski W, Dorszewska J. Mutations of PARK genes and alpha-synuclein, and parkin levels. In: Abdul Qayyum Rana, editor. A Synopsis of Parkinson's Disease. InTech, Rijeka, Croatia; 2014. pp. 1–38.

[5] Oczkowska A, Kozubski W, Lianeri M, Dorszewska J. Genetic variants in diseases of the extrapyramidal system. Current Genomics. 2014;15:18–27. doi: 10.2174/1389202914666131210213327

[6] Dorszewska J. Genetics of Parkinson's disease and other diseases of the extrapyramidal system. Current Genomics. 2014;15:1. doi: 10.2174/1389202915011403061l0937

[7] Oczkowska A, Kozubski W, Dorszewska J. Alpha-synuclein in Parkinson's disease. (Alfa-synukleina w chorobie Parkinsona). Przeglad Lekarski. 2014;71:26–32. Polish.

[8] Oczkowska A, Florczak-Wyspianska J, Permoda-Osip A, Owecki M, Lianeri M, Kozubski W, Dorszewska J. Analysis of PRKN variants and clinical features in Polish patients with Parkinson's disease. Current Genomics. 2015;16:215–223. doi: 10.2174/1389202916666150326002549

[9] Dorszewska J, Prendecki M, Lianeri M, Kozubski W. Molecular effects of L-dopa therapy in Parkinson's disease. Current Genomics. 2014;15:11–17. doi: 10.2174/1389202914666131210213042

[10] Florczak J, Dorszewska J, Owecki M, Polrolniczak A, Bugaj R, Kozubski W. Catecholamines in patients with Parkinson's disease and multiple system atrophy – preliminary report. In: 7th International Congress on Mental Dysfunctions & Other Non-Motor Features in Parkinson's Disease & Related Disorders; 9–12 December 2010; Barcelona, Spain. 2010. p. 1.

[11] Bugaj R, Wolny L, Rozycka A, Dorszewska J, Florczak J, Półrolniczak A, Owecki M, Jagodziński PP, Kozubski W. *MAO-A, COMT, NET* gene polymorphisms and the levels of catecholamines and their metabolites in patients with Parkinson's disease. In: 10th International Conference on Alzheimer's and Parkinson's Diseases; 9–13 March 2011; Barcelona, Spain. Neurodegenerative Diseases. 2011; 8(Supp. 1):P1.

[12] Dorszewska J, Prendecki M, Oczkowska A, Rozycka A, Lianeri M, Kozubski W. Polymorphism of the *COMT, MAO, DAT, NET* and *5-HTT* genes, and biogenic amines in Parkinson's disease. Current Genomics. 2013;14:518–533. doi: 10.2174/13892029114666131210210241

[13] Dorszewska J, Florczak J, Różycka A, Kempisty B, Jaroszewska-Kolecka J, Chojnacka K, Trzeciak WH, Kozubski W. Oxidative DNA damage and level of thiols as related to polymorphism of *MTHFR, MTR, MTHFD1* in Alzheimer's and Parkinson's disease. Acta Neurobiologiae Experimentalis. 2007;67:113–129.

[14] Dorszewska J, Florczak J, Kozubski W. Level of oxidative DNA damage and expression of apoptotic proteins in patients with Parkinson's disease treatment with L-dopa. In: XVIII WFN World Congress on Parkinson's Disease and Related Disorders. 13–16 December 2009; Miami Beach, FL, USA. Parkinsonism and Related Disorders. 2009;15(Suppl. 2):111.

[15] Dorszewska J, Kozubski W. Oxidative DNA damage and the level of biothiols, and L-dopa therapy in Parkinsons disease. In: Abdul Qayyum Rana, editor. Etiology and Pathophysiology of Parkinson's Disease. InTech, Rijeka, Croatia; 2011. pp. 349–372.

[16] Dorszewska J, Florczak J, Jaroszewska-Kolecka J, Kozubski W. Homocysteine and asymmetric dimethylarginine (ADMA) in the plasma of patients with Parkinson's disease. In: XVII WFN World Congress on Parkinson's Disease and Related Diso-

rders, 9–13 December 2007; Amsterdam, Holland. Parkinsonism and Related Disorders. 2007;13:34.

[17] Rozycka A, Jagodzinski PP, Kozubski W, Lianeri M, Dorszewska J. Homocysteine level and mechanisms of injury in Parkinson's disease as related to *MTHFR, MTR*, and *MTHFD1* genes polymorphisms and L-dopa treatment. Current Genomics. 2013;14: 534–542. doi: 10.2174/13892029114666131210210559

[18] Dorszewska J, Oczkowska A, Prendecki M, Lianeri M, Kozubski W. *MTHFR* and other enzymes associated with the circulation of methyl in neurodegenerative diseases. In: Roger Evans, editor. Methylenetetrahydrofolate Reductase (MTHFR) in Health and Disease. NOVA Sciences Publishers, Inc, NY, USA; 2015. pp. 1–39.

[19] Dorszewska J, Florczak J, Kozubski W. Effects of L-DOPA treatment on the level of oxidative damage to DNA and thiols in patients with Parkinson's disease. In: XVI International Congress on Parkinson's Disease and Related Disorders, 5–9 June 2005; Berlin, Germany. Parkinsonism and Related Disorders. 2005;11(Suppl. 2):133.

[20] Florczak J, Dorszewska J, Kozubski W. Influence of L-dopa treatment on the level of oxidative damage to DNA, and the concentration of thiol compounds in patients with Parkinson's disease. (Wplyw dlugosci leczenia preparatami L-dopy na poziom oksydacyjnych uszkodzen DNA i stezenie zwiazów tiolowych u pacjentów z choroba Parkinsona). Neurologia i Neurochirurgia Polska. 2008;42(Suppl. 1):36–44. Polish.

[21] Dorszewska J, Florczak J, Kozubski W. Asymmetric dimethylarginine in the plasma of patients with Alzheimer's and Parkinson's diseases. In: Alzheimer's and Parkinson's Diseases: Advances, Concepts and New Challenges. 9th International Conference AD/PD, 11–15 March 2009; Prague, Czech Republic. Neurodegenerative Diseases. 2009;6:548.

Chapter 2

Genetics of Parkinson's Disease: The Role of Copy Number Variations

Valentina La Cognata, Velia D'Agata,
Francesca Cavalcanti and Sebastiano Cavallaro

Additional information is available at the end of the chapter

http://dx.doi.org/10.5772/62881

Abstract

Parkinson's disease (PD), the second most common progressive neurodegenerative disorder, was long believed to be a non-genetic sporadic origin syndrome. The identification of distinct genetic loci responsible for rare Mendelian forms of PD has represented a revolutionary breakthrough, allowing to discover novel mechanisms underlying this debilitating still incurable condition. Along with single-nucleotide polymorphisms (SNPs), other kinds of DNA molecular defects have emerged as significant disease-causing mutations, including large chromosomic structural rearrangements and copy number variations (CNVs). Due to their size variability and to the different sensitivity and resolution of detection methodologies, CNVs constitute a particular challenge in genetic studies and the pathogenetic or susceptibility impact of specific CNVs on PD is currently under debate. In this chapter, we will review the current literature and bioinformatic data describing the involvement of CNVs on PD pathobiology. We will discuss the recently highlighted role of *PARK2* heterozygous CNVs, the possible common founder effects of PD gene rearrangements and the importance to map genetic breakpoints. We will also add a summary about the current available molecular methods and bioinformatics web resources to detect and interpret CNVs. Assessing the global genome-wide burden of large CNVs and elucidating the role of *de novo* rare structural variants on PD may reveal new candidate genes and consequently ameliorate diagnosis and counselling of mutations carriers.

Keywords: Parkinson's disease, genetics, genomics, copy number variations, DNA rearrangements, methods

1. Introduction

Parkinson's disease (PD) is a progressive debilitating movement disorder and constitutes the second most common neurologic disease after Alzheimer's disease, affecting approximately 1% of the population older than 65 years of age [1].

Clinically, most patients present resting tremor, bradykinesia, stiffness of movement and postural instability. These major symptoms derive from the profound and selective loss of dopaminergic neurons of *substantia nigra pars compacta* (SNc), although SNc seems to become involved later in the middle stage of the disease [1]. The neuropathological hallmarks of PD are round eosinophilic intracytoplasmic inclusions termed Lewy bodies (LBs) and dystrophic neurites (Lewy neurites) present in surviving neurons [1], both composed of alpha-synuclein aggregates. In more advanced stages, patients can also develop a range of non-motor symptoms, including rapid eye movement, sleep behaviour disorder, constipation, depression and cognitive decline. Although drugs such a levodopa (L-DOPA) or surgical intervention (deep brain stimulation) can alleviate the motor symptoms, they do not halt disease progression and are not effective against the non-motor aspects of the disease [2].

PD is primarily a sporadic multifactorial disorder, resulting from an elaborate interplay of numerous elements: genes, susceptibility alleles, environmental exposures, gene-environment interactions and their overall impact on developing and aging brain. Important insights have been provided during the last years through studying the genetics, epidemiology and neuropathology of PD, together with the development of experimental *in vivo* and *in vitro* models. A prominent role of common underlying pathways, such as mitochondrial dysfunctions [3], oxidative stress [4] and impairment of the ubiquitin/proteasome system (UPS) system [5], is now supported by accumulating genetic studies, which demonstrate that PD-associated genes directly or indirectly impinge on mitochondrial integrity, reactive oxygen species production and protein clearance.

In this review chapter, we will introduce the genetics of PD and then we will focus on copy number variations (CNVs), a form of DNA structural rearrangements, which are currently attracting researchers' interest for their role in PD pathobiology.

2. PD: a genetic overview

PD was long believed to be a prototypical non-genetic disorder. In the last 15 years, however, the identification of distinct genetic loci responsible for rare monogenic Mendelian forms and the discovery of numerous risk factors have revolutionized this view and have provided novel clues to understand the molecular pathogenesis of this still incurable condition [1].

The Mendelian monogenic forms of PD are well-established and collectively account for about 30% of the familial and 3–5% of the sporadic cases [6]. These rare forms are caused by mutations in specific genes, which are inherited from parents in either a dominant or recessive way.

In the autosomal-dominant inheritance, one mutated allele of the gene is sufficient to cause the disease [6]. The *SNCA* (alpha-synuclein) gene, localized in the PARK1 locus, was the first to be associated to this pattern of transmission and was identified in an Italian American family with more than 60 affected individuals distributed on five generations [7]. Among family members, the disease was caused by the Ala53Thr (A53T) missense mutation, which induces a conformational change in the protein chain and facilitates alpha-synuclein aggregation. Additional disease-causing mutations in *SNCA* are currently known, including genetic variations in the coding regions (Ala30Pro, Glu46Lys), single-nucleotide substitution in 3′ UTR and dose-dependent genomic multiplications (duplications or triplications) [8–10] that will be discussed in the next sections. A second gene clearly associated to the dominant PD inheritance is *LRRK2* (locus PARK8), which encodes a large multi-domain protein called leucine-rich repeat kinase 2. *LRRK2* harbours several genetic variants recognized as pathogenic, some of which represent the most frequent causes of Mendelian and sporadic PD identified so far (i.e. Gly2019Ser and mutations altering codon Arg1441). The precise physiological function of LRRK2 is unknown; however, it is probably implicated in different cellular functions such as neurite outgrowth, cytoskeletal maintenance, vesicle trafficking and autophagic protein degradation [11].

Some monogenic forms of PD are inherited with the autosomal recessive pattern, and frequently, symptoms have an early onset. In these disorders, mutations in both alleles (either homozygous or compound heterozygous) cause the pathological phenotype [6]. Mutations in three genes cause the recessive typical form:

- *PARKIN* (locus PARK2), the most commonly mutated gene in the juvenile Parkinsonism, responsible of 50% of cases;
- *PINK1* (locus PARK6), which is present with a frequency variable from 1 to 9% depending on the ethnic background [12];
- *DJ1* (locus PARK7), which represents the less common cause (~1%) [1, 13].

These three genes will be discussed in the next sections.

The recessive cases of Parkinsonism can clinically manifest also in an atypical form, meaning that patients have clinical features of PD, neuronal loss in the SNc and additional cell degeneration in other regions of the nervous system, such as in the striatum. The genes currently identified as responsible of this forms of Parkinsonism are the following:

- *ATP13A2* (locus PARK9), whose mutations are associated with the Kufor–Rakeb syndrome, a form of recessively levodopa-responsive inherited atypical Parkinsonism [14]. This gene belongs to the P-type superfamily of ATPases that transport inorganic cations and other substrates across cell membranes [15];
- *PLA2G6* (*phospholipase A2 group VI*), localized in the locus PARK14, which has been recently associated to a particular Parkinsonian phenotype consisting of levodopa-responsive dystonia, pyramidal signs and cognitive/psychiatric features with onset in early adulthood [16];

- *FBXO7* (*F-box only protein 7*) is harboured in the PARK15 locus and responsible of the Parkinsonian-Pyramidal Disease (PPD), an autosomal recessive neurodegenerative disease with juvenile onset and additional pyramidal signs [17]. FBXO7 is a components of modular E3 ubiquitin protein ligases called SCFs (SKP1, cullin, F-box proteins), which function in phosphorylation-dependent ubiquitination.

Despite the existence of rare monogenic forms, it is now clear that PD is a genetically heterogeneous and most likely complex disorder. The complexity of PD is underlined by the notion that we are currently aware of dozens of more or less convincing loci, genes and risk factors linked to the different inherited or sporadic forms. For the sake of completeness, we mention here just some of them: *PARK3, GBA, UCHL1, PARK10, GIGYF2, PARK12, HTRA2, PARK16, DNAJ, HLA-DR, GAK-DGKQ, SYNJ1, GBAP1* [18–20]. This list is progressively extending thanks to the evidences revealed by linkage mapping analysis, genome-wide association studies (GWAS) and high-throughput genomic biotechnologies, such as next generation sequencing and array technologies [18, 21].

However, while the detection and interpretation of some kind of DNA molecular alterations, as single-nucleotide polymorphisms (SNPs), are relatively simple, CNVs genotyping is technically more challenging, partially due to the quantitative rather than the qualitative nature of the assay. These kinds of DNA molecular defects, therefore, are in general under-represented in genetic studies. In the next paragraphs, we will introduce CNVs and then we will focus on what is currently known about their pathogenic or susceptibility impact on PD pathobiology.

3. CNVs: origin, classification and clinical relevance

The genomic sequence along human chromosomes is constantly changing, and this process enables humans to evolve and adapt. The scientific community have long been aware of genetic variation at either size extreme (i.e. cytogenetically recognizable elements and SNPs). However, about 10 years ago, scientists began to recognize abundant variations of an intermediate size class known as structural variations. Within this class, CNVs, which involves unbalanced rearrangements that increase or decrease the DNA content, represent the largest component by far. Currently, the size of CNVs is defined as larger than 50 bp [22] and can be limited to a single gene or include a contiguous set of genes. These structural variants encompass more polymorphic base pairs than SNPs and finally result in an altered DNA diploid status (i.e. gain or loss of genomic region).

DNA structural changes and CNVs originate when specific architectural genomic elements are present that render DNA regions very susceptible to rearrangements. These latter can be classified as recurrent or non-recurrent events, depending on whether the same rearrangement is identified in unrelated individuals [23].

Three major mechanisms for the generation of recurrent and non-recurrent CNVs have been proposed. The most common cause of recurrent genomic rearrangements is the non-allelic homologous recombination (NAHR), which occurs during both mitosis and meiosis between two DNA blocks of high homology, like the region-specific low-copy repeats sequences (LCRs). Specifically, CNVs generate when tracts of directly oriented LCRs recombine by unequal crossing-over leading to both deletion and duplication of the genomic fragment [23, 24] (**Figure 1**). LCRs with different orientations can recombine to produce NAHR-mediated inversions or more complex genomic rearrangements.

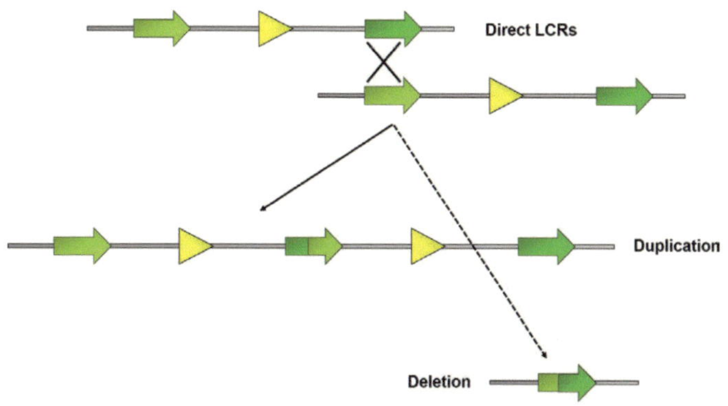

Figure 1. NAHR generates CNVs when genomic segments with high sequence similarity (direct LCRs, green arrows) recombine. This recombination can generate a duplication of the similar locus (yellow arrow) on one chromosome, while removing the copy from the other.

Non-recurrent CNVs can mainly result from non-homologous end joining (NHEJ) mechanism. NHEJ is the major cellular mechanism for double-strand break (DSB) repair. Upon DSB, NHEJ reconnects chromosome ends, very often editing them before ligation and leaving an information scar (i.e. random nucleotides added at the site of the breakage to facilitate the strands' alignment and ligation) [25] (**Figure 2**). NHEJ is more often associated with deletions and chromosomal translocations. However, complicated DNA intermediates have been proposed as origin mechanisms for duplications as well [26].

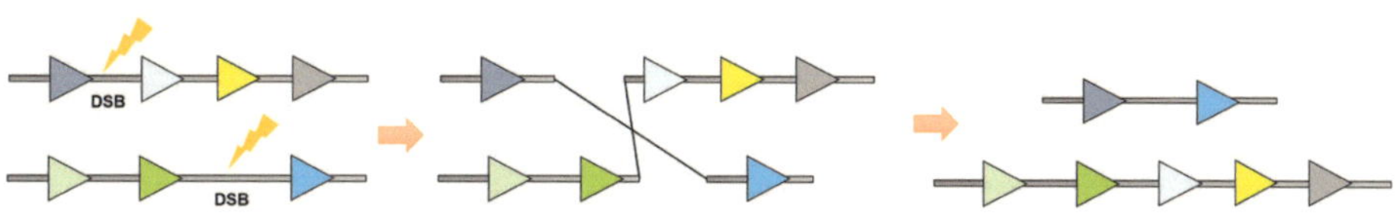

Figure 2. DBS in DNA sequence recruit NHEJ associated proteins to repair and ligate DNA strands together. First, end-repair protein replaces lost nucleotides on the double-strand break and DNA ligase associates broken DNA fragments together. If fragments from different chromosomes ligate together, duplications or deletions of sequence can occur.

The third mechanism proposed to trigger non-recurrent genomic rearrangements is fork stalling and template switching (FoSTeS) [27]. FoSTeS occurs when the DNA replication machinery pauses, the lagging strand dissociates from the polymerase holoenzyme and the template is switched with another region of the genome that is usually in physical proximity to the original replication fork. Replication continues based on a wrong template until the original fork is restored. Such template switching may occur several times before the replication process gets back to its original template, resulting in complex rearrangements (**Figure 3**) [25]. The pausing and stalling of the DNA replication machinery are common at certain nucleotide motifs and repetitive DNA sequences; however, such events can also occur due to chemical changes in DNA structure as DNA lesions or DNA alkylization [26]. CNVs generated by FoSTeS mainly originate during the S phase of the cell cycle as a consequence of DNA repair mechanisms. It should be noted that the CNVs created through FoSTeS are difficult to be distinguished from those generated by micro-homology-mediated breakpoint-induced repair (MMBIR), a mechanism of end-joining that relies on small-scale homology of DNA sequence at the ends of DSBs [26].

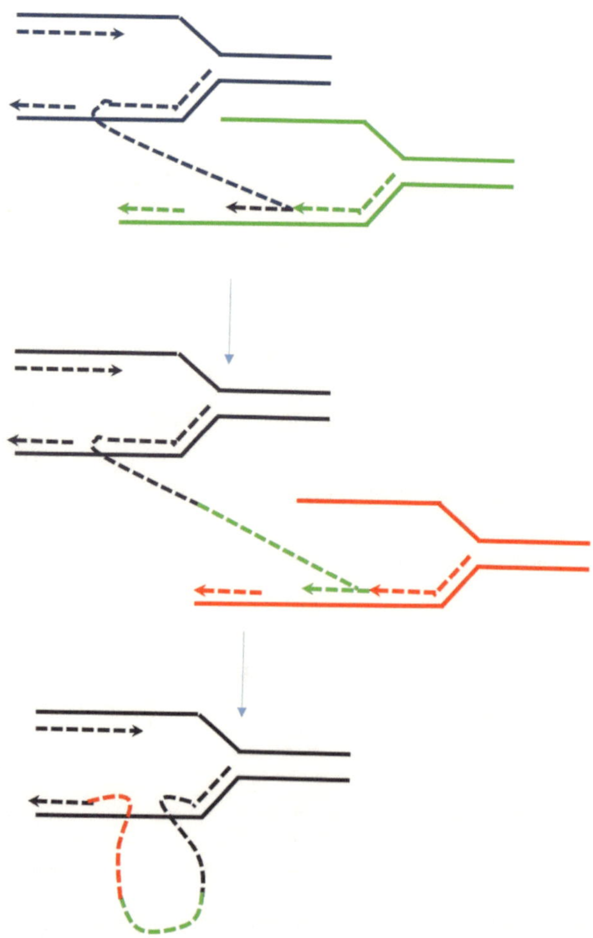

Figure 3. After the original stalling of the replication fork (dark blue lines), the lagging strand disengages and anneals to a second fork (green lines), followed by extension of the now 'primed' second fork and DNA synthesis. After the fork disengages, the tethered original fork with its lagging strand (blue and green lines) could invade a third fork (red lines). Serial replication fork disengaging and lagging strand invasion could occur several times (e.g. FoSTeS × 2, FoSTeS × 3, etc.) before resumption of replication on the original template.

CNVs are very common and constitute a prevalent source of genomic variations. These alterations may account for adaptive or behavioural traits, may have no phenotypic effects or can underlie diseases [22]. For this reason, determining the clinical significance of CNVs is very challenging and relies heavily on both frequency information from healthy control cohorts and databases with previously reported clinically relevant CNVs.

In a clinical setting, CNVs are categorized into five groups (according The American College of Medical Genetics and Genomics practice guidelines):

- Abnormal or pathogenic (e.g. well-established association with a disease);
- Likely pathogenic;
- VOUS (Variants of uncertain clinical significance – rare or private CNV);
- Likely benign;
- Benign (a polymorphic variant detected in a normal individual without clinical significance).

Specific large CNVs and single-gene dosage alterations have emerged as critical elements for the development and maintenance of the nervous system [28] and have appeared to contribute to hereditable or sporadic neurological diseases, such as neuropathies, epilepsy forms, autistic syndromes, psychiatric illnesses and also neurodegenerative diseases [23, 29–33]. In the next paragraphs, we will focus on the current evidences about the recurrence of CNVs in PD pathobiology.

4. CNVs in PD

4.1. Single-gene CNVs in familiar PD-genes

4.1.1. SNCA

Accumulating evidences show that alpha-synuclein gene (*SNCA*) copy number gains play a major role in the disease severity of PARK1. Singleton et al. [34] were the first to describe a genomic triplication of chromosome 4q21 22 containing the *SNCA* locus within a large family with PD autosomal-dominant inheritance pattern and dementia called the Spellman–Muenter family or Iowa Kindred. The size of the triplication region, confirmed with quantitative polymerase chain reaction (PCR) and fluorescence in situ hybridization (FISH) methodology, was over 2.0 Mb.

After the initial description, numerous families with *SNCA* genomic alterations have been reported. PD families with members carrying four copies of *SNCA* gene have been detected in South Africa, Iran, Japan, Pakistan and Italy [35–40]: in general, triplication generates very high expression of mRNA and protein and influences the clinical manifestations of PD, causing severe forms of Parkinsonism similar to dementia with Lewy body. Duplications have been reported in more numerous families than triplications [33, 38, 41–51]. In some of the patients with the same ethnic background (Japan), haplotype analysis revealed their derivation from common founders [43, 44]. In contrast to triplication carriers, the clinical phenotype of patients with duplicated *SNCA* resembles idiopathic PD, mainly with late age at onset, good efficacy for levodopa therapy, slower disease progression and without early development of dementia. An interesting familiar case, the Swedish-American family (named the "Lister family"), presents both duplicated and triplicated *SNCA* carriers within different branches of the pedigree (branches J and I), suggesting a primary duplication event followed later by another one and resulting in the triplication [52, 53]. A similar pedigree, the Ikeuchi family, has both heterozygote and homozygote duplication from a consanguineous marriage (producing a pseudo-triplication) [54]. The clinical features of the individual with the *SNCA* homozygote duplication showed severe Parkinsonism similar to that of a triplication carrier.

In 2007, Ahn et al. [42] firstly reported two sporadic patients with *SNCA* duplication from a large screen of PD patients. The age at onset was 65 and 50 years old for the two patients. Their clinical course was similar to typical sporadic PD without severe progression or cognitive decline. Other cases of sporadic PD carrying *de novo SNCA* duplication were later revealed by different detection assays [55–59].

The breakpoint of *SNCA* multiplication is different among families and sporadic patients. The largest multiplication detected so far is about 41.2 Mb, containing 150 genes and defined a partial trisomy 4q [55]. The smallest one sizes about 0.2 Mb and was found in a Japanese family [43]. The size and gene make-up of each multiplicated region does not seem to severely influence the clinical presentation of the carrier. The single common determining factor that appears between all patients with *SNCA* multiplications is the presence of the more than two copies of the entire gene.

Significant data regard the mosaicism of *SNCA* rearrangements, indicating the situation in which not all the body cells present the same genetic composition but specific groups of cells have a different genomic architecture. In this regard, Perandones et al. [60] have reported two interesting cases. In these patients, the exon dosage test conducted on peripheral blood revealed no alterations, while FISH analysis conducted on interphase cells from the buccal cavity (oral mucosa cells) revealed a good percentage of cells with *SNCA* triplication or duplication. It should be noted that both patients displayed a Parkinsonian clinical phenotype already described for the SNCA duplication or triplication carriers. Since usually only DNA from peripheral lymphocytic tissues are examined for *SNCA* rearrangements, it should be taken into consideration that the possibility to examine cells from other tissues in order to detect low-grade mosaicism.

4.1.2. PARK2

Although the *SNCA* story suggests a gain of function, several early-onset forms of PD have demonstrated the role of loss of function in the aetiology of the disease. The most common loss-of-function causes of early-onset PD are mutations in Parkin (or *PARK2*) gene, one of the largest known genes of our genome harboured in the long arm of chromosome 6 (6q25.2-q27) and encoding an E3 ubiquitin ligase. Mutations of *PARK2* are particularly frequent in individuals with evidence of familiar recessive inheritance and account for 50% of the cases with juvenile PD. Parkin mutations also explain ~15% of the sporadic cases with onset before 45 [61, 62] and act as susceptibility alleles for late-onset forms of PD (2% of cases) [63].

The *PARK2* gene has a high mutation rate since it is located in the *core* of FRA6E site, one of the most mutation-susceptible common fragile site of human genome [25]. For this reason, more than 200 putative pathogenic mutations have been reported worldwide, affecting numerous ethnic populations [33, 35, 59, 64–77]. The *PARK2* mutation spectrum includes homozygous or compound heterozygous missense and nonsense point mutations, as well as several exon rearrangements (both duplications and deletions) involving all 12 exons and the promoter region. The list of studies focusing on *PARK2* CNVs is such high that describing them one by one is very arduous. Overall, Parkin CNVs mutations published so far are summarized in **Figure 4** and are collected in the Parkinson Disease Mutation database (http://www.molgen.vib-ua.be/PDMutDB), whose the reader is referred for a more complete overview. Recently, our research group has outlined a complex alternative splicing mechanism regulating the expression of *PARK2* [78–80]. These data suggest the existence of five additional exons that, however, have never been considered for dosage screening.

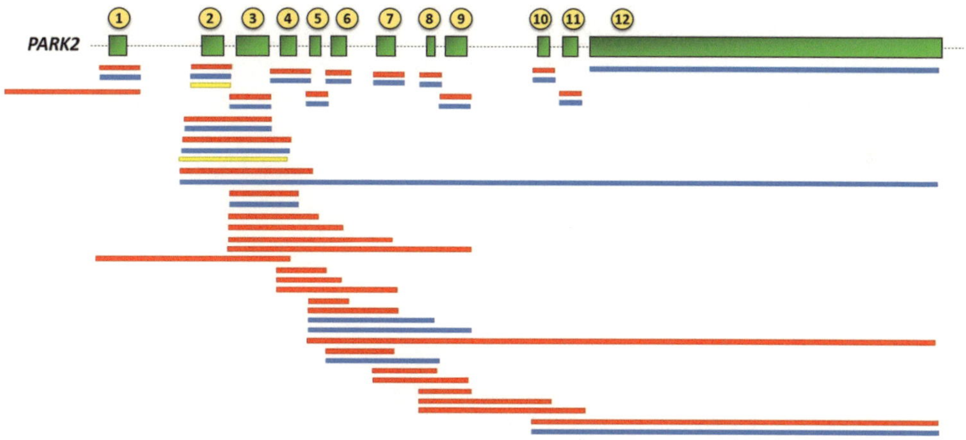

Figure 4. Schematic representation of *PARK2* genetic structure and currently identified CNVs in PD patients. All the canonical *PARK2* exons are involved in exons rearrangements. Red bars correspond to exons deletions, blue bars to duplications and yellow bars to triplications. All depicted CNVs can be found at the Parkinson Disease Mutation database (http://www.molgen.vib-ua.be/PDMutDB).

CNV rearrangements involving *PARK2* exons accounts for 50–60% of all pathogenic anomalies, rendering gene-dosage assays essential in Parkin mutational screening [81]. However, the *hot-spot* nature of this gene makes its quantitative analysis a particular challenge, and several issues need to be pointed out in this regard.

First of all, the determination of mutational phase of the rearrangements, meaning the assessment that amplified or deleted exons are really contiguous. Kim et al. [81] have showed that phase determination is a prerequisite for *PARK2* molecular diagnosis: by phase determination, several patients with apparent contiguous multi-exon deletions were re-diagnosed as compound heterozygotes. Simple gene-dosage assays seem to be not sufficient to determine the phase of rearrangements, and therefore, the true incidence of molecularly confirmed Parkin-type early-onset PD may be underestimated.

A second important point refers to breakpoint mapping which can be useful to compare exon rearrangements between patients and families and to study the possible causing event mechanism [82]. Just few papers have addressed this issue so far, but mostly report rearrangements into the region between *PARK2* exons 2 and 8 [25, 82]. In the majority of mapped cases, micro-homologies at breakpoint junctions were present, thus supporting NHEJ and FoSTeS/MMBIR as the major mechanisms responsible for *PARK2* genomic rearrangements [25].

Despite these hypotheses, it cannot be excluded that *PARK2* CNVs may arise in some minor ethnic groups from an ancient founder [83]. For example, haplotype analysis in four families from The Netherlands has showed a common haplotype of 1.2 Mb responsible for exon 7 duplication and a common haplotype of 6.3 Mb responsible for exon 4 deletion [82].

A relevant matter of ongoing debates is the pathogenic role of single-heterozygous *PARK2* CNVs. Several studies have sought to address this issue, but the findings published so far are inconsistent and conflicting. Some reports indicate that CNVs heterozygous mutations in *PARK2* associate with increased PD risk [49, 68], albeit others found no differences for an association [33, 69]. Not only association studies but also examinations of families have yielded contradictory results. Heterozygous family members of homozygous carriers have been described with mild PD signs of late onset [84, 85], whereas another group found no typical clinical signs of the disease [33]. Very recently, Huttenlocher et al. [86] have genotyped a large sample of Icelanders, observing that PD patients were more often heterozygous carriers of CNVs than controls, and confirmed these results by a meta-analysis study. These findings seem again to suggest that heterozygous carriers of *PARK2* CNVs have greater risk of developing PD than non-carriers.

4.1.3. PINK1

Pathogenic mutations in the PTEN-induced kinase (*PINK1*) gene are much less common than *PARK2* mutations with a frequency variable from 1 to 9% depending on the ethnic background [12]. The encoded protein is a putative serine/threonine kinase of 581 amino acids involved in mitochondrial response to cellular and oxidative stress [87].

Homozygous deletions involving different combination of exons 4–8 have been described in both familial and sporadic early-onset cases coming from Japan, Brazil, Sudan and Iran [38, 88–91]. Just in one of them, breakpoint analysis has been performed, revealing a complex rearrangement combining a large deletion and the insertion of a duplicated sequence from the neighbouring *DDOST* gene intron 2 [91]. As suggested by breakpoint analysis, this rearrangement may result from FoSTeS mechanism. Only one case of a sporadic patient carrying two different CNVs on *PINK1* (compound heterozygous mutations) has been reported until now, consisting of exon 2 deletion in one allele and exons 2–4 deletion in the other one [38].

The spectrum mutation of *PINK1* CNVs is enlarged by the heterozygous cases that, however, do not explain the recessive inheritance. The largest heterozygous deletion published so far includes the entire *PINK1* gene and spans for 56 kb [92]. This deletion also partly involves two neighbouring genes and two highly similar AluJo repeat sequences. It is likely that the deletion results from an unequal crossing-over between these two sequences. Further heterozygous deletions involving exons 1, 3–8 and exon 7 have been described in familial or sporadic cases of early-onset PD [72, 93, 94].

4.1.4. DJ1

The PARK7 locus on chromosome 1p36 was localized by homozygosity mapping in two consanguineous families from genetically isolated communities in the Netherlands and Italy [95, 96]. In one of the families, a 14 kb deletion involving the first five of seven exons in the *DJ-1* gene has been identified [95]. Furthermore, three siblings of Iranian origins born from consanguineous parents and carriers of a homozygous deletion of exon 5 have been described [38].

The product of *DJ-1* is a highly conserved multifunctional protein belonging to the peptidase C56 family [97]. It acts as positive regulator of transcription, redox-sensitive chaperone and sensor for oxidative stress and apparently protects neurons from ROS-induced apoptosis [98, 99]. Alu repeat elements flank the deleted sequence on both sides, suggesting that unequal crossing-over is likely at the origin of this rare genomic rearrangement [2].

Further heterozygous CNVs (both deletions and duplication) involving the exons of *DJ-1* gene have been published so far [93, 100–102], although they do not completely explain the recessive pattern of the PD phenotype.

4.1.5. ATP13A2

ATP13A2 mutations are associated with Kufor–Rakeb syndrome (KRS), a form of recessively levodopa-responsive inherited atypical Parkinsonism [14]. It encodes a large protein belonging to the ATPase transmembrane transporters, and recently, it has been identified as a potent modifier of the toxicity induced by alpha-synuclein [103].

To our knowledge, just one family from Iran with deletion of *ATP13A2* has been reported [38]. Specifically, three affected siblings born from consanguineous parents have been described as carriers of a homozygous deletion of exon 2. All three affected individuals had moderate mental retardation, aggressive behaviours, visual hallucinations, supranuclear vertical gaze paresis, slow vertical saccades and dystonia. Cognitive function deteriorated rapidly and all three affected individuals had dementia by age 10. Further clinical and genetic follow-up of KRS patients will increase the knowledge on the natural history and clinical features of this syndrome.

4.2. Rare single-gene CNVs in other PD-genes

4.2.1. TH

The tyrosine hydroxylase (*TH*) gene encodes a monooxygenase that catalyses the conversion of L-tyrosine to L-dihydroxyphenylalanine (L-DOPA), which constitutes the rate-limiting step in dopamine biosynthesis. Consistent with the essential role of TH in dopamine homeostasis, missense mutations in *TH* have been associated with severe Parkinsonism-related phenotypes, such as Segawa's syndrome, L-DOPA-responsive infantile Parkinsonism or L-DOPA-responsive dystonia (DRD) in recessive form [104].

In 2010, for the first time, Bademci et al. [105] reported a 34 kb deletion of the entire *TH* gene in a 54 years-age-at-onset PD patient, presenting no evidence for dystonia, but responsive to L-DOPA treatment. The deletion was first identified by CNV analysis in a GWAS using SNP array, then confirmed by multiple quantitative PCR assays and was not found in any of 642 controls.

More recently, Ormazabal et al. [106] reported a DRD patient with a deletion in *TH* encompassing several exons. A heterozygous exon 12 deletion was first identified by MLPA. Additional analysis with long range PCR over breakpoints confirmed the deletion encompassing a segment of 716 bp (c.1197 + 25_1391del) including exon 12 and part of exon 13. The patient also had a heterozygous mutation (c.1 – 70 G > A) at promoter region in another allele. The promoter mutation was believed to be the underlying cause for DRD phenotype, but authors recommend the inclusion of structural variant analysis for those patients with clinical and biochemical features of *TH* deficiency lacking molecular confirmation by the usual sequencing techniques.

4.2.2. *VPS35*

In 2011, two independent groups reported the identification of the same missense mutation (p.Asp620Asn) in the vacuolar protein sorting 35 (*VPS35*) gene as a novel disease-causing mutation in large autosomal-dominant PD pedigrees of Austrian and Swiss origins [107, 108]. After this discovery, Verstraeten et al. [109] performed in-depth sequence and dosage analyses of *VPS35* in an extended LBD patient group comprised of PD, PD with dementia, and dementia with LBs patients living throughout Flanders. The dosage analyses were performed using multiplex amplicon quantification, but no CNVs were detected in this patient's cohort. Despite these data, it cannot be excluded that CNVs in *VPS35* maybe occur in other PD patients groups and contribute to PD onset. It has very recently demonstrated that specific deletion of *VPS35* in dopaminergic neurons of deficient mice resulted in PD-like deficits including loss of dopaminergic neurons and accumulation of alpha-synuclein [110].

4.2.3. *PGRN*

The progranulin (*PGRN*) gene is expressed in a wide variety of tissues including neuronal and microglial populations of the central nervous system and encodes for an autocrine growth factor [111]. Its loss-of-function mutations are responsible for ubiquitin-positive frontotemporal lobar degeneration linked to chromosome 17 (FTLDU-17). A deletion of exons 1–11 of the *PGRN* has been reported in a patient with typical PGRN neuropathology, and equally, in his sister presenting PD [111]. The deletion resulted from a non-homologous recombination event and was measured by using quantitative multiplex PCR of short fluorescent fragments.

Although *PGRN* mutations are certainly not a major cause of PD, these data suggest that *PGRN* CNVs may attend to PD mechanisms.

4.2.4. HMOX1

A relevant feature of PD development is the abnormal iron deposition in the SN of PD patients [112]. The HMOX (Heme oxygenase) protein degrades heme ring to biliverdin, free ferrous iron and carbon monoxide being the rate-limiting activity in heme catabolism. The isoform HMOX1 is highly inducible in response to oxidative stress, which is considered a significant pathway altered in PD conditions. Based on these major findings, Ayuso et al. [112] analysed exon 3 dosage alterations in the *HMOX1* gene in 691 patients suffering from PD and 766 healthy control individuals. CNVs of the *HMOX1* gene were analyzed using a TaqMan assay, designed to hybridize just within the *HMOX1* exon 3. CNV analyses in the whole study group revealed the occurrence of three patients with PD and six control individuals with a single copy of the *HMOX1* gene. Thus, authors conclude that *HMOX1* CNVs exist but they do not seem to have a major association with PD risk. However, it cannot be excluded the occurrence of structural alterations in other *HMOX1* exons.

4.3. The 22q11.2 deletion

The 22q11.2 deletion syndrome (22qDS), also known as Di George or velocardiofacial syndrome, is a multi-system disorder caused by a chromosomal microdeletion most commonly involving a 3 Mb segment on the long arm of chromosome 22. Several case reports of individuals with the hemizygous deletion of chromosome 22q11.2 and some clinical features of Parkinsonism have suggested that this genetic anomaly may also confer an increased risk of early-onset PD [113–115]. Some of these cases were reported to be treated with L-DOPA, while in other case, presynaptic dopamine imaging indicated degeneration of the nigrostriatal dopamine system [113–115]. To investigate the association between 22q11.2 deletions and PD, Butcher and colleagues [116] assessed the occurrence of a clinical diagnosis of PD in a well-characterized cohort of adults with 22qDS. They also examined available brain tissue from 3 individuals with 22qDS and an ante-mortem diagnosis of PD. They reported four patients with the 22q11.2 hemizygous deletion and diagnosed of early-onset PD. Three of them also displayed typical neuropathological features with prominent LBs and Lewy neurite formations on autopsy examination. The authors concluded chromosome 22q11.2 deletions may represent a novel risk factor for early-onset PD and, with their neuropathological data, excluded that Parkinsonian clinical features can be due to adverse effects of antipsychotics.

Ogaki and Ross [117] proposed it is not the microdeletion *per se* that is responsible for the phenotype, but rather the complete loss of function of a gene at the locus due to the combination of the deletion and a mutation on the other allele. Indeed, the chromosome 22q11.2 region contains some excellent candidate genes, such as *COMT*, encoding catechol-O-methyltransferase that is involved in catecholamine catabolism including dopamine and thus plays a role in regulating dopamine levels (COMT-inhibitor has been used as a treatment for PD). The deletion region also contains *SEPT5*, encoding SEPTIN5 that functionally interacts with PARK2, and *DGCR8* that encodes a subunit of a complex which mediates the biogenesis of microRNAs, including miR-185 (also encoded within the chromosome 22q11.2 deletion) which is predicted to target *LRRK2* [117].

Very recently, a 37-year-old early-onset PD patient was found carrying the 22q11.2 deletion but lacking the more severe features of 22qDS, such as cardiac defect, palatal defect and hypocalcemia [118]. The deletion was revealed using chromosomal microarray analysis, suggesting that this genetic test should be considered as part of the evaluation for patients with early-onset PD and other features associated with 22qDS. Interestingly, very recently, Perandones et al. [119] reported a case of mosaicism of a patient from an Ashkenazi Jewish ethnic group with a history of midline defects and PD onset at 46 years. In this patient, FISH test detected a mosaicism of a 22q deletion in 24% of the analyzed blood cells, highlighting the relevance of performing individual cell-by-cell analysis, at least until single-cell sequencing becomes optimized and generally available. The pathogenesis of early-onset PD in patients with 22qDS remains unknown but, if elucidated, it may contribute to understanding the aetiology of PD and ultimately to prevention and treatment strategies.

4.4. CNVs involving the mtDNA of PD patients

Mitochondria dysfunction was implicated in the pathogenesis of idiopathic PD. Accumulated evidence of mitochondrial DNA (mtDNA) anomalies has been observed in PD patients, including increased mtDNA deletions/rearrangements in both cerebral area (SN and striatum) and peripheral tissues (skeletal muscle) [120–122]. The number and variety of mtDNA deletions/rearrangements seem to be selectively increased in the SN of PD patients compared to other disorders (multiple system atrophy and dementia with LBs) as well as patients with Alzheimer disease and age-matched controls.

More recently, Gui et al. [123] analyzed the copy number of mtDNA using quantitative real-time PCR in 414 cases with PD and 231 healthy subjects from mainland of China. The level of mtDNA was significantly decreased in PD patients' peripheral blood as compared to that of healthy controls. Furthermore, lower mtDNA copy number was more frequently detected in the older onset age group than that in the younger group, suggesting mtDNA content might be an important genetic event in PD progression. In addition, using direct sequencing, they examined the mutations in the D-loop (the region that controls replication and transcription of mtDNA) and in the genomic *POLG1* gene. The results revealed that 17% of the PD patients carried mutations in the D-loop of mtDNA and that patients carrying mutated *POLG1* had a significantly lower copy number of mtDNA than those of PD patients without *POLG1* alterations, suggesting a role of *POLG1* variations for reducing mtDNA copy number in PD.

5. Genome-wide studies to map CNVs in PD

The typical attempts to identify genetic lesions that underlie monogenic forms of disease have involved the use of linkage mapping analysis in large pedigrees of several affected individuals with known relationships. The application of genome-wide technologies assays now allows the fast production of high quality, ultra-dense genotypes, producing rapid mapping and localization of genomic deletion and duplication. However, there is still no consensus on the best approach for the detection or analysis of genome-wide CNVs, and very few studies have been conducted so far.

The first pilot analyses of structural genetic variations in a large cohort PD patients and neurologically normal controls have been carried out using the genome-wide SNP association study approach [124]. In this study, no new regions associated with PD were identified, but several deletions and duplications in *PARK2* were observed, confirmed by independent gene dosage experiments. Some months later, Kim et al. [125], tried to investigate CNVs in PD patients by array-based comparative genomic hybridization (CGH). They observed several candidate CNVs in many chromosomes, but finally conclude these did not involve any regions harbouring genes implicated in PD pathogenesis or progression.

In 2011, Pankratz et al. [49] presented the results of the first systematic genome-wide analysis of CNVs for PD using CNV calling algorithms. The final sample included 816 cases and 856 controls. They replicated the association of PD susceptibility with *PARK2* CNVs and also detected CNVs in two novel genes, *DOCK5* and *USP32*, associated with an increase in risk for PD at genome-wide significance. However, neither of these novel loci could be validated with independent molecular tests.

To identify novel CNVs and to evaluate their contribution to the risk of PD, more recently Liu et al. [126] have conducted a genome-wide scan for CNVs in a case–control dataset (268 PD cases and 178 controls), focusing on a genetic isolate, the Ashkenazi Jewish population. Using high-confidence CNVs, this research group examined the global genome wide burden of large and rare CNVs. Overall, global burden analyses did not reveal significant differences between cases and controls, but the deletions were found 1.4 times more often in cases. Interestingly, a total of 81 PD cases carried a rare genic CNV that was absent in controls. Of note, duplication of the *OVOS2* (ovostatin 2) gene on Chr. 12p11.21 was identified as significant risk factors for PD. In one PD case, sample was observed a deletion spanning *NSF* and *WNT3* genes, a region previously identified as "top-hit" in GWAS studies and physically near to *MAPT* gene. Other interesting genes include *ATXN3, FBXW7, CHCHD3, HSF1, KLC1* and *MBD3*, which participates in the disease pathways with known PD genes.

Whole-genome microarray detection was used to identify somatic CNVs in PD patients by Pamphlett et al. [127], who investigated the existence of candidate brain-situated genetic variations missing in blood DNA. In this study, a total of 45 CNVs in PD brain samples but in any control, brains were founded, including genes related to mitochondrial function (*BCL2, IMMP2L*), cellular vesicle formation (*NRSN1*) and apoptosis (*BCL2*), pathways implicated in the pathogenesis of PD. Furthermore, additional private rare CNVs observed in PD brains have been reported. This study shows that specific-brain CNVs can be detected, and raises the possibility that brain-situated mutations could underlie some cases of PD.

6. How to detect and analyse CNVs: molecular methods and bioinformatics web resources

CNVs can be detected and analysed by laboratory methods restricted to certain locations on chromosomes (locus-specific levels), or targeting the whole genome (genome-wide level). In the next sections, we will briefly describe the traditional methodologies, the currently available high-throughput biotechnologies, and the supporting bioinformatics tools to help the detection, analysis and interpretation of CNVs.

6.1. Locus-specific methods

6.1.1. RFLP—Southern blotting

The most conventional method for detecting structural rearrangements is RFLP—Southern blot, which relies on DNA digestion with rare-cut enzyme, electrophoresis separation of digested DNA fragments by pulsed field gel, membranes transfers and hybridization with appropriate probes [128]. The RFLP—Southern blot method may be a good choice to resolve large size CNVs and structural variations. However, there are some drawbacks to this method: 1) the very low resolution; 2) the higher cost per analysis compared to other methods; 3) time-consuming and laborious procedures that require more than a week; 4) the need for purified high molecular weight DNA. For these reason, the RFLP—Southern blot is not so much used in both clinical and research fields.

6.1.2. Fluorescence in situ hybridization

FISH is an extremely useful method for the detection of chromosomal abnormalities. This methods relies on the hybridization of fluorescently labelled DNA probes to metaphase chromosome spreads (resolution 1–3 Mb) or interphase nuclei (50 kb–2 Mb) [128]. The highest resolution is obtained by fibre-FISH (5–500 kb), where probes are visualized on mechanically stretched chromosome fibres, and is currently the preferred method to precisely determine the genomic structure of complex CNVs [128]. Nowadays, FISH combined with multiple probes labelled in different colours (multicolour FISH), is widely used in clinical diagnostics as a screening tool to confirm the presence of CNVs and other structural variants [128]. However, FISH has several limitations. Locus-specific probes are expensive, and the procedure is time-consuming and labour intensive. Furthermore, only a limited number of chromosomal loci can be screened in a single experiment and the identification of an abnormality is highly dependent on the DNA probe used, specifically on its size and hybridization localization.

6.1.3. PCR-based approaches

The first PCR-based technique used for targeted CNV analysis was real-time quantitative PCR (qPCR) that combines "traditional" endpoint PCR with fluorescent detection technologies to record the accumulation of amplicons during PCR cycling [128]. Fluorescence monitoring systems is based on fluorescence probes (e.g. TaqMan, Scorpions, FRET probes) or DNA-intercalating agents (SYBR green). With the accumulation of target sequences during PCR, the fluorescence signal increases. Amplicon quantification relies on the observation of the threshold cycle number (Ct), at which the amount of an amplified target amplicon is directly related to the amount of starting target. So a higher or lower starting copy number of a genomic DNA target will respectively result in a significant earlier or later increase in fluorescence, and thus, in a decreased or increased Ct. The qPCR technique offers great flexibility and adaptability, and can be carried out in a closed system, thus eliminating the risk of PCR and sample contamination and does not require post-processing of PCR products. Therefore, it has become one of the most popular methods for CNV analysis, especially for validation of results obtained by microarray tests.

Another widely used PCR-based approach is MLPA (or multiplex ligand probe amplification). MLPA consists of two oligonucleotide hemiprobes, one synthetic and one derived from the single-stranded M13 bacteriophage [128]. These oligonucleotides hybridize to adjacent sites of the target sequence. Each hemiprobe is flanked by universal PCR primer sites and one of the hemiprobes also has a "stuffer" sequence allowing each probe set to have different fragment lengths. After the hybridization to genomic DNA, the two hybridized hemiprobes are ligated resulting in a proportional relation between the number of joined primers and the target copy number. Then, PCR amplification is carried out using a single universal dye-labelled primerset. The resulting PCR products are separated by capillary gel electrophoresis followed by data analysis to identify CNVs. Since the relative quantity of each of the PCR products is proportional to the number of copies of the target sequence, results are given as allele copy numbers as compared to normal controls. MLPA is specifically developed to screen up to 50 (on average 20–40) independent loci simultaneously, with results typically available after 1–3 days.

6.2. Genome-wide high-throughput biotechnologies

As anticipated, the above-described traditional methodological approaches bear objective limits: they are time-consuming and labour-intensive, they require multiple phase steps and severe equipment costs and above all do not provide a complete genomic overview of structural imbalances at sufficiently high resolution. The recent development of the aCGH and next generation sequencing (NGS) biotechnology has dramatically improved and catalysed the detection and characterization of multiple CNVs, offering high reproducibility, high resolution and scalability for complete genome-wide mapping of imbalances [129–133].

6.2.1. CGH array

The application of the whole-genome high-resolution aCGH (comparative genomic hybridization array) platforms for detecting deletions or duplications has extensively grown. This biotechnology is now recognized as the first-tier clinical diagnostic test for individuals with developmental disabilities or congenital anomalies [134]. In addition, several customized high-density aCGH, suitably designed to focus on specific clinically relevant chromosomal locations have been developed [133, 135, 136] and aim to obtain an improved resolution. The designing of customized aCGH platforms has been already applied to different human diseases including neuromuscular diseases, cancer, autism, epilepsy, multiple sclerosis, mitochondrial and metabolic disorders [132, 137–143].

The CGH method uses two different fluorescent dyes for the test (unknown or experimental) and reference DNA samples, which contemporary hybridize on a microarray glass spotted with millions of probes. By measuring the ratio between the fluorescence signals of the two dyes and assuming that the reference sample has a normal diploid, the CNVs can be detected as either the gain or loss of signal in the test sample.

6.2.2. Next generation sequencing

In the last few years, the NGS technology is becoming more frequently used in various fields of life science. The NGS is a high-throughput technology that can output million or billion short reads from the shotgun sequencing, and thus provides high resolution mapping of genomic regions. The huge amount of data can be utilized for de novo assembly, SNPs calling, structural variations and for the detection of CNVs with high resolution. Recently, a variety of algorithm suitably projected to analyse CNVs has been proposed [144–147], and scientists are still studying to find out the best one. The application of next-generation sequencing platforms to PD genetic studies promises to improve resolution and reveal new clues to better understand its molecular causes.

6.3. Online web resources

The collection of CNVs into web databases has provided an essential tool in interpreting results for diagnostic laboratories and in helping researchers. Public available repositories are The Database of Genomic Variants (DGV—http://dgv.tcag.ca/dgv/app/home), The International

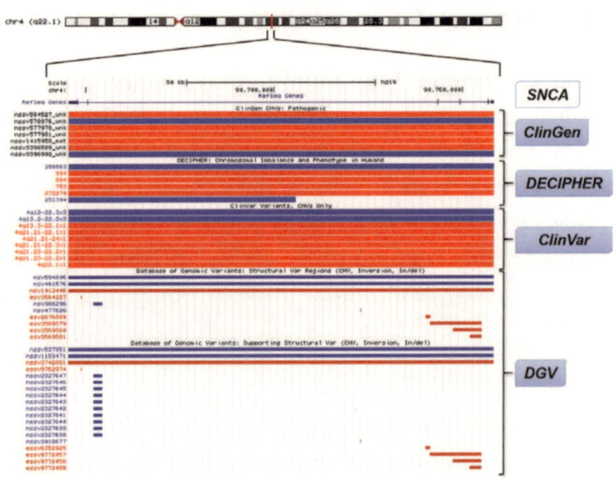

Figure 5. Representative view of the tracks data for CNVs loaded into the Human Genome Browser (https://genome-euro.ucsc.edu/index.html) database. The figure represents *SNCA* genetic structure, harboured in chromosome 4. Data deposited in the ISCA, DECIPHER, ClinVar and DGV databases are gathered here and displayed as red bars for deletions, blue bars for duplications and brown or orange bars for more complex rearrangements.

Standard for Cytogenomic Arrays (ISCA—http://www.clinicalgenome.org), The database of Chromosomal Imbalance and Phenotype in Human using Ensembl Resources (DECIPHER—http://decipher.sanger.ac.uk), and the NCBI Database of Genomic Structural Variations (dbVAR—http://www.ncbi.nlm.nih.gov/dbvar).

CNVs deposited in these databases are currently loaded into the Human Genome Browser (http://genome-euro.ucsc.edu/index.html) as searchable tracks (**Figure 5**). All together, these databases are helpful in reporting genomic reports updated information on CNVs frequencies in unaffected controls and are classified in VOUS, benign, pathogenic, likely benign or likely pathogenic.

7. Conclusive remarks

Several evidences suggest an extensive and complex genetic action of CNVs on PD etiopathogenesis. Thus far, unfortunately, only a small portion of the genetic variance has been identified; the remaining substantial components remain unknown. Assessing the global genome-wide burden of large CNVs and elucidating the role of *de novo* rare structural variants on PD may reveal new candidate genes, explain a portion of the "missing heritability" (for example, new susceptibility or causative factors that overall converge on PD syndrome) and consequently ameliorate diagnosis and counselling of mutations carriers. The forthcoming new era of genomics data promises to increase resolution and uncover new interesting perspectives.

Acknowledgements

This work was supported by the Italian Ministry of Education, Universities and Research through Grant CTN01_00177_817708 and the international Ph.D. program in Neuroscience of the University of Catania. Authors gratefully acknowledge Cristina Calì, Alfia Corsino, Maria Patrizia D'Angelo and Francesco Marino for their administrative and technical support.

Author details

Valentina La Cognata[1,2], Velia D'Agata[2], Francesca Cavalcanti[3] and Sebastiano Cavallaro[1*]

*Address all correspondence to: sebastiano.cavallaro@cnr.it

1 Institute of Neurological Sciences, Italian National Research Council, Catania, Italy

2 Department of Biomedical and Biotechnological Sciences, Section of Human Anatomy and Histology, University of Catania, Catania, Italy

3 Institute of Neurological Sciences, National Research Council, Mangone (CS), Italy

References

[1] Moore DJ, West AB, Dawson VL, Dawson TM. Molecular pathophysiology of Parkinson's disease. Annual Review of Neuroscience. 2005;28:57–87. doi:10.1146/annurev.neuro.28.061604.135718.

[2] Toft M, Ross OA. Copy number variation in Parkinson's disease. Genome Medicine. 2010;2(9):62. doi:10.1186/gm183.

[3] Winklhofer KF, Haass C. Mitochondrial dysfunction in Parkinson's disease. Biochimica et Biophysica Acta. 2010;1802(1):29–44. doi:10.1016/j.bbadis.2009.08.013.

[4] Dias V, Junn E, Mouradian MM. The role of oxidative stress in Parkinson's disease. Journal of Parkinson's Disease. 2013;3(4):461–91. doi:10.3233/JPD-130230.

[5] Betarbet R, Sherer TB, Greenamyre JT. Ubiquitin-proteasome system and Parkinson's diseases. Experimental Neurology. 2005;191 Suppl 1:S17–27. doi:10.1016/j.expneurol.2004.08.021.

[6] Klein C, Westenberger A. Genetics of Parkinson's disease. Cold Spring Harbor Perspectives in Medicine. 2012;2(1):a008888. doi:10.1101/cshperspect.a008888.

[7] Polymeropoulos MH, Higgins JJ, Golbe LI, Johnson WG, Ide SE, Di Iorio G, et al. Mapping of a gene for Parkinson's disease to chromosome 4q21-q23. Science. 1996;274(5290):1197–9.

[8] Pihlstrom L, Toft M. Genetic variability in SNCA and Parkinson's disease. Neurogenetics. 2011;12(4):283–93. doi:10.1007/s10048-011-0292-7.

[9] Stefanis L. alpha-Synuclein in Parkinson's disease. Cold Spring Harbor Perspectives in Medicine. 2012;2(2):a009399. doi:10.1101/cshperspect.a009399.

[10] Deng H, Yuan L. Genetic variants and animal models in SNCA and Parkinson disease. Ageing Research Reviews. 2014;15C:161–76. doi:10.1016/j.arr.2014.04.002.

[11] Rideout HJ, Stefanis L. The neurobiology of LRRK2 and its role in the pathogenesis of Parkinson's disease. Neurochemical Research. 2014;39(3):576–92. doi:10.1007/s11064-013-1073-5.

[12] Pogson JH, Ivatt RM, Whitworth AJ. Molecular mechanisms of PINK1-related neurodegeneration. Current Neurology and Neuroscience Reports. 2011;11(3):283–90. doi:10.1007/s11910-011-0187-x.

[13] Lockhart PJ, Lincoln S, Hulihan M, Kachergus J, Wilkes K, Bisceglio G, et al. DJ-1 mutations are a rare cause of recessively inherited early onset Parkinsonism mediated by loss of protein function. Journal of Medical Genetics. 2004;41(3):e22.

[14] Vilarino-Guell C, Soto AI, Lincoln SJ, Ben Yahmed S, Kefi M, Heckman MG, et al. ATP13A2 variability in Parkinson disease. Human Mutation. 2009;30(3):406. doi:10. 10.1002/humu.20877.

[15] Schultheis PJ, Hagen TT, O'Toole KK, Tachibana A, Burke CR, McGill DL, et al. Characterization of the P5 subfamily of P-type transport ATPases in mice. Biochemical and Biophysical Research Communications. 2004;323(3):731–8. doi:10.1016/j.bbrc. 2004.08.156.

[16] Lu CS, Lai SC, Wu RM, Weng YH, Huang CL, Chen RS, et al. PLA2G6 mutations in PARK14-linked young-onset Parkinsonism and sporadic Parkinson's disease. American Journal of Medical Genetics Part B, Neuropsychiatric Genetics. 2012;159B(2):183–91. doi:10.1002/ajmg.b.32012.

[17] Di Fonzo A, Dekker MC, Montagna P, Baruzzi A, Yonova EH, Correia Guedes L, et al. FBXO7 mutations cause autosomal recessive, early-onset Parkinsonian-pyramidal syndrome. Neurology. 2009;72(3):240–5. doi:10.1212/01.wnl.0000338144.10967.2b.

[18] Bonifati V. Genetics of Parkinson's disease—state of the art, 2013. Parkinsonism & Related Disorders. 2014;20 Suppl 1:S23–8. doi:10.1016/S1353-8020(13)70009-9.

[19] Lubbe S, Morris HR. Recent advances in Parkinson's disease genetics. Journal of Neurology. 2014;261(2):259–66. doi:10.1007/s00415-013-7003-2.

[20] Trinh J, Farrer M. Advances in the genetics of Parkinson disease. Nature Reviews Neurology. 2013;9(8):445–54. doi:10.1038/nrneurol.2013.132.

[21] Lewis PA, Cookson MR. Gene expression in the Parkinson's disease brain. Brain Research Bulletin. 2012;88(4):302–12. doi:10.1016/j.brainresbull.2011.11.016.

[22] Zarrei M, MacDonald JR, Merico D, Scherer SW. A copy number variation map of the human genome. Nature Reviews Genetics. 2015;16(3):172–83. doi:10.1038/nrg3871.

[23] Lee JA, Lupski JR. Genomic rearrangements and gene copy-number alterations as a cause of nervous system disorders. Neuron. 2006;52(1):103–21. doi:10.1016/j.neuron. 2006.09.027.

[24] Chen L, Zhou W, Zhang L, Zhang F. Genome architecture and its roles in human copy number variation. Genomics & Informatics. 2014;12(4):136–44. doi:10.5808/GI. 2014.12.4.136.

[25] Ambroziak W, Koziorowski D, Duszyc K, Gorka-Skoczylas P, Potulska-Chromik A, Slawek J, et al. Genomic instability in the PARK2 locus is associated with Parkinson's disease. Journal of Applied Genetics. 2015;56(4):451–61. doi:10.1007/s13353-015-0282-9.

[26] Bickhart DM, Liu GE. The challenges and importance of structural variation detection in livestock. Frontiers in Genetics. 2014;5:37. doi:10.3389/fgene.2014.00037.

[27] Lee JA, Carvalho CM, Lupski JR. A DNA replication mechanism for generating nonrecurrent rearrangements associated with genomic disorders. Cell. 2007;131(7): 1235–47. doi:10.1016/j.cell.2007.11.037.

[28] Gu W, Lupski JR. CNV and nervous system diseases—what's new? Cytogenetic and Genome Research. 2008;123(1–4):54–64. doi:10.1159/000184692.

[29] Kalman B, Vitale E. Structural chromosomal variations in neurological diseases. The Neurologist. 2009;15(5):245–53. doi:10.1097/NRL.0b013e3181963cef.

[30] Hoyer H, Braathen GJ, Eek AK, Nordang GB, Skjelbred CF, Russell MB. Copy number variations in a population-based study of Charcot-Marie-Tooth disease. BioMed Research International. 2015;2015:960404. doi:10.1155/2015/960404.

[31] Olson H, Shen Y, Avallone J, Sheidley BR, Pinsky R, Bergin AM, et al. Copy number variation plays an important role in clinical epilepsy. Annals of Neurology. 2014;75(6): 943–58. doi:10.1002/ana.24178.

[32] Grayton HM, Fernandes C, Rujescu D, Collier DA. Copy number variations in neurodevelopmental disorders. Progress in Neurobiology. 2012;99(1):81–91. doi:10.1016/j.pneurobio.2012.07.005.

[33] Wang L, Nuytemans K, Bademci G, Jauregui C, Martin ER, Scott WK, et al. High-resolution survey in familial Parkinson disease genes reveals multiple independent copy number variation events in PARK2. Human Mutation. 2013;34(8):1071–4. doi: 10.1002/humu.22344.

[34] Singleton AB, Farrer M, Johnson J, Singleton A, Hague S, Kachergus J, et al. α-Synuclein locus triplication causes Parkinson's disease. Science. 2003;302(5646):841. doi:10.1126/science.1090278.

[35] Keyser RJ, Lombard D, Veikondis R, Carr J, Bardien S. Analysis of exon dosage using MLPA in South African Parkinson's disease patients. Neurogenetics. 2010;11(3):305–12. doi:10.1007/s10048-009-0229-6.

[36] Sekine T, Kagaya H, Funayama M, Li Y, Yoshino H, Tomiyama H, et al. Clinical course of the first Asian family with Parkinsonism related to SNCA triplication. Movement Disorders. 2010;25(16):2871–5. doi:10.1002/mds.23313.

[37] Kojovic M, Sheerin UM, Rubio-Agusti I, Saha A, Bras J, Gibbons V, et al. Young-onset Parkinsonism due to homozygous duplication of α-synuclein in a consanguineous family. Movement Disorders. 2012;27(14):1827–9. doi:10.1002/mds.25199.

[38] Darvish H, Movafagh A, Omrani MD, Firouzabadi SG, Azargashb E, Jamshidi J, et al. Detection of copy number changes in genes associated with Parkinson's disease in Iranian patients. Neuroscience Letters. 2013;551:75–8. doi:10.1016/j.neulet.2013.07.013.

[39] Olgiati S, Thomas A, Quadri M, Breedveld GJ, Graafland J, Eussen H, et al. Early-onset Parkinsonism caused by alpha-synuclein gene triplication: Clinical and genetic

findings in a novel family. Parkinsonism & Related Disorders. 2015;21(8):981–6. doi: 10.1016/j.parkreldis.2015.06.005.

[40] Ferese R, Modugno N, Campopiano R, Santilli M, Zampatti S, Giardina E, et al. Four copies of SNCA responsible for autosomal dominant Parkinson's disease in two Italian siblings. Parkinson's Disease. 2015;2015:1–6. doi:10.1155/2015/546462.

[41] Uchiyama T, Ikeuchi T, Ouchi Y, Sakamoto M, Kasuga K, Shiga A, et al. Prominent psychiatric symptoms and glucose hypometabolism in a family with a SNCA duplication. Neurology. 2008;71(16):1289–91. doi:10.1212/01.wnl.0000327607.28928.e6.

[42] Ahn TB, Kim SY, Kim JY, Park SS, Lee DS, Min HJ, et al. α-Synuclein gene duplication is present in sporadic Parkinson disease. Neurology. 2008;70(1):43–9. doi: 10.1212/01.wnl.0000271080.53272.c7.

[43] Nishioka K, Ross OA, Ishii K, Kachergus JM, Ishiwata K, Kitagawa M, et al. Expanding the clinical phenotype of SNCA duplication carriers. Movement Disorders. 2009;24(12): 1811–9. doi:10.1002/mds.22682.

[44] Nishioka K, Hayashi S, Farrer MJ, Singleton AB, Yoshino H, Imai H, et al. Clinical heterogeneity of α-synuclein gene duplication in Parkinson's disease. Annals of Neurology. 2006;59(2):298–309. doi:10.1002/ana.20753.

[45] Chartier-Harlin MC, Kachergus J, Roumier C, Mouroux V, Douay X, Lincoln S, et al. α-Synuclein locus duplication as a cause of familial Parkinson's disease. Lancet. 2004;364(9440):1167–9. doi:10.1016/S0140-6736(04)17103-1.

[46] Ibanez P, Bonnet AM, Debarges B, Lohmann E, Tison F, Pollak P, et al. Causal relation between alpha-synuclein gene duplication and familial Parkinson's disease. Lancet. 2004;364(9440):1169–71. doi:10.1016/S0140-6736(04)17104-3.

[47] Ibanez P, Lesage S, Janin S, Lohmann E, Durif F, Destee A, et al. α-Synuclein gene rearrangements in dominantly inherited Parkinsonism: frequency, phenotype, and mechanisms. Archives of Neurology. 2009;66(1):102–8. doi:10.1001/archneurol. 2008.555.

[48] Sironi F, Trotta L, Antonini A, Zini M, Ciccone R, Della Mina E, et al. α-Synuclein multiplication analysis in Italian familial Parkinson disease. Parkinsonism & Related Disorders. 2010;16(3):228–31. doi:10.1016/j.parkreldis.2009.09.008.

[49] Pankratz N, Dumitriu A, Hetrick KN, Sun M, Latourelle JC, Wilk JB, et al. Copy number variation in familial Parkinson disease. Plos One. 2011;6(8):e20988. doi:10.1371/ journal.pone.0020988.

[50] Elia AE, Petrucci S, Fasano A, Guidi M, Valbonesi S, Bernardini L, et al. alpha-Synuclein gene duplication: marked intrafamilial variability in two novel pedigrees. Movement Disorders. 2013;28(6):813–7. doi:10.1002/mds.25518.

[51] Konno T, Ross OA, Puschmann A, Dickson DW, Wszolek ZK. Autosomal dominant Parkinson's disease caused by SNCA duplications. Parkinsonism & Related Disorders. 2016;22 Suppl 1:S1–6. doi:10.1016/j.parkreldis.2015.09.007.

[52] Farrer M, Kachergus J, Forno L, Lincoln S, Wang DS, Hulihan M, et al. Comparison of kindreds with Parkinsonism and α-synuclein genomic multiplications. Annals of Neurology. 2004;55(2):174–9. doi:10.1002/ana.10846.

[53] Fuchs J, Nilsson C, Kachergus J, Munz M, Larsson EM, Schule B, et al. Phenotypic variation in a large Swedish pedigree due to SNCA duplication and triplication. Neurology. 2007;68(12):916–22. doi:10.1212/01.wnl.0000254458.17630.c5.

[54] Ikeuchi T, Kakita A, Shiga A, Kasuga K, Kaneko H, Tan CF, et al. Patients homozygous and heterozygous for SNCA duplication in a family with Parkinsonism and dementia. Archives of Neurology. 2008;65(4):514–9. doi:10.1001/archneur.65.4.514.

[55] Garraux G, Caberg JH, Vanbellinghen JF, Jamar M, Bours V, Moonen G, et al. Partial trisomy 4q associated with young-onset dopa-responsive Parkinsonism. Archives of Neurology. 2012;69(3):398–400. doi:10.1001/archneurol.2011.802.

[56] Shin CW, Kim HJ, Park SS, Kim SY, Kim JY, Jeon BS. Two Parkinson's disease patients with α-synuclein gene duplication and rapid cognitive decline. Movement Disorders. 2010;25(7):957–9. doi:10.1002/mds.23043.

[57] Troiano AR, Cazeneuve C, Le Ber I, Bonnet AM, Lesage S, Brice A. Re: alpha-synuclein gene duplication is present in sporadic Parkinson disease. Neurology. 2008;71(16):1295; author reply doi:10.1212/01.wnl.0000338435.78120.0f.

[58] Brueggemann N, Odin P, Gruenewald A, Tadic V, Hagenah J, Seidel G, et al. Re: α-synuclein gene duplication is present in sporadic Parkinson disease. Neurology. 2008;71(16):1294; author reply doi:10.1212/01.wnl.0000338439.00992.c7.

[59] Nuytemans K, Meeus B, Crosiers D, Brouwers N, Goossens D, Engelborghs S, et al. Relative contribution of simple mutations vs. copy number variations in five Parkinson disease genes in the Belgian population. Human Mutation. 2009;30(7):1054–61. doi: 10.1002/humu.21007.

[60] Perandones C, Giugni JC, Calvo DS, Raina GB, De Jorge Lopez L, Volpini V, et al. Mosaicism of alpha-synuclein gene rearrangements: report of two unrelated cases of early-onset Parkinsonism. Parkinsonism & Related Disorders. 2014;20(5):558–61. doi: 10.1016/j.parkreldis.2013.11.014.

[61] Bonifati V. Autosomal recessive Parkinsonism. Parkinsonism & Related Disorders. 2012;18 Suppl 1:S4–6. doi:10.1016/S1353-8020(11)70004-9.

[62] Lucking CB, Durr A, Bonifati V, Vaughan J, De Michele G, Gasser T, et al. Association between early-onset Parkinson's disease and mutations in the Parkin gene. New England Journal of Medicine. 2000;342(21):1560–7. doi:10.1056/NEJM200005253422103.

[63] Oliveira SA, Scott WK, Martin ER, Nance MA, Watts RL, Hubble JP, et al. Parkin mutations and susceptibility alleles in late-onset Parkinson's disease. Annals of Neurology. 2003;53(5):624–9. doi:10.1002/ana.10524.

[64] Chaudhary S, Behari M, Dihana M, Swaminath PV, Govindappa ST, Jayaram S, et al. Parkin mutations in familial and sporadic Parkinson's disease among Indians. Parkinsonism & Related Disorders. 2006;12(4):239–45. doi:10.1016/j.parkreldis.2005.12.004.

[65] Klein C, Djarmati A, Hedrich K, Schafer N, Scaglione C, Marchese R, et al. PINK1, Parkin, and DJ-1 mutations in Italian patients with early-onset Parkinsonism. European Journal of Human Genetics: EJHG. 2005;13(9):1086–93. doi:10.1038/sj.ejhg.5201455.

[66] Shadrina MI, Semenova EV, Slominsky PA, Bagyeva GH, Illarioshkin SN, Ivanova S, II, et al. Effective quantitative real-time polymerase chain reaction analysis of the Parkin gene (PARK2) exon 1-12 dosage. BMC Medical Genetics. 2007;8:6. doi: 10.1186/1471-2350-8-6.

[67] Choi JM, Woo MS, Ma HI, Kang SY, Sung YH, Yong SW, et al. Analysis of PARK genes in a Korean cohort of early-onset Parkinson disease. Neurogenetics. 2008;9(4):263–9. doi:10.1007/s10048-008-0138-0.

[68] Pankratz N, Kissell DK, Pauciulo MW, Halter CA, Rudolph A, Pfeiffer RF, et al. Parkin dosage mutations have greater pathogenicity in familial PD than simple sequence mutations. Neurology. 2009;73(4):279–86. doi:10.1212/WNL.0b013e3181af7a33.

[69] Kay DM, Stevens CF, Hamza TH, Montimurro JS, Zabetian CP, Factor SA, et al. A comprehensive analysis of deletions, multiplications, and copy number variations in PARK2. Neurology. 2010;75(13):1189–94. doi:10.1212/WNL.0b013e3181f4d832.

[70] Wang C, Ma H, Feng X, Xie S, Chan P. Parkin dosage mutations in patients with early-onset sporadic and familial Parkinson's disease in Chinese: an independent pathogenic role. Brain Research. 2010;1358:30–8. doi:10.1016/j.brainres.2010.08.060.

[71] Guerrero Camacho JL, Monroy Jaramillo N, Yescas Gomez P, Rodriguez Violante M, Boll Woehrlen C, Alonso Vilatela ME, et al. High frequency of Parkin exon rearrangements in Mexican-mestizo patients with early-onset Parkinson's disease. Movement Disorders. 2012;27(8):1047–51. doi:10.1002/mds.25030.

[72] Moura KC, Junior MC, de Rosso AL, Nicaretta DH, Pereira JS, Jose Silva D, et al. Exon dosage variations in Brazilian patients with Parkinson's disease: analysis of SNCA, PARKIN, PINK1 and DJ-1 genes. Disease Markers. 2012;32(3):173–8. doi:10.3233/DMA-2011-0873.

[73] Yonova-Doing E, Atadzhanov M, Quadri M, Kelly P, Shawa N, Musonda ST, et al. Analysis of LRRK2, SNCA, Parkin, PINK1, and DJ-1 in Zambian patients with Parkinson's disease. Parkinsonism & Related Disorders. 2012;18(5):567–71. doi:10.1016/j.parkreldis.2012.02.018.

[74] Chu MK, Kim WC, Choi JM, Hong JH, Kang SY, Ma HI, et al. Analysis of dosage mutation in PARK2 among Korean patients with early-onset or familial Parkinson's disease. Journal of Clinical Neurology. 2014;10(3):244–8. doi:10.3988/jcn.2014.10.3.244.

[75] Al-Mubarak BR, Bohlega SA, Alkhairallah TS, Magrashi AI, AlTurki MI, Khalil DS, et al. Parkinson's disease in Saudi patients: a genetic study. Plos One. 2015;10(8):e0135950. doi:10.1371/journal.pone.0135950.

[76] Guo JF, Dong XL, Xu Q, Li N, Yan XX, Xia K, et al. Exon dosage analysis of Parkin gene in Chinese sporadic Parkinson's disease. Neuroscience Letters. 2015;604:47–51. doi: 10.1016/j.neulet.2015.07.046.

[77] Mata IF, Alvarez V, Coto E, Blazquez M, Guisasola LM, Salvador C, et al. Homozygous partial genomic triplication of the Parkin gene in early-onset Parkinsonism. Neuroscience Letters. 2005;380(3):257–9. doi:10.1016/j.neulet.2005.01.051.

[78] La Cognata V, Iemmolo R, D'Agata V, Scuderi S, Drago F, Zappia M, et al. Increasing the coding potential of genomes through alternative splicing: the case of PARK2 gene. Current Genomics. 2014;15(3):203–16. doi:10.2174/1389202915666140426003342.

[79] Scuderi S, La Cognata V, Drago F, Cavallaro S, D'Agata V. Alternative splicing generates different Parkin protein isoforms: evidences in human, rat, and mouse brain. BioMed Research International. 2014;2014:690796. doi:10.1155/2014/690796.

[80] La Cognata V, D'Agata V, Cavalcanti F, Cavallaro S. Parkin Alternative splicing: not only Parkinsonism. ARC Journal of Neuroscience. 2016;1(1):9–18.

[81] Kim SY, Seong MW, Jeon BS, Kim SY, Ko HS, Kim JY, et al. Phase analysis identifies compound heterozygous deletions of the PARK2 gene in patients with early-onset Parkinson disease. Clinical Genetics. 2012;82(1):77–82. doi:10.1111/j.1399-0004.2011.01693.x.

[82] Elfferich P, Verleun-Mooijman MC, Maat-Kievit JA, van de Warrenburg BP, Abdo WF, Eshuis SA, et al. Breakpoint mapping of 13 large Parkin deletions/duplications reveals an exon 4 deletion and an exon 7 duplication as founder mutations. Neurogenetics. 2011;12(4):263–71. doi:10.1007/s10048-011-0302-9.

[83] Periquet M, Lucking C, Vaughan J, Bonifati V, Durr A, De Michele G, et al. Origin of the mutations in the Parkin gene in Europe: exon rearrangements are independent recurrent events, whereas point mutations may result from Founder effects. American Journal of Human Genetics. 2001;68(3):617–26.

[84] Klein C, Pramstaller PP, Kis B, Page CC, Kann M, Leung J, et al. Parkin deletions in a family with adult-onset, tremor-dominant Parkinsonism: expanding the phenotype. Annals of Neurology. 2000;48(1):65–71.

[85] Farrer M, Chan P, Chen R, Tan L, Lincoln S, Hernandez D, et al. Lewy bodies and Parkinsonism in families with Parkin mutations. Annals of Neurology. 2001;50(3):293–300.

[86] Huttenlocher J, Stefansson H, Steinberg S, Helgadottir HT, Sveinbjornsdottir S, Riess O, et al. Heterozygote carriers for CNVs in PARK2 are at increased risk of Parkinson's disease. Human Molecular Genetics. 2015;24(19):5637–43. doi:10.1093/hmg/ddv277.

[87] Valente EM, Abou-Sleiman PM, Caputo V, Muqit MM, Harvey K, Gispert S, et al. Hereditary early-onset Parkinson's disease caused by mutations in PINK1. Science. 2004;304(5674):1158–60. doi:10.1126/science.1096284.

[88] Atsumi M, Li Y, Tomiyama H, Sato K, Hattori N. [A 62-year-old woman with early-onset Parkinson's disease associated with the PINKi gene deletion]. Rinsho shinkeigaku = Clinical Neurology. 2006;46(3):199–202.

[89] Li Y, Tomiyama H, Sato K, Hatano Y, Yoshino H, Atsumi M, et al. Clinicogenetic study of PINK1 mutations in autosomal recessive early-onset Parkinsonism. Neurology. 2005;64(11):1955–7. doi:10.1212/01.WNL.0000164009.36740.4E.

[90] Camargos ST, Dornas LO, Momeni P, Lees A, Hardy J, Singleton A, et al. Familial Parkinsonism and early onset Parkinson's disease in a Brazilian movement disorders clinic: phenotypic characterization and frequency of SNCA, PRKN, PINK1, and LRRK2 mutations. Movement Disorders. 2009;24(5):662–6. doi:10.1002/mds.22365.

[91] Cazeneuve C, San C, Ibrahim SA, Mukhtar MM, Kheir MM, Leguern E, et al. A new complex homozygous large rearrangement of the PINK1 gene in a Sudanese family with early onset Parkinson's disease. Neurogenetics. 2009;10(3):265–70. doi:10.1007/s10048-009-0174-4.

[92] Marongiu R, Brancati F, Antonini A, Ialongo T, Ceccarini C, Scarciolla O, et al. Whole gene deletion and splicing mutations expand the PINK1 genotypic spectrum. Human Mutation. 2007;28(1):98. doi:10.1002/humu.9472.

[93] Guo JF, Zhang XW, Nie LL, Zhang HN, Liao B, Li J, et al. Mutation analysis of Parkin, PINK1 and DJ-1 genes in Chinese patients with sporadic early onset Parkinsonism. Journal of Neurology. 2010;257(7):1170–5. doi:10.1007/s00415-010-5485-8.

[94] Samaranch L, Lorenzo-Betancor O, Arbelo JM, Ferrer I, Lorenzo E, Irigoyen J, et al. PINK1-linked Parkinsonism is associated with Lewy body pathology. Brain: a Journal of Neurology. 2010;133(Pt 4):1128–42. doi:10.1093/brain/awq051.

[95] Bonifati V, Rizzu P, Squitieri F, Krieger E, Vanacore N, van Swieten JC, et al. DJ-1(PARK7), a novel gene for autosomal recessive, early onset Parkinsonism. Neurological Sciences. 2003;24(3):159–60. doi:10.1007/s10072-003-0108-0.

[96] van Duijn CM, Dekker MC, Bonifati V, Galjaard RJ, Houwing-Duistermaat JJ, Snijders PJ, et al. Park7, a novel locus for autosomal recessive early-onset Parkinsonism, on chromosome 1p36. The American Journal of Human Genetics. 2001;69(3):629–34. doi:10.1086/322996.

[97] Lev N, Roncevic D, Ickowicz D, Melamed E, Offen D. Role of DJ-1 in Parkinson's disease. Journal of Molecular Neuroscience: MN. 2006;29(3):215–25.

[98] Ariga H, Takahashi-Niki K, Kato I, Maita H, Niki T, Iguchi-Ariga SM. Neuroprotective function of DJ-1 in Parkinson's disease. Oxidative Medicine and Cellular Longevity. 2013;2013:683920. doi:10.1155/2013/683920.

[99] Xu J, Zhong N, Wang H, Elias JE, Kim CY, Woldman I, et al. The Parkinson's disease-associated DJ-1 protein is a transcriptional co-activator that protects against neuronal apoptosis. Human Molecular Genetics. 2005;14(9):1231–41. doi:10.1093/hmg/ddi134.

[100] Hedrich K, Djarmati A, Schafer N, Hering R, Wellenbrock C, Weiss PH, et al. DJ-1 (PARK7) mutations are less frequent than Parkin (PARK2) mutations in early-onset Parkinson disease. Neurology. 2004;62(3):389–94.

[101] Djarmati A, Hedrich K, Svetel M, Schafer N, Juric V, Vukosavic S, et al. Detection of Parkin (PARK2) and DJ1 (PARK7) mutations in early-onset Parkinson disease: Parkin mutation frequency depends on ethnic origin of patients. Human Mutation. 2004;23(5): 525. doi:10.1002/humu.9240.

[102] Macedo MG, Verbaan D, Fang Y, van Rooden SM, Visser M, Anar B, et al. Genotypic and phenotypic characteristics of Dutch patients with early onset Parkinson's disease. Movement Disorders. 2009;24(2):196–203. doi:10.1002/mds.22287.

[103] Murphy KE, Cottle L, Gysbers AM, Cooper AA, Halliday GM. ATP13A2 (PARK9) protein levels are reduced in brain tissue of cases with Lewy bodies. Acta Neuropathologica Communications. 2013;1(1):11. doi:10.1186/2051-5960-1-11.

[104] Bademci G, Vance JM, Wang L. Tyrosine hydroxylase gene: another piece of the genetic puzzle of Parkinson's disease. CNS & Neurological Disorders Drug Targets. 2012;11(4): 469–81.

[105] Bademci G, Edwards TL, Torres AL, Scott WK, Zuchner S, Martin ER, et al. A rare novel deletion of the tyrosine hydroxylase gene in Parkinson disease. Human Mutation. 2010;31(10):E1767–71. doi:10.1002/humu.21351.

[106] Ormazabal A, Serrano M, Garcia-Cazorla A, Campistol J, Artuch R, Castro de Castro P, et al. Deletion in the tyrosine hydroxylase gene in a patient with a mild phenotype. Movement Disorders. 2011;26(8):1558–60. doi:10.1002/mds.23564.

[107] Vilarino-Guell C, Wider C, Ross OA, Dachsel JC, Kachergus JM, Lincoln SJ, et al. VPS35 mutations in Parkinson disease. American Journal of Human Genetics. 2011;89(1):162–7. doi:10.1016/j.ajhg.2011.06.001.

[108] Zimprich A, Benet-Pages A, Struhal W, Graf E, Eck SH, Offman MN, et al. A mutation in VPS35, encoding a subunit of the retromer complex, causes late-onset Parkinson disease. American Journal of Human Genetics. 2011;89(1):168–75. doi:10.1016/j.ajhg.2011.06.008.

[109] Verstraeten A, Wauters E, Crosiers D, Meeus B, Corsmit E, Elinck E, et al. Contribution of VPS35 genetic variability to LBD in the Flanders-Belgian population. Neurobiology of Aging. 2012;33(8):1844 e11–3. doi:10.1016/j.neurobiolaging.2012.01.006.

[110] Tang FL, Liu W, Hu JX, Erion JR, Ye J, Mei L, et al. VPS35 deficiency or mutation causes dopaminergic neuronal loss by impairing mitochondrial fusion and function. Cell Reports. 2015;12(10):1631–43. doi:10.1016/j.celrep.2015.08.001.

[111] Rovelet-Lecrux A, Deramecourt V, Legallic S, Maurage CA, Le Ber I, Brice A, et al. Deletion of the progranulin gene in patients with frontotemporal lobar degeneration or Parkinson disease. Neurobiology of Disease. 2008;31(1):41–5. doi:10.1016/j.nbd.2008.03.004.

[112] Ayuso P, Martinez C, Pastor P, Lorenzo-Betancor O, Luengo A, Jimenez-Jimenez FJ, et al. An association study between Heme oxygenase-1 genetic variants and Parkinson's disease. Frontiers in Cellular Neuroscience. 2014;8:298. doi:10.3389/fncel.2014.00298.

[113] Krahn LE, Maraganore DM, Michels VV. Childhood-onset schizophrenia associated with Parkinsonism in a patient with a microdeletion of chromosome 22. Mayo Clinic Proceedings. 1998;73(10):956–9. doi:10.4065/73.10.956.

[114] Zaleski C, Bassett AS, Tam K, Shugar AL, Chow EW, McPherson E. The co-occurrence of early onset Parkinson disease and 22q11.2 deletion syndrome. American Journal of Medical Genetics Part A. 2009;149A(3):525–8. doi:10.1002/ajmg.a.32650.

[115] Booij J, van Amelsvoort T, Boot E. Co-occurrence of early-onset Parkinson disease and 22q11.2 deletion syndrome: potential role for dopamine transporter imaging. American Journal of Medical Genetics Part A. 2010;152A(11):2937–8. doi:10.1002/ajmg.a.33665.

[116] Butcher NJ, Kiehl TR, Hazrati LN, Chow EW, Rogaeva E, Lang AE, et al. Association between early-onset Parkinson disease and 22q11.2 deletion syndrome: identification of a novel genetic form of Parkinson disease and its clinical implications. JAMA Neurology. 2013;70(11):1359–66. doi:10.1001/jamaneurol.2013.3646.

[117] Ogaki K, Ross OA. Chromosome 22q11.2 deletion may contain a locus for recessive early-onset Parkinson's disease. Parkinsonism & Related Disorders. 2014;20(9):945–6. doi:10.1016/j.parkreldis.2014.06.020.

[118] Rehman AF, Dhamija R, Williams ES, Barrett MJ. 22q11.2 deletion syndrome presenting with early-onset Parkinson's disease. Movement Disorders. 2015;30(9):1289–90. doi:10.1002/mds.26305.

[119] Perandones C, Farini VL, Pellene LA, Sáenz Farret M, Cuevas SM, et al. (2015) Parkinson's Disease in a Patient with 22q11.2 Deletion Syndrome: The Relevance of Detecting Mosaicisms by Means of Cell-By-Cell Evaluation Techniques. Single Cell Bio. 2015, Volume 4, Issue 4: 123. doi:10.4172/2168-9431.1000123

[120] Ikebe S, Tanaka M, Ohno K, Sato W, Hattori K, Kondo T, et al. Increase of deleted mitochondrial DNA in the striatum in Parkinson's disease and senescence. Biochemical and Biophysical Research Communications. 1990;170(3):1044–8.

[121] Siciliano G, Mancuso M, Ceravolo R, Lombardi V, Iudice A, Bonuccelli U. Mitochondrial DNA rearrangements in young onset Parkinsonism: two case reports. Journal of Neurology, Neurosurgery, and Psychiatry. 2001;71(5):685–7.

[122] Gu G, Reyes PE, Golden GT, Woltjer RL, Hulette C, Montine TJ, et al. Mitochondrial DNA deletions/rearrangements in Parkinson disease and related neurodegenerative disorders. Journal of Neuropathology and Experimental Neurology. 2002;61(7):634–9.

[123] Gui YX, Xu ZP, Lv W, Zhao JJ, Hu XY. Evidence for polymerase gamma, POLG1 variation in reduced mitochondrial DNA copy number in Parkinson's disease. Parkinsonism & Related Disorders. 2015;21(3):282–6. doi:10.1016/j.parkreldis.2014.12.030.

[124] Simon-Sanchez J, Scholz S, Matarin Mdel M, Fung HC, Hernandez D, Gibbs JR, et al. Genomewide SNP assay reveals mutations underlying Parkinson disease. Human Mutation. 2008;29(2):315–22. doi:10.1002/humu.20626.

[125] Kim JS, Yoo JY, Lee KS, Kim HS, Choi JS, Rha HK, et al. Comparative genome hybridization array analysis for sporadic Parkinson's disease. The International Journal of Neuroscience. 2008;118(9):1331–45. doi:10.1080/00207450802174522.

[126] Liu X, Cheng R, Ye X, Verbitsky M, Kisselev S, Mejia-Santana H, et al. Increased rate of sporadic and recurrent rare genic copy number variants in Parkinson's disease among Ashkenazi Jews. Molecular Genetics & Genomic Medicine. 2013;1(3):142–54. doi:10.1002/mgg3.18.

[127] Pamphlett R, Morahan JM, Luquin N, Yu B. An approach to finding brain-situated mutations in sporadic Parkinson's disease. Parkinsonism & Related Disorders. 2012;18(1):82–5. doi:10.1016/j.parkreldis.2011.08.024.

[128] Ceulemans S, van der Ven K, Del-Favero J. Targeted screening and validation of copy number variations. Methods in Molecular Biology. 2012;838:311–28. doi: 10.1007/978-1-61779-507-7_15.

[129] Carter NP, Fiegler H, Piper J. Comparative analysis of comparative genomic hybridization microarray technologies: report of a workshop sponsored by the Wellcome Trust. Cytometry. 2002;49(2):43–8. doi:10.1002/cyto.10153.

[130] Shaw-Smith C, Redon R, Rickman L, Rio M, Willatt L, Fiegler H, et al. Microarray based comparative genomic hybridisation (array-CGH) detects submicroscopic chromosomal deletions and duplications in patients with learning disability/mental retardation and dysmorphic features. Journal of Medical Genetics. 2004;41(4):241–8.

[131] Iafrate AJ, Feuk L, Rivera MN, Listewnik ML, Donahoe PK, Qi Y, et al. Detection of large-scale variation in the human genome. Nature Genetics. 2004;36(9):949–51. doi: 10.1038/ng1416.

[132] Inazawa J, Inoue J, Imoto I. Comparative genomic hybridization (CGH)-arrays pave the way for identification of novel cancer-related genes. Cancer Science. 2004;95(7):559–63.

[133] Ishkanian AS, Malloff CA, Watson SK, DeLeeuw RJ, Chi B, Coe BP, et al. A tiling resolution DNA microarray with complete coverage of the human genome. Nature Genetics. 2004;36(3):299–303. doi:10.1038/ng1307.

[134] Miller DT, Adam MP, Aradhya S, Biesecker LG, Brothman AR, Carter NP, et al. Consensus statement: chromosomal microarray is a first-tier clinical diagnostic test for individuals with developmental disabilities or congenital anomalies. American Journal of Human Genetics. 2010;86(5):749–64. doi:10.1016/j.ajhg.2010.04.006.

[135] Vasson A, Leroux C, Orhant L, Boimard M, Toussaint A, Leroy C, et al. Custom oligonucleotide array-based CGH: a reliable diagnostic tool for detection of exonic copy-number changes in multiple targeted genes. European Journal of Human Genetics: EJHG. 2013;21(9):977–87. doi:10.1038/ejhg.2012.279.

[136] Boone PM, Bacino CA, Shaw CA, Eng PA, Hixson PM, Pursley AN, et al. Detection of clinically relevant exonic copy-number changes by array CGH. Human Mutation. 2010;31(12):1326–42. doi:10.1002/humu.21360.

[137] Ferlini A, Bovolenta M, Neri M, Gualandi F, Balboni A, Yuryev A, et al. Custom CGH array profiling of copy number variations (CNVs) on chromosome 6p21.32 (HLA locus) in patients with venous malformations associated with multiple sclerosis. BMC Medical Genetics. 2010;11:64. doi:10.1186/1471-2350-11-64.

[138] Piluso G, Dionisi M, Del Vecchio Blanco F, Torella A, Aurino S, Savarese M, et al. Motor chip: a comparative genomic hybridization microarray for copy-number mutations in 245 neuromuscular disorders. Clinical Chemistry. 2011;57(11):1584–96. doi:10.1373/clinchem.2011.168898.

[139] Wisniowiecka-Kowalnik B, Kastory-Bronowska M, Bartnik M, Derwinska K, Dymczak-Domini W, Szumbarska D, et al. Application of custom-designed oligonucleotide array CGH in 145 patients with autistic spectrum disorders. European Journal of Human Genetics: EJHG. 2013;21(6):620–5. doi:10.1038/ejhg.2012.219.

[140] Mefford HC, Muhle H, Ostertag P, von Spiczak S, Buysse K, Baker C, et al. Genome-wide copy number variation in epilepsy: novel susceptibility loci in idiopathic generalized and focal epilepsies. PLoS Genetics. 2010;6(5):e1000962. doi:10.1371/journal.pgen.1000962.

[141] Tayeh MK, Chin EL, Miller VR, Bean LJ, Coffee B, Hegde M. Targeted comparative genomic hybridization array for the detection of single- and multiexon gene deletions and duplications. Genetics in Medicine. 2009;11(4):232–40. doi:10.1097/GIM.0b013e318195e191.

[142] Wang J, Zhan H, Li FY, Pursley AN, Schmitt ES, Wong LJ. Targeted array CGH as a valuable molecular diagnostic approach: experience in the diagnosis of mitochondrial and metabolic disorders. Molecular Genetics and Metabolism. 2012;106(2):221–30. doi:10.1016/j.ymgme.2012.03.005.

[143] Wang J, Rakhade M. Utility of array CGH in molecular diagnosis of mitochondrial disorders. Methods in Molecular Biology. 2012;837:301–12. doi: 10.1007/978-1-61779-504-6_20.

[144] Yoon S, Xuan Z, Makarov V, Ye K, Sebat J. Sensitive and accurate detection of copy number variants using read depth of coverage. Genome Research. 2009;19(9):1586–92. doi:10.1101/gr.092981.109.

[145] Duan J, Zhang JG, Deng HW, Wang YP. Detection of common copy number variation with application to population clustering from next generation sequencing data. Conference proceedings: Annual International Conference of the IEEE Engineering in Medicine and Biology Society IEEE Engineering in Medicine and Biology Society Annual Conference. 2012;2012:1246–9. doi:10.1109/EMBC.2012.6346163.

[146] Duan J, Zhang JG, Deng HW, Wang YP. Comparative studies of copy number variation detection methods for next-generation sequencing technologies. PLoS One. 2013;8(3):e59128. doi:10.1371/journal.pone.0059128.

[147] Wang H, Nettleton D, Ying K. Copy number variation detection using next generation sequencing read counts. BMC Bioinformatics. 2014;15:109. doi: 10.1186/1471-2105-15-109.

Chapter 3

Mechanisms for Neuronal Cell Death in Parkinson's Disease: Pathological Cross Talks Between Epigenetics and Various Signalling Pathways

S Meenalochani, ST Dheen and SSW Tay

Additional information is available at the end of the chapter

http://dx.doi.org/10.5772/63103

Abstract

Parkinson's disease (PD) is an incapacitating neurodegenerative disorder affecting the population over the age of 65 years. Clinically, most patients present with the symptoms of bradykinesia, resting tremor, rigidity, and postural instability. A number of patients also suffer from autonomic, cognitive, and psychiatric disturbances. The symptoms of PD result from the selective loss of dopaminergic (DA) neurons in the substantia nigra (SNc) pars compacta. However, the exact molecular mechanism that causes this cell death still remains elusive. The cross talk between various molecular signals facilitates the cell to undergo developmental and differentiation programs with such tantalizing accuracy. In recent years, epigenetic mechanisms have advanced as a regulatory driver of processes such as signal transduction, cell cycle control, and stress response. These include DNA methylation, histone modifications, and small RNA-mediated mechanisms. Increasing evidence suggests that epigenetic mechanisms play a major role in the pathogenesis of PD. Researchers are now working to comprehend the therapeutic promises of epigenetic molecules to offset age-related neurodegenerative diseases. In this chapter, we focus on some examples of the cross talk between epigenetic processes and various signal transduction pathways that underlie the pathogenesis of PD.

Keywords: Parkinson's disease, epigenetics, DNA methylation, histone modifications, non-coding RNAs

1. Introduction

Parkinson's disease (PD) is a devastating disorder of the brain characterized by continuous deterioration of motor functions owing to the loss of dopaminergic neurons in the substantia nigra of the mid brain. It is the second most common neurodegenerative disorder after Alzheimer's disease. The first clear medical explanation about PD was written in 1817 by an English physician James Parkinson in his work titled *An Essay on the Shaking Palsy* [1]. The SNc of the midbrain contains the DA neurons which produce dopamine. Dopamine is a neurotransmitter responsible for coordinating movements. Although few in number, these DA neurons play a vital role in controlling multiple brain functions including voluntary movement and a broad array of behavioural processes [2]. In PD, there is a severe depletion in the levels of dopamine due to the degeneration of DA neurons. This results in the lack of control over body movements [2]. Nevertheless, the precise cause of this neuronal cell death still remains an enigma.

The signs and symptoms of PD may vary from person to person. The symptoms have a gradual onset and usually advance simultaneously with the progression of the disease. Early signs may be mild and may go unnoticed and later tend to worsen over time. If left untreated, it may lead to disability with associated immobility. The early classic symptoms of PD include motor symptoms such as postural instability, resting tremor, bradykinesia, and rigidity [3]. These symptoms are linked to the progressive loss of dopamine and are usually improved by treatment with levodopa or dopamine agonists [4]. Nevertheless, as the disease progresses, symptoms that fail to respond to levodopa develop [5]. These symptoms include flexed posture, freezing phenomenon, and loss of postural stability [6]. Although the motor symptoms lead the clinical picture of PD, some patients are also associated with a range of non-motor symptoms such as sleep, sensation, autonomic, mood disturbances as well as cognitive disturbances such as dementia [7].

The diagnosis of PD is extremely complicated, mainly during its early stages. This is due to the fact that as the disease advances, the symptoms might mimic other ailments. Moreover, at present, there is no specific lab test available to diagnose the disease. In most cases, physical examination of the patient forms the basis for the diagnosis of PD. Levodopa continues to be the most effective treatment for PD [8]. Another feasible option is deep brain stimulation, although some patients encounter the necessity for surgery. New treatments that offer better control over the symptoms stay on developmental demand.

2. Possible pathways involved in the pathogenesis of PD

Several enthralling theories have shown that different molecular pathways are involved in the propagation of PD pathogenesis. Accumulating evidence has confirmed that mitochondrial dysfunction, impairment of the ubiquitin proteasome system (UPS), and oxidative stress may perhaps represent the prime molecular pathways that generally mitigate the pathogenesis of both sporadic and familial forms of PD [9]. In addition to these, inflammation and loss of neurotrophic factors have also been shown to play a major role in the progress of PD [9].

3. Potential risk factors in PD

Age is one of the prominent risk factors in PD [10, 11]. Studies have shown that dopaminergic neuronal populations appear selectively susceptible to loss with ageing compared to many other brain regions and those related to other neurodegenerative disorders [12]. Furthermore, studies have also shown that the dopaminergic neurons are particularly vulnerable to the mitochondrial dysfunction with advancing age [13, 14].

4. Genetic factors in PD

Although PD was long considered to be sporadic in origin, monogenic Parkinsonism disorders are gaining growing importance in recent years. Genetic factors appear to be the main cause in about 5–10% of the PD patients [15]. However, in both cases, the degeneration of nigrostriatal DA neurons remains a general overlapping characteristic [16]. Studies have shown that around 13 genetic loci are involved in the rare forms of PD [17]. Out of the 13, around 6 PARK loci genes have been identified and have been reported to carry mutations that are related to relatives who are affected by PD. Out of the six genes, four have similarly been shown to be involved in sporadic PD [17].

There is considerable evidence that, in addition to well-defined genetic mechanisms, environmental factors play a crucial role in PD pathogenesis. Nevertheless, the exact mechanism by which the environment could affect the genetic factors and contribute to PD development remains obscure. In recent years, epigenetic mechanisms such as DNA methylation, chromatin remodelling, and alterations in gene expression via non-coding RNAs (ncRNAs) are surging in importance as potential factors in the pathogenesis of PD.

5. Epigenetics

Epigenetics refers to mechanisms which can alter the expression of genes without modifying the actual DNA sequence and are heritable [18]. Epigenetic modulation exists throughout life, beginning in prenatal stages, is dependent on the lifestyle, environmental exposure, and genetic makeup of an individual and may serve as a missing link between PD risk factors and development of the disease [18].

At the molecular level, epigenetic mechanisms influence protein expression through post-translational modifications of histones (e.g. acetylation, methylation, phosphorylation, and ubiquitination), the methylation of cytosine bases and positioning of nucleosome, and by activation/deactivation of microRNAs (miRNAs). These processes act as a switch for the fate of the cell through regulating gene and miRNA expression, as well as through parental imprinting, X chromosome inactivation, suppressing transposons, and regulating developmental processes [19]. The epigenome offers the flexibility to address a fluctuating environment above the relatively rigid architecture of DNA sequence information and thus influences the formation of a phenotype without altering the genotype. The three distinct mechanisms of epigenetic regulation that are complex and interrelated are DNA methylation, histone modification, and RNA-based mechanisms.

5.1. Epigenetic mechanisms in PD

In spite of having a familial aspect, PD does not show a clear Mendelian pattern of inheritance, making it difficult to correlate the genetic variations with the disease state. In this case, an epigenetic framework would be most useful in understanding the age dependence (which is not clearly explained by the accumulation of genetic mutations) and the environmental impact on genetic predisposition to the disease. A better understanding of the complex interplay of genetic and epigenetic factors can help in improving the existing knowledge on disease mechanisms and therapeutic strategies. In diseases where age and environment play an important role, the identification of epigenetic variations contributing to the age- and environment-mediated control of disease mechanism will simplify the disease diagnosis [20]. Studying epigenetic mechanisms involved in PD can hence be a major milestone in the pursuit of understanding the disease better. In recent years, the impact of epigenetic mechanisms in PD has been increasingly studied [21]. DNA methylation, histone tail modifications, and microRNA-mediated pathways are considered to play a role in the pathogenesis of PD based on recent evidence ([22–26]).

6. DNA methylation

6.1. Principle of DNA methylation

DNA methylation is one such epigenetic modification that has been studied extensively for the past several decades since its discovery in cancer in 1983 [27]. DNA methylation involves the transfer of a methyl group to the 5′ position of a cytosine residue. This dinucleotide unit is always written as CpG (representing a cytosine followed by guanine and a phosphate group between them). Regions that are enriched with CpGs are called CpG islands. These CpG islands are usually located in the promoter region of genes. CpG islands are usually non-methylated, except in some rare cases where methylation of CPG islands is required. On the contrary, CpGs outside CpG islands are usually methylated [28, 29]. Methylation of CpG sequences can modify gene expression levels by inducing conformational changes in the chromatin. This impedes the availability of the gene promoter region for the transcriptional machinery [30]. Therefore, it is obvious that promoter hyper-methylation leads to gene silencing while hypo-methylation will augment gene expression. CpG methylation within promoter and intragenic sites has been extensively studied, and moreover, there has been surging interest regarding non-CpG methylation. This denotes the methylation that occurs at cytosine of non-CpG dinucleotides, such as CA, CT, or CC. DNA methylation works in congruence with histone modification (such as histone acetylation) to control memory formation and synaptic plasticity [31], and it also has a possible impact on genetic and neuronal function affecting behaviours [32]. Moreover, the association between DNA methylation, chromatin structure, and gene silencing has been extensively studied for many years, and gene silencing is thought to be an epigenetic intervention on neurodegenerative diseases like Alzheimer's disease (AD) [33]. Therefore, it seems justified to suggest that there is a very strong potential link between DNA methylation and neurodegenerative diseases.

6.1.1. DNA methylation in PD

Methylation can be instigated by a variety of factors, which can be the cause of many serious diseases including PD. Ageing has been shown to decrease global DNA methylation [34], while it increases methylation in specific promoters. This could be a contributing factor in PD as it is an age-related disorder.

Although there have not been many reports, there are indications of impaired methylation in PD patients [25]. DNA methylation has been widely studied in the SNCA gene. Methylation of intron 1 of the SNCA gene is associated with decreased transcription [35]. Decreased methylation of the SNCA gene and of the SNCA intron 1 has been observed in the SNc of clinical PD cases [36]. It is obvious from these results that the increased α-synuclein production (that is associated with PD) is caused by the increased SNCA gene expression, as a result of a decreased methylation state of the SNCA gene. Furthermore, it has been demonstrated that α-synuclein could sequester DNA methyltransferase 1 (which maintains DNA methylation) in the cytoplasm. DNA methyltransferase 1 is an important enzyme which is expressed copiously in the brain and maintains DNA methylation in the cytoplasm. Sequestering DNMT1 leads to global DNA hypo-methylation in PD patients with dementia and presence of neuronal Lewy body (DLB) [37]. A GWAS on methylation of candidate genes identified changes in methylation status of proximal DNA CpG sites of other genes such as PARK16/1q32, glycoprotein (transmembrane) nmb (GPNMB), and syntaxin 1b (STX1B), *ARK16*. This is indicative of the fact that other PD-related genes may possibly be susceptible to these methylation changes (International Parkinson's Disease Genomics and Welcome Trust Case Control, 2011). Nevertheless, the clear undeviating link between DNA methylation and PD still remains obscure. The epigenetic regulation of SNCA gene has also been reported in an A53T-linked familial case of PD. A recent methylation study on brain and blood samples from PD patients has revealed that there is differential methylation of CpG sites [25]. Of these, over 80% of the sites were hypo-methylated in both blood and brain. The same study has reported that genes such as major histocompatibility complex, class II (MHC II), dq alpha 1 (HLA-DQA1), glutamine-fructose-6-phosphate transaminase 2 (GFPT2), MAPT, and vault RNA2-1 (VTRNA2-1) are highly associated with PD being similarly methylated in brain and blood samples from clinical PD cases [25].

The number of methylated sites in DNA has been reported to increase with ageing [34] which is a major risk factor for PD. Results from the GWAS have already provided many novel and important perceptions for molecular mechanisms underlying the pathogenesis of complex diseases such as PD. Nevertheless, it is probable that understanding exact epigenetic modifications might be significantly assisted by knowledge of genetic susceptibility loci determined from GWAS.

7. Histone modifications

7.1. Principle behind histone modification and the different types of histone modifications

Histones are proteins that pack and order DNA into nucleosomes. Each nucleosome contains two subunits each of histones H2A, H2B, H3, and H4, known as the core histones (octomers). A 147-bp segment of DNA wrapped around the histone octamer and neighbouring nucleosomes are separated by, on average, 50 bp of free DNA. Histone H1 is termed the linker histone, and it does not form the integral part of the nucleosome. However, it binds to the linker DNA (that is, the DNA separating two histone complexes), sealing off the nucleosome at the location where DNA enters and leaves.

Histones play a crucial role in epigenetics. All histones are subject to several post-transcriptional modifications such as acetylation, methylation, phosphorylation, ubiquitination, SUMOylation, and ADP-ribosylation, among others [38]. These post-translational modifications made to histone tails can influence gene expression by altering the structure of chromatin or using histone modifiers. Histone protein modifications can alter the availability of transcriptional machinery to specific promoters leading to gene activation or silencing [39]. Histone modifications have vital roles in transcriptional regulation, DNA repair, DNA replication, alternative splicing [40], and chromosome condensation [41]. With respect to its transcriptional state, the human genome can be roughly divided into actively transcribed euchromatin and transcriptionally inactive heterochromatin. Euchromatin is characterized by high levels of histone modifications such as acetylation and trimethylated H3K4, H3K36, and H3K79. On the contrary, heterochromatin is characterized by low levels of acetylation and high levels of H3K9, H3K27, and H4K20 methylation [42]. Recent studies have demonstrated that actively transcribed genes are characterized by high levels of H3K4me3, H3K27ac, H2BK5ac, and H4K20me1 in the promoter and H3K79me1 and H4K20me1 in the gene body [43].

7.1.1. *Histone acetylation/deacetylation*

Histone modifications such as acetylation and deacetylation play important roles in gene regulation. These are associated with transcriptional activation and repression respectively [41]. Histone acetylation is a reversible process. Acetylation is catalysed by histone acetyltransferases (HATs), which are categorized into three families (GNAT, MYST, and CBP/p300) [44]. HATs catalyse acetylation via the transfer of an acetyl group from acetyl-coenzyme A to the ε-amino group of lysine side chains on the N-terminal tails of H2A, H2B, H3, and H4 [44]. It has recently been shown that HATs can catalyse acetylation at lysine 56 (K56) within the core domain of H3 [41]. Histone deacetylation is performed by a class of enzymes known as histone deacetylases (HDACs). These HDACs remove the acetyl groups from the ε-amino group of lysines. HDACs are classified into four classes based upon sequence homology and cofactor dependencies.

7.1.2. Histone methylation/demethylation

Histone methylation involves the transfer of methyl groups from S-adenosyl-L-methionine to lysine or arginine residues of histone proteins by histone methyltransferases (HMTs). As described earlier, DNA methylation and histone modifications work in association with each other. HMTs control DNA methylation through transcriptional repression or activation which is chromatin dependent. Several different histone methyltransferases exist, and each of them is specific for the lysine or arginine residue they modify. For example, on histone H3, SET1, SET7/9, Ash1, ALL-1, MLL, ALR, Trx, and SMYD3 are the histone methyltransferases that catalyse methylation of histone H3 at lysine 4 (H3-K4) in mammalian cells [45]. ESET, SUV39-h1, SUV39-h2, SETDB1, Dim-5, and Eu-HMTase are histone methyltransferases that catalyse methylation of histone H3 at lysine 9 (H3-K9) in mammalian cells [45]. G9a and polycomb group enzymes such as EZH2 are histone methyltransferases that catalyse methylation of histone H3 at lysine 27 (H3-K27) in mammalian cells [46]. Arginine methylation of histones H3 and H4 promotes transcriptional activation and is mediated by a family of protein arginine methyltransferases (PRMTs) [47]. Based on the position to which the methyl groups are added, PRMTs are classified into type I (CARM1, PRMT1, PRMT2, PRMT3, PRMT6, and PRMT8) and type II (PRMT5 and PRMT7) [47].

7.2. Histone modifications in PD

The precise role of histone modifications in the pathogenesis of PD still remains indefinable, and most of the data are obtained from experimental cell cultures and animal models of PD.

α-synuclein, the major protein involved in PD pathogenesis, is known to interact with histones and inhibit histone deacetylation [48]. Several histone deacetylase inhibitors have been reported to protect against α-synuclein-mediated toxicity in PD models [48]. Inhibition of the histone deacetylase sirtuin-2 is known to decrease α-synuclein-mediated toxicity and protect against dopaminergic neuronal death [49]. When mouse nigral neurons were treated with the herbicide paraquat, alpha-synuclein translocated into the nucleus and was able to interact directly with histones [50]. Another study in Drosophila model of PD has demonstrated that alpha-synuclein interacts directly with histones by inhibiting histone acetylation. This neurotoxic effect of alpha-synuclein was counteracted by the administration of HDAC inhibitors [51]. Together with alpha-synuclein, HDAC6 and HDAC4 are the chief components of Lewy bodies in PD [52]. It is interesting to note that HDAC6 protects dopaminergic neurons from alpha-synuclein toxicity by promoting inclusion formation [53]. This has been confirmed by various other reports on neuronal cell lines expressing mutant alpha-synuclein wherein they have reported that the neurons are rescued from alpha-synuclein toxicity by HDAC6. In PD, histones seem to be more involved in aggregate formation, than in epigenetic dysregulation of gene expression. It has also been demonstrated that α-synuclein, interact with histone H1, which is localized in the cytoplasm of neurons and astrocytes from affected brain areas in PD. This has been shown to play a role in fibril formation [54]. Although not directly linked to histone acetylation, alpha-synuclein overexpression can downregulate the expression of histone genes. Previous reports on *C. elegans* model have demonstrated that overexpressing human alpha-synuclein leads to downregulation of nine genes coding for histones H1, H2B, and H4 [55]. It is clear from these studies that most of histone PTM evidence in PD is derived from the effects of alpha-synuclein. Moreover, few other genes associated with PD pathogenesis have been linked to HDAC function. Mutations in parkin cause early onset of familial PD (AR-JP) [56]. Parkin has been shown to promote mitophagy by catalysing mitochondrial ubiquitination, which in turn employs ubiquitin-binding autophagic components, such as HDAC6 [56]. The treatment of a dopaminergic cell line with the HDAC inhibitor phenylbutyrate resulted in increased levels of DJ-1 which protected these cells from mutant alpha-synuclein toxicity. An increase in DJ-1 expression was also observed in mice treated with phenylbutyrate and protected MPP^{+}-challenged dopaminergic neurons [57]. In addition, PINK-1 is also affected by HDAC activity. Transgenic expression of sirtuin 2 in PINK-1 Drosophila mutants rescued mitochondrial defects and spared dopaminergic neurons [58]. This suggests that depending on the PD model, HDACs may have a neuroprotective role. Levodopa remains as the most effective and extensively used therapy in the treatment of PD although it is tied with some serious side effects. Prolonged treatment with levodopa leads to the development of abnormal involuntary movements, termed levodopa-induced dyskinesia (LDID). Interestingly, histone PTMs have been shown to play a role in LDID. Previous reports on primate model have demonstrated that LDID is associated with marked deacetylation of histone H4, hyperacetylation, and dephosphorylation of histone H3 in the striatum [59]. In mouse models of LDID, histone H3 exhibited decreased trimethylation [59]. Histone H3 phosphorylation changes have also been demonstrated in striatonigral medium spiny neurons, thereby linking ERK-dependent histone phosphorylation in striatal plasticity leading to dyskinesia [60]. Future studies are warranted in order to understand the underlying molecular mechanism and the direct link between histone modifications in PD. This will enhance our knowledge and light up new avenues for the identification of epigenetics-based therapeutics for the better treatment of PD.

8. Non-coding RNAs

8.1. What are microRNAs?

miRNAs are critical regulators of gene expression. Their discovery adds a new facet to our understanding of intricate gene regulatory networks. These are a family of small, ncRNAs that regulate gene expression in a sequence-specific manner. They were first identified in *Caenorhabditis elegans* as genes that were responsible for the regulation of developmental events. Since then, hundreds of microRNAs have been identified in almost all species [61]. MicroRNAs have diverse expression patterns and play a vital role in various developmental and physiological processes. These small ncRNAs are transcribed by RNA polymerase II (RNA Pol II) from two primary genomic loci: miRNA genes and intronic sequences. In the canonical biogenesis pathway, pri-miRNAs are transcribed from miRNA genes [62]. These are processed in the nucleus by the Drosha/DGCR8 microprocessor complex to produce pre-miRNAs. The processed pre-miRNAs are then exported to the cytoplasm by Exportin-5. In the cytoplasm, these pre-miRNAs are further cleaved by the RNase III enzyme Dicer to yield a mature miRNA duplex. The mature strand also termed the guide strand is 20–22 nucleotides in length and associates with Argonaute proteins, AGO 1–4, to form a functional RNA-induced silencing complex (RISC) [62]. The antisense strand, denoted by miRNA*, was previously thought to be degraded; recent evidence suggests that some of these may have biological activity. The mature miRNA functions by aligning the RISC to target mRNA by binding at complementary seed sequences in the 3′UTR. This association of target mRNA with the miRNA-containing RISC results in silencing the gene expression by translational repression and recruitment of protein complexes causing deadenylation and degradation of target mRNA [63].

9. Interaction between miRNAs and PD-related genes

Overproduction of a gene product is one of the cardinal mechanisms by which the gene contributes to PD pathogenesis (a best known example is α-synuclein). There is a strong association that miRNA-mediated gene suppression could hold prospective approaches to improve the disease phenotype.

On this ground, miR-7 was first discovered as a regulator of α-synuclein expression [64, 65]. Junn et al. [64] demonstrated that miR-7 level is 40 times higher in neurons than in other cells. Further miR-7 is higher in the substantia nigra and striatum of mice, compared to cerebral cortex and cerebellum. This provides support for endogenous miR-7 regulation of α-synuclein levels in neurons. To further this study and to understand the clear mechanistic underpinnings of miR-7 in PD, the same group investigated miR-7 levels in MPP+-treated SH-SY5Y cells, and MPTP-intoxicated mice [65]. From this study, it was demonstrated that overexpressing miR-7 reduces endogenous α-synuclein levels. Hence it seems justified to suggest that a reduction in miR-7 might be a major contributor to nigrostriatal degeneration. In addition to miR-7, Doxakis [65] described the role of miR-153. In the regulation of α-synuclein, overexpression of miR-153 in cultured cortical neurons has been shown to reduce endogenous α-synuclein levels to around 30–40%. These results advocate the potential role of miR-7 and miR-153 as promising therapeutic targets to promote neuroprotection in patients with known α-synuclein gene multiplications. Another major gene involved in the PD pathogenesis is LRRK2 gene. Although the function of the leucine-rich repeat kinase 2 (LRRK2 gene) still remains largely unknown, some recent evidence suggests that this gene could be involved in membrane trafficking [66]. Mutation in the LRRK2 gene has been implicated as a risk factor for both familial and sporadic PD [67]. Reports have demonstrated that LRRK2 gene inhibition blocks neurotoxicity *in vitro* and *in vivo* [68]. These reports provide further support for its role in PD [69]. Cho et al. [70] have demonstrated that normal LRRK2 gene levels are higher in the frontal cortex of sporadic PD and PD with dementia (PDD) patients compared to controls (NPC) . Interestingly, MiR-205 has been identified as a putative regulator of LRRK2 gene. In addition, further investigations revealed significantly lower levels of miR-205 in the frontal cortex and striatum of PD patients, compared to NPC. Inhibition of miR-205 is associated with upregulation of the LRRK2 gene protein and vice versa. DA neurons in rodent brain displayed a high level of miR-205. Reports on transgenic mice overexpressing mutant LRRK2 gene, miR-205 treatment rescued impairment of neurite outgrowth. Like miR-7 and miR153, miR 205 is a potential target for therapeutic intervention, particularly for sporadic cases in which LRRK2 gene levels were found to be elevated, and miR-205 levels were found to be low [70]. DJ1 and parkin are other genes that are regulated by miR34b and miR34c, respectively. Miñones-Moyano et al. [71] first discovered a dysregulation of miR-34b and miR-34c in the post-mortem brains of clinical PD cases. Their study demonstrated that miR-34 reduction compromises neuronal viability by mitochondrial dysfunction and production of reactive oxygen species in an SH-SY5Y neuroblastoma culture model. They further characterized that the miR-34b/c reduction is correlated with decreased expression of DJ1 and Parkin, noting that these proteins were indeed downregulated in PD brain tissue as well [71]. This provides evidence that miR-34b/c downregulation may involve DJ1 and Parkin; however, the exact molecular mechanism by which this interaction occurs remains unclear. Previous work from our group has demonstrated that downregulation of MiR124 in the MPTP-induced mouse model of PD modulates the expression of Calpain/CDK5 pathway proteins [72]. This study proves that miRNAs can serve as a powerful tool to gain in-depth knowledge about the underlying mechanism that leads to the pathogenesis of the disease, and miRNA-based therapies can be used to validate drug targets for PD.

10. Examples of cross talks between epigenetics and signalling pathways underlying PD pathogenesis

MAPK pathway has been reported to cause neurodegeneration in PD. In addition, it has also been demonstrated that cocaine induces the MAPK pathway and through MSK1 phosphorylates histone H3 at Ser10 [73]. In addition, DNA methylation has been shown to affect the stimulation of aurora-B kinase which has been reported to phosphorylate H3S10 [74]. Casein kinase II (CKII) which is a serine/threonine kinase has been reported to phosphorylate histone H4 serine 1 in response to DNA damage [75]. CKII can also phosphorylate synphilin-1, reducing its interaction with α-synuclein and formation of inclusion bodies [76]. In addition, CKII phosphorylates Ser-129 of α-synuclein in human brain and inhibits Cdk5 [77]. It is well known that α-synuclein by the activation of nitric oxide synthase (NOS) and releasing NO considerably reduces PARP-1 [78]. Activation of PARP-1 in response to DNA damage inhibits aurora-B kinase, which is required for H3S10 phosphorylation [79]. Reports on miRNAs have shed light on the fact that miRNAs regulate various signalling pathways such as checkpoint transduction cascades or transcriptional repression that are associated with PD pathogenesis [80]. An interesting study in human H4 neuroglioma cells identified a large set of putative α-synuclein target (interacting) genes which are widely used as a model for studying the molecular basis of PD, providing the first insight into the interaction of endogenous α-synuclein. Their study identified several primary targets of α-synuclein, with the glycosphingolipid biosynthesis and the protein ubiquitination pathways being common to miRNome IPA analysis. In addition, they have also shown that miR-30b, miR-30c, and miR-26a which are among the most abundant miRNAs in primary human neuronal and glial cells and are reported to be involved in the regulation of α-synuclein [81] emerged as the main modulators of these two pathways. Taken together, these reports highlight a few examples on the role of epigenetic mechanism that may act as modulators of cellular mechanisms leading to PD.

11. Conclusion

Evidence has shed light on the role of epigenetics in PD and has increased our understanding of the genetics of PD since the first report. The studies described in this chapter provide evidence that targeting the epigenome, with small drugs such as HDAC inhibitors that are able to cross the blood-brain barrier, can be one of the potential candidates to delay the onset and progression of the symptoms in animal models of PD. Further studies aiming at understanding the complex interplay between genetic and epigenetic biomarkers, lifestyles, and environmental factors are warranted in order to completely counter the progression of PD in the near future.

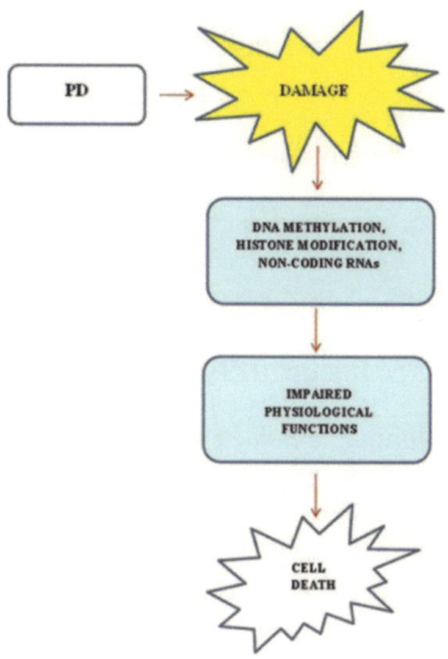

Figure 1. Epigenetics and cell death in PD.

Author details

S Meenalochani, ST Dheen and SSW Tay*

*Address all correspondence to: anttaysw@nus.edu.sg

Department of Anatomy, Yong Loo Lin school of Medicine, National University Health System, National University of Singapore, Singapore

References

[1] Parkinson, J., *An essay on the shaking palsy. 1817.* J Neuropsychiatry Clin Neurosci, 2002. 14(2): pp. 223–36; discussion 222.

[2] Chinta, S.J. and J.K. Andersen, *Dopaminergic neurons.* Int J Biochem Cell Biol, 2005. 37(5): pp. 942–946.

[3] Jankovic, J., *Parkinson's disease: clinical features and diagnosis.* J Neurol Neurosurg Psychiatry, 2008. 79(4): pp. 368–376.

[4] Katzenschlager, R. and A.J. Lees, *Treatment of Parkinson's disease: levodopa as the first choice.* J Neurol, 2002. 249 Suppl 2: pp. Ii19–24.

[5] Thanvi, B., N. Lo, and T. Robinson, *Levodopa-induced dyskinesia in Parkinson's disease: clinical features, pathogenesis, prevention and treatment.* Postgrad Med J, 2007. 83(980): pp. 384–388.

[6] Davie, C.A., *A review of Parkinson's disease.* Br Med Bull, 2008. 86: pp. 109–27.

[7] Shulman, L.M., et al., *Non-recognition of depression and other non-motor symptoms in Parkinson's disease.* Parkinsonism Rel Disord, 2002. 8(3): pp. 193–197.

[8] Gelb, D.J., E. Oliver, and S. Gilman, *Diagnostic criteria for Parkinson disease.* Arch Neurol, 1999. 56(1): pp. 33–39.

[9] Dawson, T.M. and V.L. Dawson, *Molecular Pathways of Neurodegeneration in Parkinson's disease.* Science, 2003. 302(5646): pp. 819–822.

[10] Schapira, A.H. and P. Jenner, *Etiology and pathogenesis of Parkinson's disease.* Mov Disorders, 2011. 26(6): pp. 1049–1055.

[11] Reeve, A., E. Simcox, and D. Turnbull, *Ageing and Parkinson's disease: why is advancing age the biggest risk factor?* Ageing Res Rev, 2014. 14(0): pp. 19–30.

[12] Hirsch, E.C., et al., *Neuronal loss in the pedunculopontine tegmental nucleus in Parkinson disease and in progressive supranuclear palsy.* Proc Natl Acad Sci, 1987. 84(16): pp. 5976–5980.

[13] Bender, A., et al., *High levels of mitochondrial DNA deletions in substantia nigra neurons in aging and Parkinson disease.* Nature Genet, 2006. 38(5): pp. 515–517.

[14] Kraytsberg, Y., et al., *Mitochondrial DNA deletions are abundant and cause functional impairment in aged human substantia nigra neurons.* Nature Genet, 2006. 38(5): pp. 518–520.

[15] Lesage, S. and A. Brice, *Parkinson's disease: from monogenic forms to genetic susceptibility factors.* Hum Mol Gen, 2009. 18(R1): pp. R48–R59.

[16] Hardy, J., M.R. Cookson, and A. Singleton, *Genes and parkinsonism*. Lancet Neurol, 2003. 2(4): pp. 221–8.

[17] Farrer, M.J., *Genetics of Parkinson disease: paradigm shifts and future prospects*. Nat Rev Genet, 2006. 7(4): pp. 306–18.

[18] Egger, G., et al., *Epigenetics in human disease and prospects for epigenetic therapy*. Nature, 2004. 429(6990): pp. 457–463.

[19] Ammal Kaidery, N., S. Tarannum, and B. Thomas, *Epigenetic landscape of Parkinson's disease: emerging role in disease mechanisms and therapeutic modalities*. Neurotherapeutics, 2013. 10(4): pp. 698–708.

[20] Bjornsson, H.T., M. Daniele Fallin, and A.P. Feinberg, *An integrated epigenetic and genetic approach to common human disease*. Trends Genetics, 2004. 20(8): pp. 350–358.

[21] Coppedè, F., *Genetics and epigenetics of Parkinson's disease*. Sci World J, 2012. 2012.

[22] Filatova, E., et al., *MicroRNAs: possible role in pathogenesis of Parkinson's disease*. Biochemistry (Moscow), 2012. 77(8): pp. 813–819.

[23] Kaut, O., I. Schmitt, and U. Wüllner, *Genome-scale methylation analysis of Parkinson's disease patients' brains reveals DNA hypomethylation and increased mRNA expression of cytochrome P450 2E1*. Neurogenetics, 2012. 13(1): pp. 87–91.

[24] Mouradian, M.M., *MicroRNAs in Parkinson's disease*. Neurobiol Dis, 2012. 46(2): pp. 279–84.

[25] Masliah, E., et al., *Distinctive patterns of DNA methylation associated with Parkinson disease: identification of concordant epigenetic changes in brain and peripheral blood leukocytes*. Epigenetics, 2013. 8(10): pp. 1030–8.

[26] Pena-Altamira, L.E., E. Polazzi, and B. Monti, *Histone post-translational modifications in Huntington's and Parkinson's diseases*. Curr Pharm Des, 2013. 19(28): pp. 5085–92.

[27] Weinhold, B., *Epigenetics: the science of change*. Environ Health Perspect, 2006. 114(3): pp. A160–7.

[28] Reik, W., et al., *Age at onset in Huntington's disease and methylation at D4S95*. J Med Genet, 1993. 30(3): pp. 185–8.

[29] Bird, A., *DNA methylation patterns and epigenetic memory*. Genes Dev, 2002. 16(1): pp. 6–21.

[30] Curradi, M., et al., *Molecular mechanisms of gene silencing mediated by DNA methylation*. Mol Cell Biol, 2002. 22(9): pp. 3157–73.

[31] Miller, C.A., S.L. Campbell, and J.D. Sweatt, *DNA methylation and histone acetylation work in concert to regulate memory formation and synaptic plasticity*. Neurobiol Learn Mem, 2008. 89(4): pp. 599–603.

[32] Day, J.J. and J.D. Sweatt, *DNA methylation and memory formation*. Nat Neurosci, 2010. 13(11): pp. 1319–23.

[33] Scarpa, S., et al., *Gene silencing through methylation: an epigenetic intervention on Alzheimer disease*. J Alzheimers Dis, 2006. 9(4): pp. 407–14.

[34] Hernandez, D.G., et al., *Distinct DNA methylation changes highly correlated with chronological age in the human brain*. Hum Mol Genet, 2011. 20(6): pp. 1164–72.

[35] Jowaed, A., et al., *Methylation regulates alpha-synuclein expression and is decreased in Parkinson's disease patients' brains*. J Neurosci, 2010. 30(18): pp. 6355–9.

[36] Matsumoto, L., et al., *CpG demethylation enhances alpha-synuclein expression and affects the pathogenesis of Parkinson's disease*. PLoS One, 2010. 5(11): pp. e15522.

[37] Desplats, P., et al., *Alpha-synuclein sequesters Dnmt1 from the nucleus: a novel mechanism for epigenetic alterations in Lewy body diseases*. J Biol Chem, 2011. 286(11): pp. 9031–7.

[38] Maze, I., K.M. Noh, and C.D. Allis, *Histone regulation in the CNS: basic principles of epigenetic plasticity*. Neuropsychopharmacology, 2013. 38(1): pp. 3–22.

[39] Cheung, P., et al., *Synergistic coupling of histone H3 phosphorylation and acetylation in response to epidermal growth factor stimulation*. Mol Cell, 2000. 5(6): pp. 905–15.

[40] Luco, R.F., et al., *Regulation of alternative splicing by histone modifications*. Science, 2010. 327(5968): pp. 996–1000.

[41] Kouzarides, T., *Chromatin modifications and their function*. Cell, 2007. 128(4): pp. 693–705.

[42] Li, B., M. Carey, and J.L. Workman, *The Role of Chromatin during Transcription*. Cell, 2007. 128(4): pp. 707–719.

[43] Karlić, R., et al., *Histone modification levels are predictive for gene expression*. Proc Natl Acad Sci, 2010. 107(7): pp. 2926–2931.

[44] Roth, S.Y., J.M. Denu, and C.D. Allis, *Histone acetyltransferases*. Annu Rev Biochem, 2001. 70: pp. 81–120.

[45] Trievel, R.C., *Structure and function of histone methyltransferases*. Crit Rev Eukaryot Gene Expr, 2004. 14(3): pp. 147–69.

[46] Greer, E.L. and Y. Shi, *Histone methylation: a dynamic mark in health, disease and inheritance*. Nat Rev Genet, 2012. 13(5): pp. 343–357.

[47] Morales, Y., et al., *Biochemistry and regulation of the protein arginine methyltransferases (PRMTs)*. Arch Biochem Biophys, 2015. 590: pp. 138–152.

[48] Kontopoulos, E., J.D. Parvin, and M.B. Feany, *Alpha-synuclein acts in the nucleus to inhibit histone acetylation and promote neurotoxicity*. Hum Mol Genet, 2006. 15(20): pp. 3012–23.

[49] Outeiro, T.F., et al., *Sirtuin 2 inhibitors rescue alpha-synuclein-mediated toxicity in models of Parkinson's disease*. Science, 2007. 317(5837): pp. 516–9.

[50] Goers, J., et al., *Nuclear localization of alpha-synuclein and its interaction with histones.* Biochemistry, 2003. 42(28): pp. 8465–71.

[51] Abel, T. and R.S. Zukin, *Epigenetic targets of HDAC inhibition in neurodegenerative and psychiatric disorders.* Curr Opin Pharmacol, 2008. 8(1): pp. 57–64.

[52] Simoes-Pires, C., et al., *HDAC6 as a target for neurodegenerative diseases: what makes it different from the other HDACs?* Mol Neurodegener, 2013. 8(1): p. 7.

[53] Du, G., et al., *Drosophila histone deacetylase 6 protects dopaminergic neurons against {alpha}-synuclein toxicity by promoting inclusion formation.* Mol Biol Cell, 2010. 21(13): pp. 2128–37.

[54] Duce, J.A., et al., *Linker histone H1 binds to disease associated amyloid-like fibrils.* J Mol Biol, 2006. 361(3): pp. 493–505.

[55] Vartiainen, S., et al., *Identification of gene expression changes in transgenic* C. elegans *overexpressing human alpha-synuclein.* Neurobiol Dis, 2006. 22(3): pp. 477–86.

[56] Lee, J.Y., et al., *Disease-causing mutations in parkin impair mitochondrial ubiquitination, aggregation, and HDAC6-dependent mitophagy.* J Cell Biol, 2010. 189(4): pp. 671–9.

[57] Sharma, S. and R. Taliyan, *Targeting histone deacetylases: a novel approach in Parkinson's disease.* Parkinson's Disease, 2015. 2015: p. 11.

[58] Koh, H., et al., *Silent information regulator 2 (Sir2) and Forkhead box O (FOXO) complement mitochondrial dysfunction and dopaminergic neuron loss in Drosophila PTEN-induced kinase 1 (PINK1) null mutant.* J Biol Chem, 2012. 287(16): pp. 12750–8.

[59] Nicholas, A.P., et al., *Striatal histone modifications in models of levodopa-induced dyskinesia.* J Neurochem, 2008. 106(1): pp. 486–94.

[60] Santini, E., et al., *L-DOPA activates ERK signaling and phosphorylates histone H3 in the striatonigral medium spiny neurons of hemiparkinsonian mice.* J Neurochem, 2009. 108(3): pp. 621–33.

[61] Almeida, M.I., R.M. Reis, and G.A. Calin, *MicroRNA history: Discovery, recent applications, and next frontiers.* Mut Res/Fund Mol Mech Mut, 2011. 717(1–2): pp. 1–8.

[62] Ha, M. and V.N. Kim, *Regulation of microRNA biogenesis.* Nat Rev Mol Cell Biol, 2014. 15(8): pp. 509–524.

[63] Wahid, F., et al., *MicroRNAs: Synthesis, mechanism, function, and recent clinical trials.* Biochimica et Biophysica Acta (BBA) - Molecular Cell Research, 2010. 1803(11): pp. 1231–1243.

[64] Junn, E., et al., *Repression of alpha-synuclein expression and toxicity by microRNA-7.* Proc Natl Acad Sci U S A, 2009. 106(31): pp. 13052–7.

[65] Doxakis, E., *Post-transcriptional regulation of alpha-synuclein expression by mir-7 and mir-153.* J Biol Chem, 2010. 285(17): pp. 12726–34.

[66] Gandhi, P.N., S.G. Chen, and A.L. Wilson-Delfosse, *Leucine-rich repeat kinase 2 (LRRK2): a key player in the pathogenesis of Parkinson's disease*. J Neurosci Res, 2009. 87(6): pp. 1283–1295.

[67] Kett, L.R., et al., *LRRK2 Parkinson disease mutations enhance its microtubule association*. Hum Mol Gen, 2012. 21(4): pp. 890–899.

[68] Martin, I., et al., *LRRK2 Pathobiology in Parkinson's Disease*. J Neurochem, 2014. 131(5): pp. 554–565.

[69] Skibinski, G., et al., *Mutant LRRK2 Toxicity in Neurons Depends on LRRK2 Levels and Synuclein But Not Kinase Activity or Inclusion Bodies*. J Neurosci, 2014. 34(2): pp. 418–433.

[70] Cho, H.J., et al., *MicroRNA-205 regulates the expression of Parkinson's disease-related leucine-rich repeat kinase 2 protein*. Hum Mol Genet, 2013. 22(3): pp. 608–20.

[71] Minones-Moyano, E., et al., *MicroRNA profiling of Parkinson's disease brains identifies early downregulation of miR-34b/c which modulate mitochondrial function*. Hum Mol Genet, 2011. 20(15): pp. 3067–78.

[72] Kanagaraj, N., et al., *Downregulation of miR-124 in MPTP-treated mouse model of Parkinson's disease and MPP iodide-treated MN9D cells modulates the expression of the calpain/cdk5 pathway proteins*. Neuroscience, 2014. 272: pp. 167–179.

[73] Renthal, W. and E.J. Nestler, *Chromatin regulation in drug addiction and depression*. Dialogues in Clinical Neuroscience, 2009. 11(3): pp. 257–268.

[74] Latham, J.A. and S.Y. Dent, *Cross-regulation of histone modifications*. Nat Struct Mol Biol, 2007. 14(11): pp. 1017–24.

[75] Cheung, W.L., et al., *Phosphorylation of histone H4 serine 1 during DNA damage requires casein kinase II in S. cerevisiae*. Curr Biol, 2005. 15(7): pp. 656–60.

[76] Lee, G., et al., *Casein kinase II-mediated phosphorylation regulates alpha-synuclein/synphilin-1 interaction and inclusion body formation*. J Biol Chem, 2004. 279(8): pp. 6834–9.

[77] Cavallarin, N., M. Vicario, and A. Negro, *The role of phosphorylation in synucleinopathies: focus on Parkinson's disease*. CNS Neurol Disord-Dr Targets (Formerly Current Drug Targets-CNS & Neurological Disorders), 2010. 9(4): pp. 471–481.

[78] Adamczyk, A. and A. Kazmierczak, *Alpha-synuclein inhibits poly (ADP-ribose) polymerase-1 (PARP-1) activity via NO-dependent pathway*. Folia Neuropathol, 2009. 47(3): pp. 247–51.

[79] Monaco, L., et al., *Inhibition of Aurora-B kinase activity by poly(ADP-ribosyl)ation in response to DNA damage*. Proc Natl Acad Sci U S A, 2005. 102(40): pp. 14244–8.

[80] Saijo, K., et al., *A Nurr1/CoREST pathway in microglia and astrocytes protects dopaminergic neurons from inflammation-induced death*. Cell, 2009. 137(1): pp. 47–59.

[81] Sethi, P. and W.J. Lukiw, *Micro-RNA abundance and stability in human brain: specific alterations in Alzheimer's disease temporal lobe neocortex*. Neurosci Lett, 2009. 459(2): pp. 100–104.

Chapter 4

Inflammation: Role in Parkinson's Disease and Target for Therapy

Patrick Flood, Naik Arbabzada and Monika Sharma

Additional information is available at the end of the chapter

http://dx.doi.org/10.5772/63027

Abstract

Evidence is now overwhelming that inflammation is a central process in the pathogenesis of progressive Parkinson's disease (PD). The hallmark of this neuroinflammation is the activation of microglial cells and the secondary role of adaptive immunity in both the familial and idiopathic forms of PD, leading to the loss of dopamine-producing cells within the Substantia nigra. This activation is characterized by the oxidative stress response, production of inflammatory mediators, recruitment and activation of immune effector cells which create a toxic environment for dopaminergic neurons, and in forming a continuous cycle of inflammatory responses that result in chronic neuroinflammation and progressive neurodegeneration. This chapter focuses on the different components of the inflammatory response that are involved in Dopamine-neurodegeneration, the evidence for inflammation in different forms of PD, and the role of inflammation in the various animal models of PD. Finally, we provide current evidence that targeting this inflammation with a number of anti-inflammatory therapies can be an effective way to halt the progression of chronic neuroinflammation-induced PD.

Keywords: Inflammation, Microglia, Cytokines, Therapeutics, Neurodegeneration

1. Introduction

Recently accumulated evidence suggests that neuroinflammation and chronic inflammation of the central nervous system (CNS) may play a critical role in the development of a number of neurodegenerative diseases. Particularly, in Parkinson's disease (PD), neuroinflammation has been proposed as a major contributing factor that plays a role in the initiation and progression of the dopaminergic neuronal loss that is the hallmark of the disease. Evidence to support neuroinflammation as the mode of pathogenesis for PD originates from postmortem studies in patients and animal models. The proliferation and activation of microglial cells, as well as increased levels of pro-inflammatory mediators such as tumor necrosis factor (TNF)-α, interleukin (IL)-6, IL-1β, nitric oxide (NO), and reactive oxygen species (ROS), are present in postmortem analysis of brains and in the cerebrospinal fluid (CSF) of PD patients [1]. These findings suggest that pro-inflammatory cytokines, specifically TNF-α, may be involved in neuronal cell death. Likewise, neuronal cell death can release mediators that activate microglial cells— thereby potentiating a vicious cyclical inflammatory-mediated neuronal cell death. PD is unique in that the clinical symptoms appear after a loss of approximately 70–80% of striatal nerve terminals and 50–60% of dopaminergic cells in the Substantia nigra pars compacta (SNpc), the region of the brain that is responsible for controlling movement [2, 3]. This recent scientific understanding is vital to developing potential early biomarkers and/or therapeutic strategies to help with better diagnosis and disease management. We discuss various components of neuroinflammation, focusing on the role of the innate and adaptive immune responses as they relate to PD. In addition, we briefly summarize the inflammatory pathology seen in the genetic and toxin-induced models of this disease, as well as discuss several anti-inflammatory therapies currently being used or tested as potential treatments for PD.

2. Innate immune response and PD

The innate immune response serves as the first line of defense to both infiltrating pathogens and/or endogenous insults. As such, it primarily functions to initiate an immediate and nonspecific response to any compound it deems unnecessary and/or a potential threat. Pathogen-associated molecular patterns (PAMPS) and/or endogenous damage-associated molecular patterns (DAMPs) can trigger an innate immune response. In the case of CNS, the innate immune system has several components: cells that mediate an immune response, such as microglia and astroglia, the complement system, and the physical obstruction imparted by the blood-brain barrier (BBB). For centuries, the CNS was thought to be immune privileged because the BBB did not allow various compounds to enter the CNS through the circulatory system. However, as we are beginning to appreciate the intricacy of the immune-nervous system interaction, the notion of immune privilege no longer holds [4].

In PD, the various components of the innate immune system are activated and the integrity of the BBB is compromised, allowing for the innate-mediated recruitment and activation of the adaptive arm of the immune system. While PD is not among other immune-dependent degenerative diseases, Parkinsonian symptoms have been shown to develop after infectious inflammatory diseases such as Epstein-Barr virus (EBV)-induced encephalitis. Likewise, many anti-inflammatory therapeutic agents have served protective functions in PD models [5]. As such, while the role of the immune system is not clear and/or extensively studied in the etiology of the disease, it is well established that the immune system is critical for the progression of the disease. Initial activation of the innate immune cells as well as the complement proteins may serve protective roles, but when these innate defense mechanisms become unregulated and maladaptive, it leads to disease progression. As immediate responders, cells of the innate immune system play an important role in initiating an inflammatory response against various nonspecific components of endogenous DAMPS and/or PAMPs. The innate cells, astrocytes and microglia, play an active role in the pathological mechanism responsible for the progression of the disease.

2.1. Astrocytes

Astrocytes make up about 20–40% of the glial cell population in the CNS. Their functions include, but are not limited to, maintaining the integrity of the BBB, facilitating repair and scar formation, and maintaining the extracellular ion homeostasis. The expression of receptors that are critical for innate immunity such as Toll-like receptors (TLRs), nucleotide-binding oligomerization domains, double-stranded RNA-dependent protein kinase, scavenger receptors, mannose-binding lectin receptor, and complement system components has implicated a role for astrocytes in innate immunity [6]. The role of astrocytes in PD is debatable and not well understood. Studies are inconclusive as to whether astrocytes have a neuroprotective effect and/or a neurotoxic effect in PD. However, astrocytosis, the activation of astrocytes, has been reported in some cases of PD as demonstrated by an increase in the glial fibrillary acid proteins (GFAP) [7, 8]. GFAP is an intermediate filament needed by astrocytes to synthesize cytoskeletal structures and is a well-established biomarker for astrocytosis [8]. Furthermore, activated astrocytes are reported in postmortem brains of PD patients; however, this activation is not confined to the SNpc and its function therefore still remains elusive [9]. In contrast, astrocyte activation is not only well documented in the 1-methyl-4-phenyl-1,2,3,6-tetrahydropyridine (MPTP) and 6-hydroxydopamine (6-OHDA) models of PD, but it has been reported to precede neuronal cell death [10–12]. In the MPTP model, astrocytosis and dopaminergic cell death are synchronized. In the 6-OHDA model, several laboratories demonstrate that astrocytosis occurs in a time-dependent manner, peaking at 4 days post injection and remaining in the brain for about a month. There are also studies that contradict the presence of astrocytosis post 6-OHDA injection [13]. Therefore, while astrocytes are an important cell type in the CNS, their role in inflammation and PD is not yet well established.

2.2. Microglia

In contrast to astrocytes, consistent microglial activation and the accompanying inflammatory response have been reported in both patient and animal models of PD. As the resident CNS macrophage, microglia cells are responsible for scavenging the CNS milieu for potential infiltrating pathogens and/or endogenous insults. Consequently, the phagocytic, cytotoxic, and antigen-presenting capabilities of these cells enable them to protect the CNS from various insults. Activated microglia targets infiltrating pathogens and damaged cells by releasing toxic ROS, free radicals, and phagocytosis. Evidence of microglial activation and its role in PD pathogenesis is indisputable. Knott et al. [9] and others [14] have reported activated amoeboid-shaped microglia in postmortem brain of PD patients. These activated microglia cells are densely located and confined to the SNpc with a limited presence in the vasculature of the caudate and putamen regions. Additionally, in determining the role of microglia in PD pathogenesis, our results as well as those from other groups [15–17] have shown that in various PD models, microglial cells are needed for the pathogenesis of PD. For example, we have shown that high doses of the β2-adrenergic receptor agonist salmeterol can induce dopaminergic cell toxicity. However, microglial cells are indispensable in the β2-AR-mediated toxicity, as high-dose salmeterol has no effect on neuron-only cultures [15]. In PD, the expression of ROS, free radicals, and the enzymes responsible for the production of these species such as NADPH oxidase (NOX or PHOX), induced nitric oxide synthase (iNOS), and myeloperoxidase (MPO) are elevated in the SNpc. These reactive species can activate microglial cells, and these activated microglia release pro-inflammatory cytokines TNF-α, IL-1β, and IL-6 to recruit additional lymphocytes in the process of inflammation. Additionally, these cytokines can cause cytotoxicity in a direct, receptor-mediated manner, and/or in an indirect manner by inducing the further production of ROS and pro-inflammatory cytokines [18]. For example, dopaminergic cells express receptors for TNF-α, which, upon binding the TNF-α ligand, can cause cell death through Fas ligand-mediated apoptosis, and Tumor Necrosis Factor Receptor (TNFR) knockout is protective in the MPTP model of PD [19]. Indirectly, TNF-α can also activate additional microglia to release ROS and a variety of pro-inflammatory cytokines. This leads to a cyclical pathway whereby activation of a few cells can amplify the initial insult to a greater magnitude. This process has been termed reactive microgliosis and is now a leading working model for understanding and targeting neuroinflammation in PD [20].

3. Adaptive immune response and PD

Adaptive immune response is a highly specific response to injurious agents mediated by B- and T-lymphocytes, which is characterized by the humoral and cell-mediated response, respectively. These cells are activated by specific antigens and directly induce toxicity and cell death to the antigen-expressing cell. It is important to note that the adaptive immune cells require an antigen-presenting cell to prime the B- and/or T-cell to recognize a specific antigen. In PD, innate immune activation leads to an increased BBB permeability, allowing for the infiltration of peripheral T-cells and B-cells [21]. These infiltrating cells are activated by active microglia expressing MHC 1/II through presentation of endocytosed peptides to the respective cells. Evidence to suggest the involvement of adaptive immune system is that single-nucleotide polymorphism (SNP) in the MHC Class II predisposes individuals to PD, implying the role of both the innate and adaptive immune response in PD pathogenesis. Recent genome-wide association studies (GWAS) have highlighted alleles HLA-DRA (for Class I) and HLA-DRB5 (for Class II) as risk factors for PD [22]. Furthermore, MHC Class I proteins are typically used by CD8 T-cells and require β2-microglublin, a protein required for the structural stability of MHC Class I, and in PD, the expression of β2-microglublin is found to be increased on microglial cells [21]. Additionally, an increase in the number of cytotoxic CD8 and CD4 T-cells infiltrating into the SNpc of PD patients is accompanied by a decrease in the cytotoxicity-suppressing capacity of regulatory T-cells (T_{reg}) [23, 24]. Therefore, it suggests that toxicity of these effector T-cells is not properly regulated and can exacerbate neuronal cell death in the SN. With regard to B-cells, antibodies (Ab) to dopaminergic neurons have been found in the CSF of a proportion of the PD patients, thus implicating the involvement of the peripheral humoral arm of the adaptive immune response [25, 26]. Furthermore, immunization, which uses B-cells to generate antibodies against an antigen, with bovine mesencephalic homogenates [27] and hybrid dopaminergic cell line homogenates [25], can cause selective DA neuron damage in a microglia-dependent manner. The adaptive immune system has a delayed contribution to the pathology of PD but, nevertheless, is important to understand in order to develop therapies that can mitigate and counter the pathology induced by this system.

4. Neuroinflammation and overlapping vulnerability of Substantia nigra (SN) neurons

The oxidative stress hypothesis focuses on the role that reactive oxygen and nitrogen species play in the neurodegeneration seen in PD. Reviews by Fahn and Cohen [28] as well as by Zigmond and Burke [29] discuss four characteristics of SNpc dopaminergic neurons that support the oxidative stress hypothesis as one of the major mechanisms responsible for the pathology of PD. However, understanding these characteristics can help explain the chronic, self-perpetuating inflammatory pathology that is responsible for disease progression in PD. While inflammation involves activated immune cells and the release of a multitude of pro-inflammatory cytokines, the cycle does require a start point. The etiology of PD is unknown as is what gives rise to the chronic inflammatory pathogenesis seen in PD. Two different explanations of the chronic etiology of PD suggest that neuronal cell death leading to activated immune cells and the resulting uncontrolled inflammation further exacerbates cell death, or that activated immune cells cause cell death which results in the activation of additional immune cells resulting in a vicious cycle of immune cell-mediated inflammation and neuronal death. The characteristics of SNpc dopaminergic cells make them vulnerable to ROS, subsets of which are important pro-inflammatory cytokines. First, dopamine degradation occurs by oxidative deamination, resulting in the production of H_2O_2 that then react with iron present in the neurons to form reactive radicals. Second, superoxides and free radicals are by-products of the reaction between dopamine and the readily available oxygen to form reactive quinones. Third, the SNpc particularly rich in iron and hence the neurons found therein are more vulnerable to cell death via oxidative stress. Fourth, the SNpc neurons contain neuromelanin, which is formed by the auto-oxidation of DA, and the by-product of this reaction is ROS. These characteristics make SNpc neurons particularly sensitive to a cyclical process of oxidative stress contributing to inflammation that that leads to furthermore neuronal damage.

5. Genetic causes of PD and neuroinflammation

Although PD is typically a sporadic disease, approximately 10% of PD cases have been linked to several specific genes. These genes are α-synuclein, Parkin, UCH-L1 (ubiquitin C-terminal hydrolase L1), PINK1 (PTEN-induced kinase 1, NB for mitochondrial function), DJ-1, LRRK2 (leucine rich repeat kinase2), Pael-R, and glucocerebrosidase [21, 30, 31]. These genes and their products have a role in the degradation of α-synuclein and/or in the control of the oxidative milieu. Mutations in genes encoding α-synuclein, Parkin, and/or UCH-L1 result in the accumulation of misfolded α-synuclein protein and are accompanied by neuronal cell death [21]. Additionally, a pathological feature of PD is the Lewy body cytoplasmic inclusion bodies, which primarily consist of α-synuclein, tau, ubiquitin, and Parkin. These genes were identified in familial PD, as risk factors for sporadic PD, and further verified by a GWAS. Therefore, understanding the role of these genes and their products in mediating inflammation can help not only in developing more holistic model(s) of PD but also for therapy development.

5.1. LRRK2

Leucine-rich repeat kinase 2 (LRRK2) is an enzyme that is commonly expressed on multiple immune cells such as B-cells, monocytes, dendritic cells, and microglia [32]. Mutations in LRRK2 are associated with autosomal dominant form of PD with high resemblance to the idiopathic PD phenotype and other inflammatory-mediated diseases as Crohn's disease [33] with a high predisposition to leprosy infection [34]. LRRK2 is a member of the receptor-interacting protein kinase (RIPK) family. The RIPK family has important roles in immunity as well as regulating of cell death [35]. Furthermore, TLRs are an important activator of microglial cells. In the TLR-signaling pathway, LRRK2 is phosphorylated [36], and Kim et al. [37] as well as other groups [38] have reported a decrease in NF-κB-mediated transcription, specifically of TNF-α, post LRRK2 phosphorylation. NF-κB is a major transcription factor for many of the pro-inflammatory cytokines that are reported to play a role in the pathogenesis of PD, such as TNF-α, IL-1β, and IL-6; LRRK2 modulation of NF-κB will have important cellular effects on the inflammatory state of the activated microglial cells. Furthermore, a mutation in LRRK2, specifically R1442G, is reported to alter the phenotype of activated microglial cells to produce higher amounts of inflammatory cytokines with a decrease in the production of anti-inflammatory cytokines [39]. Gillardon et al. [39] tested the neurotoxicity of these microglial cells on cortical neurons by exposing neurons to conditioned medium from LPS-activated microglial cells, compared to conditioned medium from LPS-activated wild-type (WT) microglia, conditioned media from LPS-activated LRRK2 mutant significantly increased cell death. In addition, Kim et al. [37] have shown that LRRK2 deficiency mitigates LPS-mediated increase in the mRNA of iNOS, TNF-α, IL-1β, and IL-6. By itself, overexpression of the mutant LRRK2 *in vivo* and *in vitro* causes neurotoxicity [40]. These data support a role for LRRK2 in regulating the inflammatory response of microglial cells and the resulting effect on neuronal viability.

5.2. Parkin

Parkin is an important component of the multi-protein E3 ubiquitin ligase complex that is responsible for the ubiquitin-proteasome-mediated degradation of α-synuclein in the brain. Mutations resulting in loss of function of Parkin are responsible for autosomal recessive form of juvenile PD [41]. Parkin not only regulates mitochondrial health but also is involved in the regulation of the NF-κB signaling pathway [42]. Parkin ubiquitinates damaged mitochondria and subjects it to mitophagy and clearance from the cell [43]. Similarly, activated Parkin catalyzes ubiquitination of the IkB kinase (IKK) subunit IKKγ, resulting in the downstream activation of NF-κB [42, 44]. In this NF-κB signaling pathway, TNF-receptor-associated factor-6 (TRAF6) also plays a role in regulating IKK activity. Loss-of-function mutation in Parkin increases the expression of TRAF6 [45], thereby activating transforming growth factor-1 (TAK1) that activates IKK and ultimately NF-κB and its associated transcriptional activity [44]. With regard to Parkin and mitochondria, while mitophagy and PD have not yet been linked, damaged mitochondria are a source of ROS that can activate microglial cells through TLR-PAMP/DAMP pathways [30].

5.3. α-Synuclein

α-synuclein is an 18-kDa protein found in high concentrations in the CNS compared to other areas. While the function of α-synuclein is unclear, it is thought to be important for the release of neurotransmitters and vesicle trafficking [46, 47]. Mutations in the *SCNA*, gene coding for α-synuclein, is implicated in inherited forms of PD. Similarly, α-synuclein aggregation is a critical component of Lewy bodies in both sporadic and genetic PD. With regards to inflammation, α-synuclein is thought to activate microglial cells through the nonspecific DAMP-TLR2/4 pathway [48,49]. An emerging link between gut microbiota and peripheral inflammation and PD is of interest to note. A study by Forsyth and colleagues [50] reported increased gut permeability and *Escherichia coli (E. coli)*, a Gram negative bacterium, staining in early onset PD patients. The implication of this study is that *E. coli*-dependent inflammatory processes resulted in an increased iNOS that then nitrosylated α-synuclein. WT, mutant, aggregated forms of α-synuclein can all trigger microglial activation by acting as a TLR-ligand. Conditioned media from dopaminergic cell line SH-SY5Y that either overexpressed WT or A53T mutant α-synuclein activated BV-2 microglial cell line, with the conditioned media from the neurons overexpressing mutant α-synuclein caused a more robust increase in TNF-α, IL-1α, and IL-1β [51]. More importantly, mutant and aggregated fibrils of α-synuclein are reported to have cell-to-cell transmission capacity, thereby causing neuronal toxicity in a prion-like mechanism as well [52]. Moreover, nitrated α-synuclein can activate peripheral immune activation, especially T-cells and initiate the involvement of the adaptive immune response. Lastly, Tran and colleagues [53] have recently reported that antibodies to α-synuclein can offer a promising protective effect by inhibiting the entry of α-synuclein fibrils into neurons and causing neuronal death.

5.4. PINK1

PINK1 is a mitochondrial serine/threonine protein kinase implicated in providing cellular protection against mitochondrial-associated oxidative stress. As such, it is reported to regulate stressed mitochondria by enabling the binding of Parkin to stressed mitochondria and inducing autophagy. The role of PINK1 in inflammation is somewhat unclear; as evidence suggests that in PINK1 null animals injected with LPS, IL-1β, IL-12, and TNF-α are increased [54]. However, in PINK1-deficient embryonic fibroblasts, there is no increase in pro-inflammatory cytokine production post LPS injection because of decreased NF-κB activity [54, 55]. As such, experiments aimed at understanding the role of PINK1 in inflammation should be investigated in microglial cells which are known to propagate the inflammatory response in PD.

5.5. DJ-1

DJ-1, or Parkinson's disease Protein 7, inhibits the aggregation of α-synuclein, thereby acting as an oxidative stress sensor. PINK1 and DJ-1 deletion causes disruption of other genes involved in mitogen-associated protein kinase (MAPK)/NF-κB signaling pathway and thereby alters the innate immune response of the microglia and other inflammatory cascades [6]. MAPKs are signaling proteins that mediate various intracellular signals in response to external stimuli. Several important MAPKs play an essential role in the integrity of the cell as well as modulating inflammation such as p38, C-Jun N-terminal kinase (JNK), and extracellular signal-regulated kinases (ERKs). In astrocytes, DJ-1 loss of function primes astrocyte to release increased pro-inflammatory cytokines post LPS challenge [56]. This response was mediated through p38 and JNK, thereby DJ-1 may have a pivotal role in regulating TLR4-MAPK signaling and downstream transcriptional responses [57]. LPS-mediated activation of macrophages increases DJ-1 expression [58], which is aligned with the associated TLR/MAPK-mediated signaling in microglial cells challenged with LPS.

6. Inflammation and PD models

There are several models of PD, both toxin based and gene based, used to study disease progression and/or therapeutic development. In many of these models, inflammatory mechanisms are reported to play roles in the pathogenesis and manifestation of the disease in various animal models. In the remainder of this chapter, we will focus on characterizing the inflammatory response seen in the various models.

6.1 Toxin-based models

6.1.1. MPTP

1-methyl-4-phenyl-1,2,3,6-tetrahydropyridine (MPTP) is a dopaminergic neurotoxin selective for the dopaminergic cells of the SNpc. It is a lipophilic compound capable of crossing the BBB, and once it has crossed the BBB, it is oxidized to MPP+ by MAO-B. MPP+ interrupts the mitochondrial complex I of the electron transport chain (ETC) and results in cell death and release of ROS [23]. The MPTP model is a widely used model to develop animal models of the disease, as PD progression post MPTP administration is similar in both humans and monkeys [59]. In the MPTP model, microglial activation accompanied with an increased endothelial expression of adhesion molecules on the BBB to enable infiltration of T-cells is reported [21]. Additionally, there are an increased number of activated microglial cells which are amoeboid in shape representative of activated cells [23]. Astroglial cells are activated late in the disease, and their role is unclear. Infiltrated CD8 and CD4 T-cells have lymphocyte function-associated antigen-1 (LFA-1), a protein expressed for recruitment and these infiltrated T-cells are primarily located it the SNpc and striatum. Furthermore, an increased expression of MHC I and MHC II and microglial iNOS expression are observed [23]. In conjunction with anti-inflammatory therapies, minocycline, a potent inhibitor of microglial activation and iNOS knockout mice, is protective against MPTP-induced neuronal cell death.

6.1.2. 6-OHDA

Oxidopamine, commonly known as 6-hydroxydopamine (6-OHDA), is another dopaminergic neurotoxin capable of inducing PD symptomatology in animal models. In the 6-OHDA model, inflammatory pathology is propagated by activated microglial cells which occurs 1–3 days post intranigral injection of 6-OHDA and DA neuronal loss occurring 1 week post injection [23]. As part of the inflammatory milieu, there is an increase in TNF-α, a pro-inflammatory cytokine capable of inducing cell death through TNFR.

6.1.3. LPS/rotenone

Lipopolysaccharide (LPS) is an endotoxin derived from Gram negative bacteria and another widely used toxin to induce PD in animal models. The LPS model is different from MPTP and the 6-OHDA toxin-based models, as LPS will activate microglial cells through the TLR2/4 receptors. Activated microglial will upregulate NO, superoxide, TNF-α, and IL-1β production and release [60]. These pro-inflammatory mediators can cause neuronal cell death. In animal models, intranigral injection of LPS induces microglial activation prior to neuronal loss [32]. Rotenone is another lipophilic herbicide that disrupts the mitochondrial complex 1 causing cell death and associated upregulation in ROS. In the rotenone animal models of PD, fibrillary cytoplasmic inclusions equivalent of Lewy bodies is found in the SNpc. In addition, rotenone injection in neuronal-only culture does not cause DA cell death, but in a mixed neuronal-microglial culture, DA neuron cell death is observed. This suggests that rotenone requires microglial cells for its toxicity [23, 61]. Lastly, inhibition of superoxide is protective against rotenone-induced DA neuron degeneration. These two models suggest that while the etiology of disease is unknown, microglial cells are indispensable for the progression of disease and the resulting neuronal degeneration is seen in PD.

6.2. Gene-based models

6.2.1. α-synuclein

Genetic model of PD is very rare and not all as consistent and reproducible as the toxin-based models. While many genes are implicated in the PD etiology, α-synuclein is the most widely used gene-based model so far [62]. The α-synuclein models include a transgenic knockout and overexpression of mutant or WT α-synuclein [63]. Viral vectors expressing human α-synuclein injected into adult brains have also been used to increase α-synuclein in the respective brain regions. α-synuclein models have been developed in monkeys, rats, mice, and in flies. Bae et al. [63] as well as Watson et al. [64] reported astroglia and microglia activation accompanied with increased mRNA transcripts of TNF-α and several TLRs (1, 4, and 8) in SNpc [65]. α-synuclein can act as a DAMP and activate microglia via TRLs, thereby suggesting a primed microglial sensitivity. In the knockout transgenic models of α-synuclein, little neuronal loss and behavioral changes are reported. In addition, transgenic null mice can offer a degree of protection against MPTP intoxication and cell death [66, 67]. In contrast, viral overexpression models of α-synuclein in brain of adult animals show DA neurotoxicity accompanied by the activation of both the innate and adaptive immune response [68]. Learning from these models includes and further verifies a gain of function of α-synuclein as ablation of α-synuclein features no neuropathological changes [62]. Furthermore, in a recent study, Van der Perren et al. [69] reported the immunophilin ligand FK506 in a rAAV2/7 α-synuclein overexpression rat model to have anti-inflammatory therapeutic potential. Specifically, the group [69] reported a decrease in the infiltration of CD4+ and CD8+ T cells as well as in the number of activated microglial cells. This further supports neuroinflammation as a key to the progression of the disease and efficacy for therapeutic development.

6.2.2. LRRK2

LRRK2 mutations are implicated in an autosomal dominant form of PD with similar phenotypic expression as idiopathic PD. To study the role of LRRK2 in PD pathogenesis, LRRK2 knockout animals were developed. Several groups [70,71] report no DA degeneration in LRRK2 deficient rat and mice models. Lee et al. [72] developed herpes simplex virus (HSV) amplicon-based mouse model of LRRK2 dopaminergic neurotoxicity. Overexpression of the LRRK2 G2019S resulted in significant loss of tyrosine hydroxylase (TH+) neurons. Thereby these data suggest that knockout of LRRK2 may provide neuroprotection, and similarly, Lee et al. [72] used LRRK2 inhibitors and found that it protected the overexpressed LRRK2 mice from developing PD [72]. Most notably, the mechanism of protection seems to be dependent on the activation and proliferation of microglial cells [70], implicating LRRK2 in the inflammatory etiology for PD. Therefore, it appears LRRK2 is critical in PD pathology and plays a significant role in regulating cellular inflammation, thereby supporting the notion that neuroinflammation is critical to PD pathogenesis.

7. Anti-inflammatory therapies in PD

While evidence strongly suggests that inflammation plays a major role in the etiology of a number of different forms of PD, emerging evidence also demonstrates that therapies used to lessen inflammation, including those directed against immune cells or inflammatory mediators, can play a positive role in halting the degeneration of DA neurons in several models of PD. Many studies suggest that inflammatory mediators such as TNFα, PGE_2, NO, free radicals, and other immune mediators play a role in the pathogenesis of PD and degeneration of dopamine-producing neurons, and that the use of specific reagents that target these mediators, inhibition of cellular signaling mechanisms that regulate the production of these mediators, or the use of neurotrophic factors that help protect against the neurotoxicity induced by these mediators hold significant promise as therapeutic treatments for PD. In addition, epidemiological and observational studies already suggest that use of anti-inflammatory drugs lower the risk of developing PD [73].

Observations which demonstrate that inflammation in SNpc plays a role in PD led many investigators to initially study the potential use of steroidal and nonsteroidal anti-inflammatory drugs for the treatment of PD. Steroidal anti-inflammatory drugs (SAIDs) such as dexamethasone showed neuroprotective effects and LPS-induced neurotoxicity in Substantia nigra [74]. Nonsteroidal anti-inflammatory drugs (NSAIDs) are used as analgesics and anti-pyretics to suppress the adverse effects of inflammation. NSAIDs as a group normally reduce the production of prostaglandins by inhibiting cyclooxygenase (COX, an enzyme that catalyzes specific prostaglandin synthesis) and also reduce the synthesis of nitric oxide. In addition, it has been found that a subset of NSAIDs called as selective Aβ42 lowering agents (SALAs) reduces the risk of Alzheimer dementia (AD) [75] and consequently may be effective in PD as well. Neuroprotective effects of ibuprofen have been studied in PD pathogenesis, and these studies show that it can protect dopaminergic neurons against glutamate toxicity *in vitro* [76, 77]. It is interesting to note that some neurologic drugs used to treat PD have been found to result in changes to immune system. One such drug, amantadine (Symmetrel, Endo Pharmac
LPS induced mice and mesencephalic culture
6-OHDA induced euticals) which functions as an antagonist of the NMDA-type glutamate receptor leading to increased dopamine release and dopamine reuptake, also increases the CD4:CD8 ratio [78] and enhances IL-2 levels in PD patients. In contrast, L-DOPA monotherapy does not show similar effects [79]. In the next sections, we discuss the effectiveness of a number of anti-inflammatory treatments in preventing dopaminergic cell death in animal models of PD (section summarized in **Table 1**).

Therapy	Compounds	Study design	Outcomes	Reference
SAIDs and NSAIDs	Dexamethasone	Intra-nigral injection of LPS in rats	↑ TH activity in striatum.	[73]
	Ibuprofen	Primary mesencephalic culture from rats treated with ibuprofen	↑dopamine uptake, protected neurons against excitotoxicity.	[76]
	Amantadine	Peripheral blood mononuclear cells from idiopathic PD patients	↑ $CD3^+$ $CD4^+$ cells, improves T-cell mediated immunity.	[77]
Antibiotics	Rifampicin	LPS induced BV2 microglia	↓ in NFkB activation, ↓ expression of iNOS, COX2, TNF-α, IL-1β ↓production of NO, PGE_2.	[81]
		MPP induced PC12 cells	↓MPP induced neuronal death, ↓expression of α-syn multimer.	[83]
	Ceftriaxone	PC12 cells exposed to neurotoxin 6-OHDA	Binds with α-syn and blocks its polymerization *in vitro*	[85]
		6-OHDA induced PD rat model	↑GLT-1 expression, reduces striatal TH loss.	[86]

Therapy	Compounds	Study design	Outcomes	Reference
	D-cycloserine	MPTP induced PD rat model	Improved behavioral deficits restored IL-2 level ↓microglial activation.	[87]
	Rapamycin	In PC12 cells and MPTP induced mouse model	↓neuronal death, regulate Akt phosphorylation at Thr308.	[89]
	Minocycline	In MPTP induced mouse model, primary mesencephalic culture	↓expression of iNOS, caspase-1, inhibited NO induced neurotoxicity, ↓phosphorylation of p38.	[90]
		In differentiated LUHMES cells induced by reactive oxygen species	Specific scavenger of peroxynitrite, ↓microglia activation.	[91]
Neuropeptides	PACAP	MPP^+ induced SHSY-5Y neuroblastoma	↓cell death, ↑ cAMP	[98]
		Oxygen and glucose deprived BV2 microglia	↓TRL4, MyD88, NFkB ↓production of pro-inflammatory cytokines	[95]
		MPTP induced mice	↑TH expression, ↓caspase-3, IL-6, TNF-a	[98]
	VIP	LPS induced mice and mesencephalic culture 6-OHDA induced	↓pro-inflammatory cytokine, ↓NO	[99]
Polyphenols	Pinocembrin	6-OHDA SHSY-5Y	↓apoptosis, ↓ROS	[101]
	Naringenin	6-OHDA induced mice and SHSY-5Y	↑Nrf2. ↑neuroprotection, ↓ROS	[102]
	Flavonoids from *Selaginella* extract	Rotenone induced Drosophila PD model	↑anti-oxidant enzyme activity, ↓oxidative stress	[103, 104]
	Curcumin	6-OHDA induced SHSY-5Y	↓p-p38, ↓caspase-3	[105]
	Baicalein	MPTP induced mice and primary rat astrocytes	↓NFkB nuclear translocation, ↓microglia and astrocyte activation, ↓COX2, ↓phosphorylation of JNK and ERK	[106]
	Theaflavin	MPTP with probenecid induced mice	↑TH expression, ↓caspase-3,8,9, ↓COX2, IL-1β, TNF-α, IL-6	[109]
	Resveratrol	MPTP induced mice	↑TH protein and mRNA, ↑SOCS-1, ↓TNF-α, IL-1β,IL-6, ↓TNF-αR1, IL-1βR1, IL-Rα	[110]

Therapy	Compounds	Study design	Outcomes	Reference
		Rotenone or MPP^+ induce primary rat astrocytes/ microglia, mesencephalic culture, BV2	↓NO, ROS, MPO, ↓iNOS, COX2, TNF-a, IL-1b mRNA, ↓phagocytic activity	[111]
Anti-inflammatory Cytokines	IL-10	LPS induced mesencephalic culture	↓TNF-α, NO, ↓extracellular superoxide, inhibit PHOX activity	[112]
		Hu-IL-10 gene transfer in 6-OHDA induced rats.	↑TH-positive neurons, ↓ glial activation	[113]
	TGF-β	Retrograde model of PD induced with 6-OHDA and treated with TGF-β alone and in combination with GDNF.	Reduce dopamine receptor hypersensitivity, ↑TH-positive neurons, induce synaptogenesis	[114]
		LPS and MPTP induced mice	↓ROS, ↓PHOX $p47^{phox}$ activity, ↓LPS activated phosphorylation of ERK and $p47^{phox}$	[116]
Insulin therapy	Pioglitazone	MPTP induced mice	↓microglial activation, ↓GFAP positive cells in SN, ↑ IkBα, ↓NFkB activation	[121]
		LPS induced rat microglial cells	↓NO, iNOS, TNF-α, IL-1β, IL-6, ↓phosphorylation of p38.	[119]
	GLP-1 receptor agonist: Exenatide	MPTP mice and 6-OHDA induced mesencephalic culture	↓neurotoxicity, improve motor functions, ↑TH-positive cells, ↑cAMP ↓TNF-α, superoxide, NO	[122]
Beta2-adrenergic receptor agonists	Salmeterol	LPS and MPTP induced mice	↓phosphorylation of MAPK, p65 NFkB.	[16]
Morphinan compounds	L-morphine	LPS and MPP^+ induced rat mesencephalic culture	↓PHOX activity, ↓pro-inflammatory cytokines, ↓ERK phosphorylation.	[127]
	Sinomenine	LPS and MPP^+ induced rat mesencephalic culture	↓TNF-α, PGE_2, ROS ↓PHOX activity.	[128]
	3-HM	Rat mesencephalic culture stimulated with LPS	↓NO, TNF-α, PGE_2, ROS ↓microglia activation	[129]
		LPS and MPTP models	↑expression of neurotrophic factors ↑acetylation of histone H3 ↓reactive microgliosis ↓ROS	[130]
Therapy against NFkB	NBD	MPTP induced mice	↓NFkB activation, ↓iNOS, ↓TNF-α, IL-1β ↓CD11b, ↓neuronal death	[132]

Therapy	Compounds	Study design	Outcomes	Reference
	Compound A (IKK inhibitor)	LPS induced rats and mesencephalic culture	↓neurotoxicity, ↓TNF-α, IL-1β, ↓NO, iNOS, ↓IKKβ phosphorylation and NFkB activation ↓phosphorylation of ERK, p38, JNK, ↓ROS, ↓superoxide	[133]
Anti-oxidants	DPI (NADPH oxidase inhibitor)	LPS induced midbrain neuron-glia culture	↓neurotoxicity ↓NOX2 activation.	[135]
		LPS induced rats and mesencephalic culture	↓ROS, ↓TNF-α, NO ↓ERK phosphorylation, ↓PHOX activity	[136]
	Coenzyme Q10	MPTP model	↓ROS, ↓free radicals production, ↓neurotoxicity	[137]
	NAC	Intravenous infusion of NAC in PD patients MPP^+ induced PC12 cells	↑glutathione level in blood	[140]
	Edaravone		↓oxidative stress, ↓ROS ↑Heme-oxygenase-1 expression	[142]

Table 1. Neuroprotective effects of anti-inflammatory therapies.

7.1. Antibiotics in neuroprotection in PD

Antibiotics are routinely used to kill or inhibit the growth of microorganisms at low concentrations. In addition to their antimicrobial activity, antibiotics can either directly or indirectly regulate the expression of many inflammatory gene transcripts [80], and a number of antibiotics such as tetracycline and β-lactams have been shown to have significant anti-inflammatory properties [81]. Antibiotics now appear to have protective effects against neurodegeneration and the neuroinflammatory process [82]. These properties of antibiotics make them suitable for the development of effective therapies against neurodegenerative diseases such as PD. Rifampicin, a macrocyclic antibiotic, upregulates Ab clearance in brain, and it is also neuroprotective in other chronic neurodegenerative diseases and cerebral ischemia [83]. Pretreatment with Rifampicin increases cell viability and reduces α-synuclein expression and its aggregation. Moreover, in MPP^+-induced PC12 cells, Rifampicin prevents the formation of α-synuclein oligomer [84]. It can also block the release of pro-inflammatory cytokines such as NO, PGE_2 TNF-α, and IL-1β from LPS-stimulated BV-2 microglial cells [85]. Similarly, β-lactam also has protective role against neurodegeneration and can cross BBB. β-lactam antibiotic ceftriaxone has demonstrated neuroprotective activity as well as high binding affinity with α-synuclein and can block its *in vitro* polymerization [86]. Ceftriaxone also increases the expression of glutamate transporter-1 (GLT-1) which enhances glutamate uptake and therefore reduces excitotoxicity in 6-OHDA model of PD [87]. D-cycloserine (DCS), an antibiotic prescribed for Mycobacterium tuberculosis, also acts as an NMDA receptor antagonist that prevents excitotoxicity damage induced by MPTP [88] and inhibits the

http://dx.doi.org/10.5772/63027

production of MMP3 and MMP9 in LPS stimulate microglial cells. In addition, Rapamycin was able to prevent mitochondrial dysfunction in PINK1/Parkin Drosophila mutants [89]. Furthermore, it enhances the expression of neuronal survival promoting kinase Akt, antioxidant enzymes and anti-apoptotic markers [90]. Similarly, Minocycline has shown neuroprotective effects in PD models [91]. Minocycline suppresses α-synuclein aggregation and its toxicity [92], as well as microglial activation of p38 the MAPK signaling pathway resulting in the suppression of pro-inflammatory mediator release [93]. These results support the potential of antibiotics as neuroprotective and therapeutic agents in PD.

7.2. The role of anti-inflammatory compounds in neuroinflammation and PD

Neurotrophic factors are essential for neural growth and development, and these factors normally signal through Trk receptors. Adenosine and pituitary adenylate cyclase-activating peptide (PACAP) act as ligands and induces activation of Trk receptors through adenosine (A_{2A}) receptor and PAC1 receptors, respectively [94]. Recent studies reported the antioxidant and anti-inflammatory properties of PACAP [95, 96]. It can inhibit the release of several pro-inflammatory mediators from LPS-activated microglial cells by inhibiting the transcriptional activity of NF-kB [97], as well as the production of several chemokines like MIP-1α, -1β, MCP-1, and RANTES [98]. A synthetic analog of PACAP showed neuroprotection in MPP^+-induced SHSY-5Y cells and MPTP-injected mice. It restored the expression of tyrosine hydroxylase in Substantia nigra and modulated the inflammatory response [99]. Another peptide, called vasoactive intestinal peptide (VIP), can also inhibit the expression of pro-inflammatory cytokines from LPS-activated cultured microglia [100]. These studies suggest these peptides can serve as promising molecules for the development of anti-inflammatory and neuroprotective drugs in the treatment of PD.

7.2.1. Neuroprotective and anti-inflammatory role of polyphenols

Several traditional medicinal plants and herbs are rich in polyphenol, and their neuroprotective effects have been studied extensively. These compounds have neuroprotective properties against oxidative stress, neuroinflammation, mitochondrial dysfunction, and protein fibrillization. Kong et al. reported that polyphenols reduce the intracellular level of ROS in DA neurons [101]. Recently, it has been found that pretreatment with flavonoids such as pinocembrin [102] and naringenin [103] reduces the formation of ROS, in 6-OHDA-challenged human neuroblastoma SHSY-5Y cells. This effect was due to an increase in Nrf2 protein level and by activating ARE pathway genes. In addition, flavonoids from *Selaginella* species have the ability to increase the expression and activity of anti-oxidative enzymes endogenously [104], and the aqueous extract of *Selaginella* suppresses rotenone induced neurotoxicity, attenuated locomotor dysfunction, oxidative stress, and mitochondrial dysfunction in *Drosophila melanogaster* [105]. Polyphenols may also target MAPK pathways and apoptosis, since phosphorylation of MAPK and expression of cleaved caspase 3 were reduced in 6-OHDA induced SHSY-5Y cells by curcumin [106]. Similarly, the phosphorylation of NF-kB, JNK, and ERK was inhibited by flavone baicalein in MPP^+-induced primary astrocytes and indicated its implication in the treatment of PD [107]. Several other polyphenols have been shown to reduce the expression of pro-inflammatory cytokine such as IL-1β, TNF-α, and IL-6 [108, 109]. Furthermore, theaflavin treatment in MPTP mice model of PD increases the expression of anti-inflammatory cytokines such as IL-4 and IL-10 by the modulation of the suppressor of cytokine signaling 1 (SOCS1). Oral administration of resveratrol in MPTP mouse model upregulated the expression of SOCS1 in striatum and Substantia nigra and suppresses the production of pro-inflammatory cytokines [110] and also improved cell survival in rotenone-induced primary mesencephalic culture. Resveratrol also diminished the level of MPO (MPO; an enzyme produces hypochlorous acid and tyrosyl radical during microglial respiratory burst) and ROS in MPP^+-induced BV2 microglia cells [111, 112]. Many polyphenol compounds have been studied to test their neuroprotective and anti-inflammatory properties, but further research will be needed to understand the signaling mechanism of how these compounds act to offset neuroinflammation.

7.2.2. Anti-inflammatory cytokine therapies in PD

The use of anti-inflammatory cytokine serves as a potent approach for the development of anti-parkinsonian drugs. Two major anti-inflammatory cytokines, IL-10 and transforming growth factor beta 1 (TGFβ1), produced by T_{reg} cells, have been studied in PD models. Pre- and posttreatment of rat mesencephalic neuron glia culture with IL-10 showed neuroprotective effects against LPS-induced neurotoxicity by inhibiting the production of TNF-α, nitric oxide, and extracellular superoxide [113]. Gene delivery of human IL-10 by using adeno-associated viral type-2 (AAV2) in 6-OHDA rat model of PD also showed neuroprotection by suppressing the 6-OHDA-induced loss of TH-positive neurons [114]. Similarly, TGFβ1 also shows protective effects against neurotoxicity. TGFβ1 in combination with GDNF reduces progressive cell death and enhances the expression of TH in surviving nigral neurons in retrograde model of Parkinsonism in rats [115]. It has also been shown that TGFβ1 protects from neuronal death induced by glutamate excitotoxicity [116]. The neuroprotective effect of TGFβ1 is primarily due to its ability to inhibit the production of ROS from microglia during activation. Additionally, after LPS activation, ERK phosphorylation and subsequent serine phosphorylation on $p47^{phox}$ were significantly inhibited by pretreatment with TGFβ1 [117]. Recently, it also has been reported that overexpression of fractalkine (CX3CL1) reduces neuronal loss in 6-OHDA model of PD and suppresses α-synuclein-mediated neurodegeneration [118]. The use of these anti-inflammatory mediators therapeutically to suppress represents a new therapeutic avenue for the treatment of PD.

7.2.3. Regulatory T-cell therapy

T_{reg} cells have the capability to mitigate inflammation and serve as an attractive therapeutic target. T_{reg} cell therapy can be used for neuroprotection in PD as these cells also utilize immunosuppressive mechanisms including the production of anti-inflammatory cytokines. The neuroprotective effects of bee venom is associated with the deactivation of microglia and suppression of $CD4^+$ T cell infiltration, and it also increases the proportion of $CD4^{+,}$ $CD25^+$ and $Foxp3^+$ T_{reg} cells in MPTP mouse model of PD. Several studies have been shown that T_{reg} cell responses inhibit microglial activation and enhance neuronal survival in MPTP mouse model of PD [24, 119]. In addition, another type of T_{reg} cell, Th2 cells also inhibit microglial activation by the production of IL-4 and IL-10 against MPTP-induced neurotoxicity. What signals suppress the T_{reg} cell functions and how to improve anti-inflammatory activity are yet to be determined.

7.2.4. *Insulin as potent therapeutic agent for treatment in PD*

Insulin is the enzyme most responsible for lowering the blood glucose, but it has also been found to have potent anti-inflammatory effects. Insulin signaling regulates a number of cellular processes such as neurotransmission, vesicle trafficking cell survival, and inflammatory mediator production. Recent evidence has shown that insulin signaling is impaired in Alzheimer and, to some degree to, Parkinson's patients. Preclinical studies suggest that the application of insulin or long-lasting analogs of incretin peptides in transgenic animal model of PD, and AD reduces neurodegeneration and neuronal and synaptic functionality [120, 121]. Pioglitazone is generally prescribed for type 2 diabetes mellitus and reduces insulin resistance and acts on peroxisome proliferator-activated receptor γ (PPARγ) receptors. It also functions to reduce microglial activation and induction of iNOS positive cells by enhancing inhibitory protein kappa B (IkBα) and inhibition of NF-kB subunit p65 in MPTP mouse model of PD [122]. In LPS model of PD, Pioglitazone showed neuroprotection by inhibiting microglia-mediated oxidative stress [120]. Another anti-diabetic agent, GLP-1 (glucagon-like peptide), is a hormone which maintains homeostasis between insulin and glucose. Exenatide is a synthetic agonist for the GLP-1 receptor and shows significant promise as neuroprotective in PD animal models [123]. These studies describe the potent impact of insulin or anti-diabetic treatments as possible anti-inflammatory neuroprotective therapies for PD.

7.2.5. *Use of β-adrenergic receptor agonists as an anti-inflammatory agent in the treatment of PD*

Beta2-adrenergic receptors (β2AR) are seven transmembrane G-protein-coupled receptors found on numerous cell types, including inflammatory cells and neurons. β2AR agonists are FDA approved for the treatment of chronic obstructive pulmonary disorders (COPD), and their use as treatment for neurodegenerative diseases such as PD represents a new and potentially very productive therapeutic approach. In the CNS, microglia expresses high levels of β2AR, and it has been demonstrated that long-acting β2AR agonists such as salmeterol (Advair, GlaxoSK) protect against DA neuronal death from microglia-mediated neuroinflammation [16]. In addition to inhibiting the production of inflammatory mediators and oxidative stress responses by microglial cells, several *in vivo* studies also reported neuroprotective roles of long-acting β2AR agonists by inducing neurotrophic growth factors and astrocyte activation [124, 125]. Long-acting agonist such as salmeterol showed neuroprotective effects by pretreatment in LPS-stimulated long-term mouse model and also by the treatment with salmeterol after MPTP injection. Low dose of salmeterol treatment in these models suppressed the NF-kB activation and its nuclear translocation. Similarly, it also reduces phosphorylation of MAPK such as ERK1/2, p38, and JNK [126]. Furthermore, it has been shown that low dose of salmeterol also inhibits TGF-beta-activated kinase 1 (TAK1), which is a common upstream regulatory molecule for MAPK and NF-kB activation, and involves in various inflammatory signaling pathways [127]. This suggests the anti-inflammatory effects of salmeterol by reducing phosphorylation of MAPK and NF-kB activation via inhibition of TAK1. The activation of β2AR stimulates MAPK signaling also via β-arrestin-dependent and G-protein-independent mechanism [126]. Overall, these agonists can inhibit inflammatory response and have potential to regulate inflammation in chronic inflammatory disorders of CNS. These results suggest that β2AR agonists can be developed as anti-inflammatory therapy to subside the progressive loss of dopaminergic neurons in PD patients.

7.2.6. Use of morphinan-related anti-inflammatory compounds in PD

Several morphinan analogs such as naloxone, dextromethorphan, or naltrexone have been described as anti-inflammatory and neuroprotective. Morphine isomers (L-morphine and its D stereoenantiomer) can inhibit microglial activation and LPS- or MPP^+-induced neurotoxicity in rat primary mesencephalic cultures. Furthermore, it also suggests that morphinan compounds bind to the catalytic subunit of PHOX and inhibits its activity leading to the reduced production of superoxide and other pro-inflammatory cytokines [128]. Similar results were observed with sinomenine, a dextrorotatory isomer of morphine and protective effects of sinomenine mediated through the inhibition of microglial PHOX activity [129]. Similarly, 3-hydroxymorphinan (3-HM), a metabolite of dextromethorphan, recently emerged as a potent therapeutic agent for the treatment of PD. These compounds show neuroprotection by two different pathways; one through a neurotrophic effect mediated by astrocytes and another by their anti-inflammatory effect mediated by the suppression of microglial activation. When the 3-HM compound was studied for its mechanistic effects *in vivo*, it was found that it attenuated the depletion of striatal levels of dopamine and showed neuroprotection against LPS- and MPTP-elicited neurotoxicity [130]. These effects were observed even when drug was administered post MPTP injections [131]. Collectively, these findings offer a different yet highly potent new therapeutic direction for the treatment of neuroinflammation in PD.

7.2.7. Pro-inflammatory transcription factor, NF-kB as a therapeutic target in PD

Nuclear transcription factor NF-kB plays an important role in inflammation. It regulates the expression of various genes involved in immune function and cell survival. NF-kB activation has been reported in Substantia nigra of PD patients and in animal models of PD. The inhibition of NF-kB activation can suppress oxidative stress and production of pro-inflammatory cytokines and chemokines in microglia [132]. Ghosh et al. [133] reported that intraperitoneal injection of NBD (NF-kB essential modifier-binding domain) peptide reduces nigral activation of NF-kB, inhibits microglial activation in Substantia nigra, and improves motor function in MPTP mouse model of PD. Selective inhibitors against IKK-β also reduce microglial n and neuronal death in SNpc in MPTP-intoxicated PD mice [133] and in LPS-induced neurodegeneration by inhibiting NF-kB activation and decreasing the production of pro-inflammatory cytokines. It also suppresses the activity of microglial NADPH oxidase and reduces the production of ROS [134]. These reports suggest the suppression of NF-kB signaling pathway in microglia is neuroprotective and represent NF-kB as a strong potential target for anti-inflammatory therapy in the treatment of PD.

http://dx.doi.org/10.5772/63027

7.2.8. Antioxidants as neuroprotective agents in PD

Oxidative stress and generation of free radicals have been reported to be a major effector of neuronal death seen in neurodegeneration in PD. This can also be linked to other processes such as nitric oxide toxicity, excitotoxicity, mitochondrial dysfunction, and inflammation. Oxidative stress impairs cell viability by damaging lipid, proteins, and nucleic acids [135]. The development of therapies against oxidative stress and free radicals may be beneficial in PD by inhibiting the onset of apoptotic cell death and degeneration of nigrostriatal dopaminergic neurons. The neurotoxin MPTP inhibits the mitochondrial electron transport chain and suppresses the activity of mitochondrial complex I and eventually elevates oxidative stress within DA neurons. MPTP also increases the production of free radicals and ROS by microglial cells, ultimately leading to the death of dopamine producing neurons. It has been found that mice lacking the NADPH oxidase complex do not exhibit DA neurotoxicity from MPTP- or LPS-induced neurodegeneration, and that the administration of NADPH oxidase inhibitor DPI can prevent DA neurotoxicity [136, 137]. Several other antioxidants have been investigated in the treatment of PD, and it has been found that coenzyme Q10 is a potent antioxidant and electron acceptor for mitochondrial complex I and II, can enhance activity of complex I, and reduce oxidative stress [138]. Clinical trial with randomized, parallel group, placebo controls, and double-blind with multiple doses of CoQ10 (300, 600, or 1200 mg/day) in 80 early PD patients showed that CoQ10 is well tolerated at doses up to 1200 mg/day, less disability was developed in PD subjects, and symptomatic relief was higher in subjects receiving the highest dose [139]. In contrast, a recent phase III, randomized, double-blind, placebo-controlled clinical trial concluded that CoQ10 is safe and well tolerated but showed no evidence of clinical benefits [140]. Another antioxidant and a pro-drug of amino acid cysteine called N-acetyl-cysteine (NAC) also showed neuroprotective effects. Preclinical data suggest NAC is neuroprotective and can reduce oxidative stress and ROS accumulation. Recently, a clinical trial with NAC intravenous infusion concludes that NAC enhances the level of glutathione (a potent antioxidant) in blood and brain in PD patients [141]. Similarly, Edaravone (MCI-186, 3-methyl-1-phenyl-2-pyrozolin-5-one) is a neuroprotective antioxidant, generally prescribed for recovery of acute brain ischemia and cerebral infraction [142]. It showed neuroprotective effects in MPP-induced PC12 cells by reducing oxidative stress and enhancing expression heme oxygenase-1 expression (a cellular stress response protein) [143], but clinical trials are yet to be done.

8. Conclusion

Inflammation plays an important role in the etiology of a number of different forms of PD, and anti-inflammatory drugs hold much promise as a therapeutic treatment for patients with mild and moderate forms of PD. The continued evaluation of these drugs, including their efficacy, target, and mechanism of action, hold much promise for the future treatment of PD.

Author details

Patrick Flood*, Naik Arbabzada and Monika Sharma

*Address all correspondence to: pflood@ualberta.ca

University of Alberta, Edmonton, Canada

References

[1] Hirsch EC, Hunot S, Damier P, Faucheux B. Glial cells and inflammation in Parkinson's disease: a role in neurodegeneration? Ann Neurol. 1998 Sep;44(3 Suppl 1):S115–20.

[2] Bernheimer H, Birkmayer W, Hornykiewicz O, Jellinger K, Seitelberger F. Brain dopamine and the syndromes of Parkinson and Huntington. Clinical, morphological and neurochemical correlations. J Neurol Sci. 1973 Dec;20(4):415–55.

[3] Bezard E, Dovero S, Prunier C, Ravenscroft P, Chalon S, Guilloteau D, et al. Relationship between the appearance of symptoms and the level of nigrostriatal degeneration in a progressive 1-methyl-4-phenyl-1,2,3,6-tetrahydropyridine-lesioned macaque model of Parkinson's disease. J Neurosci Off J Soc Neurosci. 2001 Sep 1;21(17):6853–61.

[4] Elenkov IJ, Wilder RL, Chrousos GP, Vizi ES. The sympathetic nerve--an integrative interface between two supersystems: the brain and the immune system. Pharmacol Rev. 2000 Dec;52(4):595–638.

[5] Huang Y, Halliday GM. Aspects of innate immunity and Parkinson's disease. Front Pharmacol. 2012;3:33.

[6] Farina C, Aloisi F, Meinl E. Astrocytes are active players in cerebral innate immunity. Trends Immunol. 2007 Mar;28(3):138–45.

[7] Damier P, Hirsch EC, Zhang P, Agid Y, Javoy-Agid F. Glutathione peroxidase, glial cells and Parkinson's disease. Neuroscience. 1993 Jan;52(1):1–6.

[8] Wilhelmsson U, Bushong EA, Price DL, Smarr BL, Phung V, Terada M, et al. Redefining the concept of reactive astrocytes as cells that remain within their unique domains upon reaction to injury. Proc Natl Acad Sci U S A. 2006 Nov 14;103(46):17513–8.

[9] Knott C, Wilkin GP, Stern G. Astrocytes and microglia in the substantia nigra and caudate-putamen in Parkinson's disease. Parkinsonism Relat Disord. 1999 Sep;5(3): 115–22.

[10] Teismann P, Schulz JB. Cellular pathology of Parkinson's disease: astrocytes, microglia and inflammation. Cell Tissue Res. 2004 Oct;318(1):149–61.

[11] Kohutnicka M, Lewandowska E, Kurkowska-Jastrzebska I, Członkowski A, Członkowska A. Microglial and astrocytic involvement in a murine model of Parkinson's disease induced by 1-methyl-4-phenyl-1,2,3,6-tetrahydropyridine (MPTP). Immunopharmacology. 1998 Jun;39(3):167–80.

[12] Nomura T, Yabe T, Rosenthal ES, Krzan M, Schwartz JP. PSA-NCAM distinguishes reactive astrocytes in 6-OHDA-lesioned substantia nigra from those in the striatal terminal fields. J Neurosci Res. 2000 Sep 15;61(6):588–96.

[13] Depino AM, Earl C, Kaczmarczyk E, Ferrari C, Besedovsky H, del Rey A, et al. Microglial activation with atypical proinflammatory cytokine expression in a rat model of Parkinson's disease. Eur J Neurosci. 2003 Nov;18(10):2731–42.

[14] McGeer PL, Itagaki S, Boyes BE, McGeer EG. Reactive microglia are positive for HLA-DR in the substantia nigra of Parkinson's and Alzheimer's disease brains. Neurology. 1988 Aug;38(8):1285–91.

[15] Qian L, Hu X, Zhang D, Snyder A, Wu H-M, Li Y, et al. beta2 Adrenergic receptor activation induces microglial NADPH oxidase activation and dopaminergic neurotoxicity through an ERK-dependent/protein kinase A-independent pathway. Glia. 2009 Nov 15;57(15):1600–9.

[16] Qian L, Wu H, Chen S-H, Zhang D, Ali SF, Peterson L, et al. β2-adrenergic receptor activation prevents rodent dopaminergic neurotoxicity by inhibiting microglia via a novel signaling pathway. J Immunol Baltim Md. 1950. 2011 Apr 1;186(7):4443–54.

[17] Mount MP, Lira A, Grimes D, Smith PD, Faucher S, Slack R, et al. Involvement of interferon-gamma in microglial-mediated loss of dopaminergic neurons. J Neurosci Off J Soc Neurosci. 2007 Mar 21;27(12):3328–37.

[18] Xing B, Bachstetter AD, Van Eldik LJ. Microglial p38α MAPK is critical for LPS-induced neuron degeneration, through a mechanism involving TNFα. Mol Neurodegener. 2011;6:84.

[19] Sriram K, Matheson JM, Benkovic SA, Miller DB, Luster MI, O'Callaghan JP. Mice deficient in TNF receptors are protected against dopaminergic neurotoxicity: implications for Parkinson's disease. FASEB J Off Publ Fed Am Soc Exp Biol. 2002 Sep;16(11): 1474–6.

[20] Peterson L, Ismond KP, Chapman E, Flood P. Potential benefits of therapeutic use of β2-adrenergic receptor agonists in neuroprotection and Parkinson's disease. J Immunol Res. 2014;2014:103780.

[21] Kannarkat GT, Boss JM, Tansey MG. The role of innate and adaptive immunity in Parkinson's disease. J Parkinsons Dis. 2013;3(4):493–514.

[22] Ahmed I, Tamouza R, Delord M, Krishnamoorthy R, Tzourio C, Mulot C, et al. Association between Parkinson's disease and the HLA-DRB1 locus. Mov Disord Off J Mov Disord Soc. 2012 Aug;27(9):1104–10.

[23] Orr CF, Rowe DB, Halliday GM. An inflammatory review of Parkinson's disease. Prog Neurobiol. 2002 Dec;68(5):325–40.

[24] Reynolds AD, Banerjee R, Liu J, Gendelman HE, Mosley RL. Neuroprotective activities of CD4+CD25+ regulatory T cells in an animal model of Parkinson's disease. J Leukoc Biol. 2007 Nov;82(5):1083–94.

[25] Le WD, Engelhardt J, Xie WJ, Schneider L, Smith RG, Appel SH. Experimental autoimmune nigral damage in guinea pigs. J Neuroimmunol. 1995 Mar;57(1-2):45–53.

[26] McRae-Degueurce A, Rosengren L, Haglid K, Bööj S, Gottfries CG, Granérus AC, et al. Immunocytochemical investigations on the presence of neuron-specific antibodies in the CSF of Parkinson's disease cases. Neurochem Res. 1988 Jul;13(7):679–84.

[27] Appel SH, Le WD, Tajti J, Haverkamp LJ, Engelhardt JI. Nigral damage and dopaminergic hypofunction in mesencephalon-immunized guinea pigs. Ann Neurol. 1992 Oct; 32(4):494–501.

[28] Fahn S, Cohen G. The oxidant stress hypothesis in Parkinson's disease: evidence supporting it. Ann Neurol. 1992 Dec;32(6):804–12.

[29] Zigmond MJ. and Burke RE. Pathophsiology of Parkinson's disease. In: Kenneth L. Davis, Dennis Charney, Joseph T. Coyle, and Charles Nemeroff, editors. Neuropsychopharmacology: The Fifth Generation of Progress. American College of Neuropsychopharmacology; 2002. pp. 1781–1793.

[30] Dzamko N, Geczy CL, Halliday GM. Inflammation is genetically implicated in Parkinson's disease. Neuroscience. 2015 Aug 27;302:89–102.

[31] Wood-Kaczmar A, Gandhi S, Wood NW. Understanding the molecular causes of Parkinson's disease. Trends Mol Med. 2006 Nov;12(11):521–8.

[32] Su X, Federoff HJ. Immune responses in Parkinson's disease: interplay between central and peripheral immune systems. BioMed Res Int. 2014;2014:275178.

[33] Van Limbergen J, Wilson DC, Satsangi J. The genetics of Crohn's disease. Ann Rev Genomics Hum Genet. 2009;10:89–116.

[34] Cardoso CC, Pereira AC, de Sales Marques C, Moraes MO. Leprosy susceptibility: genetic variations regulate innate and adaptive immunity, and disease outcome. Future Microbiol. 2011 May;6(5):533–49.

[35] Green DR, Oberst A, Dillon CP, Weinlich R, Salvesen GS. RIPK-dependent necrosis and its regulation by caspases: a mystery in five acts. Mol Cell. 2011 Oct 7;44(1):9–16.

[36] Dzamko N, Inesta-Vaquera F, Zhang J, Xie C, Cai H, Arthur S, et al. The IkappaB kinase family phosphorylates the Parkinson's disease kinase LRRK2 at Ser935 and Ser910 during Toll-like receptor signaling. PLoS One. 2012;7(6):e39132.

[37] Kim JS, Cho JW, Shin H, Lee WY, Ki C-S, Cho AR, et al. A Korean Parkinson's disease family with the LRRK2 p.Tyr1699Cys mutation showing clinical heterogeneity. Mov Disord Off J Mov Disord Soc. 2012 Feb;27(2):320–4.

[38] Moehle MS, Webber PJ, Tse T, Sukar N, Standaert DG, DeSilva TM, et al. LRRK2 inhibition attenuates microglial inflammatory responses. J Neurosci Off J Soc Neurosci. 2012 Feb 1;32(5):1602–11.

[39] Gillardon F, Schmid R, Draheim H. Parkinson's disease-linked leucine-rich repeat kinase 2(R1441G) mutation increases proinflammatory cytokine release from activated primary microglial cells and resultant neurotoxicity. Neuroscience. 2012 Apr 19;208:41–8.

[40] Russo I, Bubacco L, Greggio E. LRRK2 and neuroinflammation: partners in crime in Parkinson's disease? J Neuroinflammation. 2014;11:52.

[41] Frank-Cannon TC, Tran T, Ruhn KA, Martinez TN, Hong J, Marvin M, et al. Parkin deficiency increases vulnerability to inflammation-related nigral degeneration. J Neurosci Off J Soc Neurosci. 2008 Oct 22;28(43):10825–34.

[42] Sha D, Chin L-S, Li L. Phosphorylation of parkin by Parkinson disease-linked kinase PINK1 activates parkin E3 ligase function and NF-kappaB signaling. Hum Mol Genet. 2010 Jan 15;19(2):352–63.

[43] Narendra D, Tanaka A, Suen D-F, Youle RJ. Parkin is recruited selectively to impaired mitochondria and promotes their autophagy. J Cell Biol. 2008 Dec 1;183(5):795–803.

[44] Chen ZJ. Ubiquitin signalling in the NF-kappaB pathway. Nat Cell Biol. 2005 Aug;7(8): 758–65.

[45] Chung J-Y, Park HR, Lee S-J, Lee S-H, Kim JS, Jung Y-S, et al. Elevated TRAF2/6 expression in Parkinson's disease is caused by the loss of Parkin E3 ligase activity. Lab Investig J Tech Methods Pathol. 2013 Jun;93(6):663–76.

[46] Marques O, Outeiro TF. Alpha-synuclein: from secretion to dysfunction and death. Cell Death Dis. 2012;3:e350.

[47] Recchia A, Debetto P, Negro A, Guidolin D, Skaper SD, Giusti P. Alpha-synuclein and Parkinson's disease. FASEB J Off Publ Fed Am Soc Exp Biol. 2004 Apr;18(6):617–26.

[48] Fellner L, Irschick R, Schanda K, Reindl M, Klimaschewski L, Poewe W, et al. Toll-like receptor 4 is required for α-synuclein dependent activation of microglia and astroglia. Glia. 2013 Mar;61(3):349–60.

[49] Kim C, Ho D-H, Suk J-E, You S, Michael S, Kang J, et al. Neuron-released oligomeric α-synuclein is an endogenous agonist of TLR2 for paracrine activation of microglia. Nat Commun. 2013;4:1562.

[50] Forsyth CB, Shannon KM, Kordower JH, Voigt RM, Shaikh M, Jaglin JA, et al. Increased intestinal permeability correlates with sigmoid mucosa alpha-synuclein staining and endotoxin exposure markers in early Parkinson's disease. PLoS One. 2011;6(12):e28032.

[51] Alvarez-Erviti L, Couch Y, Richardson J, Cooper JM, Wood MJA. Alpha-synuclein release by neurons activates the inflammatory response in a microglial cell line. Neurosci Res. 2011 Apr;69(4):337–42.

[52] Lema Tomé CM, Tyson T, Rey NL, Grathwohl S, Britschgi M, Brundin P. Inflammation and α-synuclein's prion-like behavior in Parkinson's disease--is there a link? Mol Neurobiol. 2013 Apr;47(2):561–74.

[53] Tran HT, Chung CH-Y, Iba M, Zhang B, Trojanowski JQ, Luk KC, et al. A-synuclein immunotherapy blocks uptake and templated propagation of misfolded α-synuclein and neurodegeneration. Cell Rep. 2014 Jun 26;7(6):2054–65.

[54] Akundi RS, Huang Z, Eason J, Pandya JD, Zhi L, Cass WA, et al. Increased mitochondrial calcium sensitivity and abnormal expression of innate immunity genes precede dopaminergic defects in Pink1-deficient mice. PLoS One. 2011;6(1):e16038.

[55] Lee HJ, Chung KC. PINK1 positively regulates IL-1β-mediated signaling through Tollip and IRAK1 modulation. J Neuroinflammation. 2012;9:271.

[56] Waak J, Weber SS, Waldenmaier A, Görner K, Alunni-Fabbroni M, Schell H, et al. Regulation of astrocyte inflammatory responses by the Parkinson's disease-associated gene DJ-1. FASEB J Off Publ Fed Am Soc Exp Biol. 2009 Aug;23(8):2478–89.

[57] Trudler D, Weinreb O, Mandel SA, Youdim MBH, Frenkel D. DJ-1 deficiency triggers microglia sensitivity to dopamine toward a pro-inflammatory phenotype that is attenuated by rasagiline. J Neurochem. 2014 May;129(3):434–47.

[58] Mitsumoto A, Nakagawa Y. DJ-1 is an indicator for endogenous reactive oxygen species elicited by endotoxin. Free Radic Res. 2001 Dec;35(6):885–93.

[59] Jackson-Lewis V, Przedborski S. Protocol for the MPTP mouse model of Parkinson's disease. Nat Protoc. 2007;2(1):141–51.

[60] Gayle DA, Ling Z, Tong C, Landers T, Lipton JW, Carvey PM. Lipopolysaccharide (LPS)-induced dopamine cell loss in culture: roles of tumor necrosis factor-alpha, interleukin-1beta, and nitric oxide. Brain Res Dev Brain Res. 2002 Jan 31;133(1):27–35.

[61] Gao H-M, Hong J-S, Zhang W, Liu B. Distinct role for microglia in rotenone-induced degeneration of dopaminergic neurons. J Neurosci Off J Soc Neurosci. 2002 Feb 1;22(3): 782–90.

[62] Dauer W, Przedborski S. Parkinson's disease: mechanisms and models. Neuron. 2003 Sep 11;39(6):889–909.

[63] Bae E-J, Lee H-J, Rockenstein E, Ho D-H, Park E-B, Yang N-Y, et al. Antibody-aided clearance of extracellular α-synuclein prevents cell-to-cell aggregate transmission. J Neurosci Off J Soc Neurosci. 2012 Sep 26;32(39):13454–69.

[64] Watson MB, Richter F, Lee SK, Gabby L, Wu J, Masliah E, et al. Regionally-specific microglial activation in young mice over-expressing human wildtype alpha-synuclein. Exp Neurol. 2012 Oct;237(2):318–34.

[65] Cebrián C, Loike JD, Sulzer D. Neuroinflammation in Parkinson's disease animal models: a cell stress response or a step in neurodegeneration? Curr Top Behav Neurosci. 2015;22:237–70.

[66] Fernagut P-O, Chesselet M-F. Alpha-synuclein and transgenic mouse models. Neurobiol Dis. 2004 Nov;17(2):123–30.

[67] Dauer W, Kholodilov N, Vila M, Trillat A-C, Goodchild R, Larsen KE, et al. Resistance of alpha-synuclein null mice to the parkinsonian neurotoxin MPTP. Proc Natl Acad Sci U S A. 2002 Oct 29;99(22):14524–9.

[68] Theodore S, Cao S, McLean PJ, Standaert DG. Targeted overexpression of human alpha-synuclein triggers microglial activation and an adaptive immune response in a mouse model of Parkinson disease. J Neuropathol Exp Neurol. 2008 Dec;67(12):1149–58.

[69] Van der Perren A, Macchi F, Toelen J, Carlon MS, Maris M, de Loor H, et al. FK506 reduces neuroinflammation and dopaminergic neurodegeneration in an α-synuclein-based rat model for Parkinson's disease. Neurobiol Aging. 2015 Mar;36(3):1559–68.

[70] Daher JPL, Volpicelli-Daley LA, Blackburn JP, Moehle MS, West AB. Abrogation of α-synuclein-mediated dopaminergic neurodegeneration in LRRK2-deficient rats. Proc Natl Acad Sci U S A. 2014 Jun 24;111(25):9289–94.

[71] Hinkle KM, Yue M, Behrouz B, Dächsel JC, Lincoln SJ, Bowles EE, et al. LRRK2 knockout mice have an intact dopaminergic system but display alterations in exploratory and motor co-ordination behaviors. Mol Neurodegener. 2012;7:25.

[72] Lee BD, Shin J-H, VanKampen J, Petrucelli L, West AB, Ko HS, et al. Inhibitors of leucine-rich repeat kinase-2 protect against models of Parkinson's disease. Nat Med. 2010 Sep;16(9):998–1000.

[73] Manthripragada AD, Schernhammer ES, Qiu J, Friis S, Wermuth L, Olsen JH, et al. Non-steroidal anti-inflammatory drug use and the risk of Parkinson's disease. Neuroepidemiology. 2011;36(3):155–61.

[74] Castaño A, Herrera AJ, Cano J, Machado A. The degenerative effect of a single intranigral injection of LPS on the dopaminergic system is prevented by dexamethasone, and not mimicked by rh-TNF-alpha, IL-1beta and IFN-gamma. J Neurochem. 2002 Apr;81(1):150–7.

[75] Szekely CA, Green RC, Breitner JCS, Østbye T, Beiser AS, Corrada MM, et al. No advantage of A beta 42-lowering NSAIDs for prevention of Alzheimer dementia in six pooled cohort studies. Neurology. 2008 Jun 10;70(24):2291–8.

[76] Gao X, Chen H, Schwarzschild MA, Ascherio A. Use of ibuprofen and risk of Parkinson disease. Neurology. 2011 Mar 8;76(10):863–9.

[77] Casper D, Yaparpalvi U, Rempel N, Werner P. Ibuprofen protects dopaminergic neurons against glutamate toxicity in vitro. Neurosci Lett. 2000 Aug 11;289(3):201–4.

[78] Tribl GG, Wöber C, Schönborn V, Brücke T, Deecke L, Panzer S. Amantadine in Parkinson's disease: lymphocyte subsets and IL-2 secreting T cell precursor frequencies. Exp Gerontol. 2001 Nov;36(10):1761–71.

[79] Gangemi S, Basile G, Merendino RA, Epifanio A, Di Pasquale G, Ferlazzo B, et al. Effect of levodopa on interleukin-15 and RANTES circulating levels in patients affected by Parkinson's disease. Mediators Inflamm. 2003 Aug;12(4):251–3.

[80] Yim G, Wang HH, Davies J. Antibiotics as signalling molecules. Philos Trans R Soc Lond B Biol Sci. 2007 Jul 29;362(1483):1195–200.

[81] Gordon RA, Mays R, Sambrano B, Mayo T, Lapolla W. Antibiotics used in nonbacterial dermatologic conditions. Dermatol Ther. 2012 Feb;25(1):38–54.

[82] Bi W, Zhu L, Wang C, Liang Y, Liu J, Shi Q, et al. Rifampicin inhibits microglial inflammation and improves neuron survival against inflammation. Brain Res. 2011 Jun 13;1395:12–20.

[83] Yulug B, Hanoglu L, Kilic E, Schabitz WR. RIFAMPICIN: an antibiotic with brain protective function. Brain Res Bull. 2014 Aug;107:37–42.

[84] Xu J, Wei C, Xu C, Bennett MC, Zhang G, Li F, et al. Rifampicin protects PC12 cells against MPP+-induced apoptosis and inhibits the expression of an alpha-Synuclein multimer. Brain Res. 2007 Mar 30;1139:220–5.

[85] Bi W, Zhu L, Jing X, Zeng Z, Liang Y, Xu A, et al. Rifampicin improves neuronal apoptosis in LPS-stimulated co-cultured BV2 cells through inhibition of the TLR-4 pathway. Mol Med Rep. 2014 Oct;10(4):1793–9.

[86] Ruzza P, Siligardi G, Hussain R, Marchiani A, Islami M, Bubacco L, et al. Ceftriaxone blocks the polymerization of α-synuclein and exerts neuroprotective effects in vitro. ACS Chem Neurosci. 2014 Jan 15;5(1):30–8.

[87] Chotibut T, Davis RW, Arnold JC, Frenchek Z, Gurwara S, Bondada V, et al. Ceftriaxone increases glutamate uptake and reduces striatal tyrosine hydroxylase loss in 6-OHDA Parkinson's model. Mol Neurobiol. 2014 Jun;49(3):1282–92.

[88] Ho Y-J, Ho S-C, Pawlak CR, Yeh K-Y. Effects of D-cycloserine on MPTP-induced behavioral and neurological changes: potential for treatment of Parkinson's disease dementia. Behav Brain Res. 2011 Jun 1;219(2):280–90.

[89] Tain LS, Mortiboys H, Tao RN, Ziviani E, Bandmann O, Whitworth AJ. Rapamycin activation of 4E-BP prevents parkinsonian dopaminergic neuron loss. Nat Neurosci. 2009 Sep;12(9):1129–35.

[90] Malagelada C, Jin ZH, Jackson-Lewis V, Przedborski S, Greene LA. Rapamycin protects against neuron death in in vitro and in vivo models of Parkinson's disease. J Neurosci Off J Soc Neurosci. 2010 Jan 20;30(3):1166–75.

[91] Du Y, Ma Z, Lin S, Dodel RC, Gao F, Bales KR, et al. Minocycline prevents nigrostriatal dopaminergic neurodegeneration in the MPTP model of Parkinson's disease. Proc Natl Acad Sci U S A. 2001 Dec 4;98(25):14669–74.

[92] Schildknecht S, Pape R, Müller N, Robotta M, Marquardt A, Bürkle A, et al. Neuroprotection by minocycline caused by direct and specific scavenging of peroxynitrite. J Biol Chem. 2011 Feb 18;286(7):4991–5002.

[93] Matsui T, Svensson CI, Hirata Y, Mizobata K, Hua X-Y, Yaksh TL. Release of prostaglandin E(2) and nitric oxide from spinal microglia is dependent on activation of p38 mitogen-activated protein kinase. Anesth Analg. 2010 Aug;111(2):554–60.

[94] Aron L, Klein R. Repairing the parkinsonian brain with neurotrophic factors. Trends Neurosci. 2011 Feb;34(2):88–100.

[95] Miyamoto K, Tsumuraya T, Ohtaki H, Dohi K, Satoh K, Xu Z, et al. PACAP38 suppresses cortical damage in mice with traumatic brain injury by enhancing antioxidant activity. J Mol Neurosci MN. 2014 Nov;54(3):370–9.

[96] Qin X, Sun Z-Q, Dai X-J, Mao S-S, Zhang J-L, Jia M-X, et al. Toll-like receptor 4 signaling is involved in PACAP-induced neuroprotection in BV2 microglial cells under OGD/reoxygenation. Neurol Res. 2012 May;34(4):379–89.

[97] Delgado M, Leceta J, Ganea D. Vasoactive intestinal peptide and pituitary adenylate cyclase-activating polypeptide inhibit the production of inflammatory mediators by activated microglia. J Leukoc Biol. 2003 Jan;73(1):155–64.

[98] Delgado M, Jonakait GM, Ganea D. Vasoactive intestinal peptide and pituitary adenylate cyclase-activating polypeptide inhibit chemokine production in activated microglia. Glia. 2002 Aug;39(2):148–61.

[99] Lamine A, Létourneau M, Doan ND, Maucotel J, Couvineau A, Vaudry H, et al. Characterizations of a synthetic pituitary adenylate cyclase-activating polypeptide analog displaying potent neuroprotective activity and reduced in vivo cardiovascular side effects in a Parkinson's disease model. Neuropharmacology. 2015 May 22;108:440–450.

[100] Delgado M, Ganea D. Vasoactive intestinal peptide prevents activated microglia-induced neurodegeneration under inflammatory conditions: potential therapeutic role in brain trauma. FASEB J Off Publ Fed Am Soc Exp Biol. 2003 Oct;17(13):1922–4.

[101] Kong AN, Owuor E, Yu R, Hebbar V, Chen C, Hu R, et al. Induction of xenobiotic enzymes by the MAP kinase pathway and the antioxidant or electrophile response element (ARE/EpRE). Drug Metab Rev. 2001 Nov;33(3-4):255–71.

[102] Jin X, Liu Q, Jia L, Li M, Wang X. Pinocembrin attenuates 6-OHDA-induced neuronal cell death through Nrf2/ARE pathway in SH-SY5Y cells. Cell Mol Neurobiol. 2015 Apr; 35(3):323–33.

[103] Lou H, Jing X, Wei X, Shi H, Ren D, Zhang X. Naringenin protects against 6-OHDA-induced neurotoxicity via activation of the Nrf2/ARE signaling pathway. Neuropharmacology. 2014 Apr;79:380–8.

[104] Chandran G, Muralidhara null. Insights on the neuromodulatory propensity of Selaginella (Sanjeevani) and its potential pharmacological applications. CNS Neurol Disord Drug Targets. 2014 Feb;13(1):82–95.

[105] Girish C, Muralidhara null. Propensity of *Selaginella delicatula* aqueous extract to offset rotenone-induced oxidative dysfunctions and neurotoxicity in *Drosophila melanogaster*: Implications for Parkinson's disease. Neurotoxicology. 2012 Jun;33(3):444–56.

[106] Meesarapee B, Thampithak A, Jaisin Y, Sanvarinda P, Suksamrarn A, Tuchinda P, et al. Curcumin I mediates neuroprotective effect through attenuation of quinoprotein formation, p-p38 MAPK expression, and caspase-3 activation in 6-hydroxydopamine treated SH-SY5Y cells. Phytother Res PTR. 2014 Apr;28(4):611–6.

[107] Lee E, Park HR, Ji ST, Lee Y, Lee J. Baicalein attenuates astroglial activation in the 1-methyl-4-phenyl-1,2,3,4-tetrahydropyridine-induced Parkinson's disease model by downregulating the activations of nuclear factor-kB, ERK, and JNK. J Neurosci Res. 2014 Jan;92(1):130–9.

[108] Siddique YH, Khan W, Singh BR, Naqvi AH. Synthesis of alginate-curcumin nanocomposite and its protective role in transgenic Drosophila model of Parkinson's disease. ISRN Pharmacol. 2013;2013:794582.

[109] Jantaratnotai N, Utaisincharoen P, Sanvarinda P, Thampithak A, Sanvarinda Y. Phytoestrogens mediated anti-inflammatory effect through suppression of IRF-1 and pSTAT1 expressions in lipopolysaccharide-activated microglia. Int Immunopharmacol. 2013 Oct;17(2):483–8.

[110] Anandhan A, Tamilselvam K, Radhiga T, Rao S, Essa MM, Manivasagam T. Theaflavin, a black tea polyphenol, protects nigral dopaminergic neurons against chronic MPTP/probenecid induced Parkinson's disease. Brain Res. 2012 Jan 18;1433:104–13.

[111] Lofrumento DD, Nicolardi G, Cianciulli A, De Nuccio F, La Pesa V, Carofiglio V, et al. Neuroprotective effects of resveratrol in an MPTP mouse model of Parkinson's-like disease: possible role of SOCS-1 in reducing pro-inflammatory responses. Innate Immun. 2014 Apr;20(3):249–60.

[112] Chang CY, Choi D-K, Lee DK, Hong YJ, Park EJ. Resveratrol confers protection against rotenone-induced neurotoxicity by modulating myeloperoxidase levels in glial cells. PloS One. 2013;8(4):e60654.

[113] Qian L, Block ML, Wei S-J, Lin C-F, Reece J, Pang H, et al. Interleukin-10 protects lipopolysaccharide-induced neurotoxicity in primary midbrain cultures by inhibiting the function of NADPH oxidase. J Pharmacol Exp Ther. 2006 Oct;319(1):44–52.

[114] Johnston LC, Su X, Maguire-Zeiss K, Horovitz K, Ankoudinova I, Guschin D, et al. Human interleukin-10 gene transfer is protective in a rat model of Parkinson's disease. Mol Ther J Am Soc Gene Ther. 2008 Aug;16(8):1392–9.

[115] Gonzalez-Aparicio R, Flores JA, Fernandez-Espejo E. Antiparkinsonian trophic action of glial cell line-derived neurotrophic factor and transforming growth factor β1 is enhanced after co-infusion in rats. Exp Neurol. 2010 Nov;226(1):136–47.

[116] Zhu Y, Yang G-Y, Ahlemeyer B, Pang L, Che X-M, Culmsee C, et al. Transforming growth factor-beta 1 increases bad phosphorylation and protects neurons against damage. J Neurosci Off J Soc Neurosci. 2002 May 15;22(10):3898–909.

[117] Qian L, Wei S-J, Zhang D, Hu X, Xu Z, Wilson B, et al. Potent anti-inflammatory and neuroprotective effects of TGF-beta1 are mediated through the inhibition of ERK and p47phox-Ser345 phosphorylation and translocation in microglia. J Immunol Baltim Md 1950. 2008 Jul 1;181(1):660–8.

[118] Nash KR, Moran P, Finneran DJ, Hudson C, Robinson J, Morgan D, et al. Fractalkine over expression suppresses α-synuclein-mediated neurodegeneration. Mol Ther J Am Soc Gene Ther. 2015 Jan;23(1):17–23.

[119] Reynolds AD, Stone DK, Hutter JAL, Benner EJ, Mosley RL, Gendelman HE. Regulatory T cells attenuate Th17 cell-mediated nigrostriatal dopaminergic neurodegeneration in a model of Parkinson's disease. J Immunol Baltim Md 1950. 2010 Mar 1;184(5):2261–71.

[120] Ji H, Wang H, Zhang F, Li X, Xiang L, Aiguo S. PPARγ agonist pioglitazone inhibits microglia inflammation by blocking p38 mitogen-activated protein kinase signaling pathways. Inflamm Res Off J Eur Histamine Res Soc Al. 2010 Nov;59(11):921–9.

[121] Hölscher C. Insulin, incretins and other growth factors as potential novel treatments for Alzheimer's and Parkinson's diseases. Biochem Soc Trans. 2014 Apr;42(2):593–9.

[122] Dehmer T, Heneka MT, Sastre M, Dichgans J, Schulz JB. Protection by pioglitazone in the MPTP model of Parkinson's disease correlates with I kappa B alpha induction and block of NF kappa B and iNOS activation. J Neurochem. 2004 Jan;88(2):494–501.

[123] Li Y, Perry T, Kindy MS, Harvey BK, Tweedie D, Holloway HW, et al. GLP-1 receptor stimulation preserves primary cortical and dopaminergic neurons in cellular and rodent models of stroke and Parkinsonism. Proc Natl Acad Sci U S A. 2009 Jan 27;106(4): 1285–90.

[124] Culmsee C, Junker V, Thal S, Kremers W, Maier S, Schneider HJ, et al. Enantio-selective effects of clenbuterol in cultured neurons and astrocytes, and in a mouse model of cerebral ischemia. Eur J Pharmacol. 2007 Dec 1;575(1-3):57–65.

[125] Culmsee C, Stumm RK, Schäfer MK, Weihe E, Krieglstein J. Clenbuterol induces growth factor mRNA, activates astrocytes, and protects rat brain tissue against ischemic damage. Eur J Pharmacol. 1999 Aug 20;379(1):33–45.

[126] Shenoy SK, Drake MT, Nelson CD, Houtz DA, Xiao K, Madabushi S, et al. beta-arrestin-dependent, G protein-independent ERK1/2 activation by the beta2 adrenergic receptor. J Biol Chem. 2006 Jan 13;281(2):1261–73.

[127] Sakurai H. Targeting of TAK1 in inflammatory disorders and cancer. Trends Pharmacol Sci. 2012 Oct;33(10):522–30.

[128] Qian L, Tan KS, Wei S-J, Wu H-M, Xu Z, Wilson B, et al. Microglia-mediated neurotoxicity is inhibited by morphine through an opioid receptor-independent reduction of NADPH oxidase activity. J Immunol Baltim Md 1950. 2007 Jul 15;179(2):1198–209.

[129] Qian L, Xu Z, Zhang W, Wilson B, Hong J-S, Flood PM. Sinomenine, a natural dextrorotatory morphinan analog, is anti-inflammatory and neuroprotective through inhibition of microglial NADPH oxidase. J Neuroinflammation. 2007;4:23.

[130] Zhang W, Qin L, Wang T, Wei S-J, Gao H, Liu J, et al. 3-hydroxymorphinan is neurotrophic to dopaminergic neurons and is also neuroprotective against LPS-induced neurotoxicity. FASEB J Off Publ Fed Am Soc Exp Biol. 2005 Mar;19(3):395–7.

[131] Zhang W, Shin E-J, Wang T, Lee PH, Pang H, Wie M-B, et al. 3-Hydroxymorphinan, a metabolite of dextromethorphan, protects nigrostriatal pathway against MPTP-elicited damage both in vivo and in vitro. FASEB J Off Publ Fed Am Soc Exp Biol. 2006 Dec; 20(14):2496–511.

[132] Anrather J, Racchumi G, Iadecola C. NF-kappaB regulates phagocytic NADPH oxidase by inducing the expression of gp91phox. J Biol Chem. 2006 Mar 3;281(9):5657–67.

[133] Ghosh A, Roy A, Liu X, Kordower JH, Mufson EJ, Hartley DM, et al. Selective inhibition of NF-kappaB activation prevents dopaminergic neuronal loss in a mouse model of Parkinson's disease. Proc Natl Acad Sci U S A. 2007 Nov 20;104(47):18754–9.

[134] Zhang F, Qian L, Flood PM, Shi J-S, Hong J-S, Gao H-M. Inhibition of IkappaB kinase-beta protects dopamine neurons against lipopolysaccharide-induced neurotoxicity. J Pharmacol Exp Ther. 2010 Jun;333(3):822–33.

[135] Jenner P. Oxidative stress in Parkinson's disease. Ann Neurol. 2003;53 Suppl 3:S26–36; discussion S36–8.

[136] Wang Q, Chu C-H, Oyarzabal E, Jiang L, Chen S-H, Wilson B, et al. Subpicomolar diphenyleneiodonium inhibits microglial NADPH oxidase with high specificity and

shows great potential as a therapeutic agent for neurodegenerative diseases. Glia. 2014 Dec;62(12):2034–43.

[137] Qian L, Gao X, Pei Z, Wu X, Block M, Wilson B, et al. NADPH oxidase inhibitor DPI is neuroprotective at femtomolar concentrations through inhibition of microglia overactivation. Parkinsonism Relat Disord. 2007;13 Suppl 3:S316–20.

[138] Przedborski S, Jackson-Lewis V. Mechanisms of MPTP toxicity. Mov Disord Off J Mov Disord Soc. 1998;13 Suppl 1:35–8.

[139] Shults CW, Oakes D, Kieburtz K, Beal MF, Haas R, Plumb S, et al. Effects of coenzyme Q10 in early Parkinson disease: evidence of slowing of the functional decline. Arch Neurol. 2002 Oct;59(10):1541–50.

[140] Parkinson Study Group QE3 Investigators, Beal MF, Oakes D, Shoulson I, Henchcliffe C, Galpern WR, et al. A randomized clinical trial of high-dosage coenzyme Q10 in early Parkinson disease: no evidence of benefit. JAMA Neurol. 2014 May;71(5):543–52.

[141] Holmay MJ, Terpstra M, Coles LD, Mishra U, Ahlskog M, Öz G, et al. N-Acetylcysteine boosts brain and blood glutathione in Gaucher and Parkinson diseases. Clin Neuropharmacol. 2013 Aug;36(4):103–6.

[142] Lapchak PA. A critical assessment of edaravone acute ischemic stroke efficacy trials: is edaravone an effective neuroprotective therapy? Expert Opin Pharmacother. 2010 Jul;11(10):1753–63.

[143] Cheng B, Guo Y, Li C, Ji B, Pan Y, Chen J, et al. Edaravone protected PC12 cells against MPP(+)-cytoxicity via inhibiting oxidative stress and up-regulating heme oxygenase-1 expression. J Neurol Sci. 2014 Aug 15;343(1-2):115–9.

Chapter 5

Chronic Inflammation Connects the Development of Parkinson's Disease and Cancer

Zhiming Li and Chi-Meng Tzeng

Additional information is available at the end of the chapter

http://dx.doi.org/10.5772/63215

Abstract

Increasing number of genetic studies suggest that the pathogenesis of Parkinson's disease (PD) and cancer may involve similar genes, pathways, and mechanisms. The differences in the pathological and cellular mechanisms, and the associated genetic mutations, may result in two such divergent diseases. However, the links between the molecular mechanisms that cause PD and cancer remain to be elucidated. This article appraises the overlapping molecular features of these diseases and discusses the implications for prevention and treatment. We propose that chronic inflammation (CI) in neurons and tumors contributes to a microenvironment that favors the amassing of DNA mutations and facilitating disease formation. CI may therefore play a key role in the development of PD and cancer, and provide a link between these two diseases.

Keywords: Parkinson's disease, cancer, chronic inflammation, neurodegenerative disease, genetic mutation

1. Introduction

Parkinson's disease (PD) is the second most common neurodegenerative disease, after Alzheimer's disease [1]. Typical symptoms include static tremors, muscle rigidity, and bradykinesia. These are caused by the premature death of dopaminergic neurons in the midbrain. The motor symptoms can be treated with dopaminergic drugs; however, the effectiveness diminishes as the severity of the clinical symptoms increases due to the development of the primary neuro-degeneration [2]. In contrast, cancer is a type of selectively advantageous cells with clonal proliferation. Although the two may appear distinctive, early epidemiological surveys have shown a connection between them. In 1954, Doshay [3] reported that the cancer incidence rate was lower among PD patients, but the reason for this was undistinguishable. Later, several epidemiological studies of cancer showed that the incidence of cancer was generally low among PD patients, regardless of whether they smoke or not [4]. However, the incidence of thyroid cancer, breast cancer, and melanoma was relatively high [5]. A recent study covering 219,194 people with PD displayed that the rate ratio (RR) for all subsequent primary malignant cancers combined was 0.92 [95% confidence interval (CI): 0.91–0.93], including increased RRs ($p < 0.05$) of breast cancer and melanoma cancer, and decreased RRs of 11 cancers [6]. This has been the most commanding epidemiological evidence for a connection between PD and cancer. Surely, there is a difference between association and causality, and it has been proposed that the association between PD and skin cancer could be linked to the way of therapy, such as Levodopa treatment, rather than with the disease itself. However, some observations did not support the causality [7, 8]. Moreover, some people thought that the low incidence of cancer in PD patients comes from the negative relationship between PD and smoking [4]. This may widely explain the decrease of smoking-related cancers, but the reduction of non-smoking-related cancers cannot be resolved.

The unusual epidemiological relation between PD and cancer has drawn the attention of many investigators. The genetic assessment encouraged an additional understanding: most of these familial PD genes had been found and summarized to be associated with cancer (**Table 1**). Mutations found in *parkin* (*PARK2*), *PINK1* (*PARK6*), *DJ-1* (*PARK7*), and *LRRK2* (*PARK8*) might cause distinctive significances and consequences of PD and cancer, respectively, in different types of cells [9]. PD and cancer have been discovered to share a PI3K/AKT/mTOR pathway, which is a central mechanism of cell growth and proliferation that mainly functions through modulating protein synthesis and responding both intrinsic and environmental stress promptly [10]. Currently, more than 12 loci were found to be related to familial PD [11]. Among these, six genes have been cloned. The monogenic forms of PD display both autosomal dominant and recessive modes of inheritance, and account for 1–3% of late-onset disease and approximately 20% of young-onset disease [1, 12]. PD-related genes are involved in a series of cellular mechanisms including misfolding and degradation of proteins, mitochondrial damage, oxidative stress response, cell cycle control, and DNA repair. These all play a vital role in both PD and cancer. Understanding of the functions of these genes in cell survival and cell death might help to reveal the connection between the two diseases.

Gene	PD locus	Chromosome location	Inheritance in PD*	Expression in cancer	Proliferation in Cancer†	Cancer
α-Synuclein	*PARK1/ PARK4*	4q21–q23	AD	Overexpressed (not express in normal tissue)	+	Brain tumors [74] Melanoma [75] Ovary cancer [76]
Parkin	*PARK2*	6q25.2–q27	AR	Decreased§	–	Glioblastoma [9] Colon cancer [9] Lung cancer [9]
UCHL1	*PARK5*	4p14	AD	Silenced	–	Nasopharyngeal carcinoma [77]

http://dx.doi.org/10.5772/63215

Gene	PD locus	Chromosome location	Inheritance in PD*	Expression in cancer	Proliferation in Cancer†	Cancer
				(via CpG methylation)		Colorectal cancer [78]
PINK1	*PARK6*	1p35–p36	AR	Decreased§	–	Breast cancer [79]
DJ-1	*PARK7*	1p36	AR	Overexpressed	+	Non-small-cell lung cancer [80]
LRRK2	*PARK8*	12p11.2–q13.1	AD	Overexpressed	+	Papillary renal cell carcinoma [64], Thyroid cancer [64]

*AD, autosomal dominant; AR, autosomal recessive
§The telomeric end of chromosome 1p is subject to frequent deletion and rearrangement in many cancers
† +/− denotes proliferation and antipoliferation.

Table 1. Parkinson's disease involved genes identified in cancer.

If genetic defect was "the match that lights the fire" of PD and cancer, chronic inflammation (CI) might supply "the fuel that feeds the flames." Over the past decades, the insight on cytokine and chemokine network has contributed to invention of a series of cytokine/chemokine antagonists used for inflammatory diseases. The first clinic practice, tumor necrosis factor antagonists, has shown encouraging efficacy [13]. CI is considered as a driving force behind many chronic diseases including cancerization and neurodegeneration. In PD, there are many activated microglia surrounding the lost neuron, and experiments have shown that inflammatory reaction does help killing neurons [14]. Epidemiological surveys have shown that taking non-steroidal anti-inflammatory drugs (NSAIDs) can reduce the risk of PD development. CI has long been known to mediate a wide variety of illnesses, including neurodegenerative disease and malignant tumors [15]. In 1863, Rudolf Virchow noticed leucocytes in neoplastic tissues and proposed a connection between inflammation and cancer. The role for inflammation in tumorigenesis is now mostly accepted, and it has become an evident that an inflammatory microenvironment is an essential piece for most tumors [16]. Inflammatory mediators in the microenvironment of CI not only benefit cancer cells proliferation and escape from immunological surveillance but also cause a large number of random mutations [17]. Amassing research evidence supports the view that inflammatory mediators, some of that are direct mutagens, directly or indirectly downregulate DNA repair pathways and cell cycle checkpoints, consequently destabilizing cell genome and contributing to the accumulation of random genetic alterations. Thus, inflammation is considered as the seventh most important sign of cancer [18].

The cellular pathways and its associated mechanisms (**Figure 1**) that involve genes common to PD and cancer have been discussed in our previous paper [19]. In this manuscript, we further explain the environmental factors that cause PD and cancer from the perspective of CI and related genes to provide a better understanding and treatment options of these two diseases.

To emphasize the multiple pathological functions of these gene mutations, they are discussed separately.

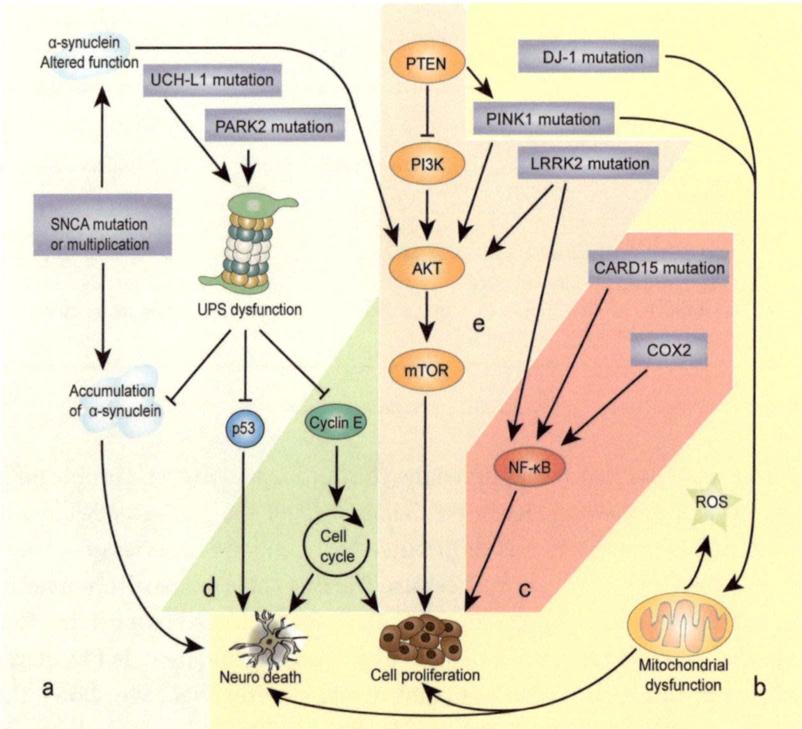

Figure 1. Overlapping genes and cellular pathways between PD and cancer.The biological connection of PD and cancer mainly includes five fields: (a) misfolding and degradation of proteins, (b) mitochondrial damage and oxidative stress response, (c) CI, (d) cell cycle control and DNA repair, and (e) PI3K/AKT/mTOR pathway regulation. The α-synuclein polymer attributed to *SNCA* multiplication is the main component of LBs. *SNCA* mutations alter the normal function of α-synuclein, which activates the PI3K/AKT/mTOR pathway and promotes cell proliferation. Under the cascade of phosphorylating AKT, PINK1, and LRRK2 can also activate mTOR. *PARK2* and *UCH-L1* mutations disrupt the degradation function of ubiquitin proteasome system (UPS) for the misfolded and aggregated α-synuclein, cyclin E, and p53. *PINK1* and *DJ-1* mutations result in the overproduction of ROS and oxidative stress in mitochondria, damaging neurons, and stimulating cell proliferation. *COX2* and *CARD15* mutations activate the NF-kB pathway and induce CI, leading to genetic mutations and oxidative stress. The different cellular backgrounds of cancer cells and neurons (mitotic vs. post-mitotic cells) bring completely distinct reactions to external stimuli and internal changes: some undergo cell proliferation and others neuron death. The final results are two serious diseases: cancer and Parkinson's disease.

2. Chronic inflammation

The blood–brain barrier (BBB) prevents the lymphatic infiltration and neurotoxins diffusion from the blood to the CNS. Conventionally, the CNS was regarded as the immunological restriction due to its limited inflammatory reaction and lymphatic infiltration. Nonetheless, accumulating evidence indicates that the CNS actually is the immunological specialization by the resident innate immune cell in the brain: microglia. Activated microglia could prevent the CNS injury from pathogenic factors (physiological disrupt and toxic insult) through releasing a number of cytokines and chemokines [20]. These inflammatory mediators could trigger or modulate the remove of neurotoxins and inhibit their detrimental effects. Thus, acute inflammatory responses are consider to be beneficial, but long-term, high-level CI can severely damage the body. Two of the pathological characteristics of PD are loss of dopaminergic neurons and accumulation of LBs in the nigrostriata of the midbrain. LBs are abnormal intracytoplasmic filamentous aggregates of α-synuclein present, respectively, in neurons and axons. Recent studies have shown that neurons able to release α-synuclein oligomers, which can bind to toll-like receptors (TLR) to activate microglia, activating the nuclear factor kappa B (NF-kB) pathway, and releasing of inflammatory factors. These immune factors not only act directly on dopaminergic neurons to cause neuronal death but also aggravate the inflammatory reaction and continue to activate microglia. Activated microglia surround dead neurons in the substantia nigra pars compacta (SNc) of PD patients. Studies have shown that inhibition of microglia cascade reactions can prevent degradation of neurons [21]. Increasing studies demonstrated that there was a positive correlation between SNc cell loss and microglia activation in both animal models and PD patients. Timing analysis displayed that reduce microglial activation can rescue SNc neurons loss in animal models, suggesting an active effect of microglia in killing SNc cell following a range of stimuli. It is increasingly clear that activation of microglia is a highly localized inflammatory reaction rather than generalized. Even though the degenerating neuronal terminals of SNc cell cannot stimulate the similar response but only the dopaminergic neurons in the SNc [22]. Therefore, cell death of PD directly relates to a substantial increase of microglia activation. At the same time, overproduction of free radicals (superoxide and peroxynitrite) damages the balance of the redox potential of neurons and acts on biomacromolecules to modulate their roles, or causes lipid peroxidation leading to cell death eventually. Alternatively, microglia might kill SNc cells by producing other noxious compounds including cytokines and proinflammatory prostaglandins. Patients with PD have selective degeneration of neurons in the SNc accompanied by microglial activation and a challenged immune system.

The presence of activated microglia in PD might reflect a scavenging role in the wake of a primary pathologic process. However, evidence for a more sinister role comes from animal models of PD. MPTP, 6-OHDA, lipopolysaccharide, rotenone, viruses, and SNc extracts all can lead to degeneration of the dopaminergic neurons and loss of striatal dopamine in primates, rodents, and other species [23]. Each of them can cause an inflammatory response that associated with the enhancement of microglia activation in the SNc. The best evidence for the significance of inflammation during neoplastic progression maybe come from study of cancer risk among long-term users of aspirin and NSAIDs. A big prospective study of hospital workers indicated that the incidence of PD in chronic users of over-the-counter NSAIDs which scavenge free oxygen radicals and inhibit cyclooxygenase (COX) activity was 46% lower than that of age-matched non-users [24]. Inhibition of COX-mediated dopaminergic neurons oxidation, as well as inhibition of microglial-derived toxic mediator production, is likely to be among the mechanisms that contribute to decreased incidence of PD in chronic NSAIDs users [25]. Therapeutically, these findings raise the possibility that early involvement with NSAIDs or similar anti-inflammatory therapy may be neuroprotective and could delay or prevent onset of PD. That anti-inflammatory medications downregulate microglial responses to a toxic insult and directly reduce neuronal loss strongly, which indicates that localized inflammation is pathogenic in the SNc rather than merely a late response to neuronal death.

3. NOD2

Crohn's disease (CD), also known as regional enteritis, is a type of inflammatory bowel disease. In 2001, three laboratories found CD associate with genetic variants. Nucleotide-binding oligomerization domain protein 2 (NOD2) also known as caspase recruitment domain protein 15 (CARD15) is a protein that in humans which is encoded by the *CARD15* gene located on human chromosome 16q12 [26–28]. Approximately 40% of CD patients in the Western countries carry at least one of these three SNPs: R702W, G908R, and L1007fsinsC, and heterozygous mutation of any of these SNPs increases CD risk 2–4 times, whereas multiple-locus heterozygous mutations or homozygous mutations may lead to a CD risk higher than 20 times. However, it has been reported that none of these three SNPs was involved in CD among Chinese (Han) [29], Korean [30], and Japanese patients [31]. NOD2, encoded by *CARD15*, is the receptor of muramyl peptides (MDP), a component of bacterial peptidoglycan. Binding of MDP and NOD2 activates NF-kB, and inflammatory reaction occurs. It has also been shown that *CARD15* mutation plays a role in innate immune system and pathogen recognition in terms of other complex polygenic diseases. In 2007, Bialecka [32] showed that the three SNPs of *CARD15* (R702W, G908R, and L1007fsinsC) were significantly correlated with PD in the Polish population. Using RFLP, our group found P268S, another SNP of *CARD15*, to be a risk factor for Chinese PD. In addition, Crane et al. [33] reported that P268S was related to susceptibility of ankylosing spondylitis. Proell et al. [34] performed sequence comparison and found that NOD2 shared a high degree of similarity with apoptotic protease activating factor 1 (Apaf-1). They simulated the homologous structure of NOD2 based on Apaf-1 structure and found that P268S was located at the connexon (ligand-binding position) before the first helix of the NOD. Replacing Pro with Ser changed the conformation of the connexon and affected its binding to the substrate.

Whether the CD's-associated *CARD15* mutations lead to a loss or gain of function of the NOD2 receptor is subject to controversy, and by which mechanisms, this change in function might increase the susceptibility to CD which is still under investigation. Patients with CD are known to have an increased risk of developing colorectal cancer [35]. *CARD15* mutations may also increase the susceptibility of developing colorectal cancer in Caucasians without CD [36, 37]. These observations suggested that immune system mechanisms were involved in the pathogenesis of cell damage in CD and also provided evidence for an ongoing active pathologic process. Inflammation can be triggered by invading microbes and also be initiated from within the organism, by diseases affecting the nervous system. There are three common outcomes of inflammation. The offending agent or process is inactivated and the injury repaired. The host loses the battle and dies or suffers irreparable tissue damage. Neither the organism nor the injurious process prevails, resulting in a prolonged battle that provides fertile ground for the development of chronic inflammatory conditions. The last outcome may relate closely to neurodegenerative diseases and cancer, two of the greatest public health problems of this century [38].

4. COX2

COX is the central enzyme in prostaglandin biosynthesis. There are two different isoforms of COX: COX-1 and COX-2. Constitutive expression of COX-1 is commonly found in many tissues. Because COX-1 is responsible for the biosynthesis of prostaglandins which regulate some physiological homeostasis, including modulation of renal blood flow and preservation of the gastric mucosa. Normally, COX-2 could not be discovered in most tissues except for stimulating by some mitogenic and inflammatory mediators [39]. COX2 is not only key to the synthesis of prostaglandin in inflammatory reactions but also an important contributor to the degradation of neurons in PD. Inhibiting COX2 activity in mice and rats can alleviate neuronal death caused by MPTP [40] and 6-ODHA [41], respectively. Macrophages, neurons, and glial cells in the central nervous system can all express COX2. Unlike COX1, which is constitutively expressed, COX2 expression is induced by inflammatory conditions. The COX2 level in the dopaminergic neurons of PD patients is elevated, and prostanoid and ROS produced by COX2 can directly act on dopaminergic neurons causing cell toxicity [42]. The role of COX2 in inflammation and neuronal degradation has yet to be verified. However, it has been shown that NSAIDs nonselectively inhibit the activities of COX1 and COX2, thus reducing prostaglandin production and promoting clearance of ROS. An epidemiological survey has revealed that individuals who take NSAIDs have a lower risk of PD than those who do not [25]. However, there has not been any report on the effects of specific COX2 inhibitors on the occurrence and development of PD.

COX-2, the inducible isoform of prostaglandin H synthase, has been implicated in the growth and progression of a variety of human cancers [43]. There are many evidence support that COX-2 is involved in the development of cancer. Because the overexpression of COX-2 is commonly found in the premalignant and malignant tissues. The most powerful findings from genetic studies support the view that it exists a cause-and-effect relationship between COX-2 and tumorigenesis. Multiple lines of evidence indicate that COX-2 is a *bona fide* pharmacological target for anticancer therapy. Epidemiologic studies have shown a 40–50% reduction in mortality from colorectal cancer in individuals who take NSAIDs on a regular basis compared with those not taking these agents [44]. COX-2, an inducible enzyme with expression regulated by NF-kB, mediates tumorigenesis. COX2 can activate not only the NF-kB pathway, but also p38 and Jnk in the MAPK pathway [45]. High levels of COX2 have been found in many cancers, particularly colon cancer [46]. COX-2 is also expressed in 93% of melanomas, with a moderate-to-strong expression in 68% [47]. COX2 can decrease the level of arachidonic acid and inhibit cell apoptosis. It can also increase prostaglandin production and promote cell growth and differentiation. These phenomena were also observed in the clinical effect of selective COX2 inhibitors in the market [48, 49].

5. LRRK2

Leucine-rich-repeat kinase 2 (*LRRK2*) is a large gene, 144 kb in length, containing 51 exons and encoding a multi-domain kinase composed of 2527 amino acids. LRRK2 is expressed in many organs and tissues, including the brain. In 2004, two laboratories reported that *LRRK2* mutations were related to PD [50, 51]. More than 40 *LRRK2* mutations, almost all missense, have been found [52]. However, the nosogeneses of many mutations remain unclear. *LRRK2* mutations account for 10% of familial PD and 3.6% of sporadic PD, suggesting strong modifiers of *LRRK2* disease [53]. LRRK2 is a large protein (280KDs). It can activate AKT, an upstream element of the mTOR pathway, thus decreasing the anti-apoptosis activity mediated by AKT and promoting neuronal death [54]. Gene structure studies showed that LRRK2 protein was consist of five conserved domains, including a leucine-rich repeat (LRR) domain, a Roc GTPase domain, a C terminal of Roc (COR) domain, a MAPKKK mixed-lineage protein kinase domain, and a WD40 domain [55, 56]. LRRK2 contains multiple sets of internal repeats, each of which is predicted to adopt a distinct structure. Such repeats, which occur in 14% of all prokaryotic and eukaryotic proteins, commonly serve as platforms for protein interactions [57]. *LRRK2* gene was discovered as part of an evolutionarily conserved family of proteins marked by GTPase (Guanosine triphosphatase) domains usually encoded together with kinase domains [55]. The G2019S mutation in the *LRRK2* is the single most common autosomal dominantly inherited PD gene defect. The LRRK2 protein is a scaffolding-type protein kinase, and G2019S is thought to lead to the disease by increasing the LRRK2 kinase activity resulting in increased phosphorylation of as yet mostly hypothetical targets, although whether all mutations in LRRK2 have the same biochemical mechanism is uncertain [58]. Missense mutations in both the kinase and GTPase domain in LRRK2 cause late-onset PD with clinical and pathological phenotypes nearly indistinguishable from idiopathic disease, possibly through the upregulation of LRRK2 kinase activity [59]. Because the clinical phenotype ensuing from LRRK2 mutations resembles idiopathic PD, LRRK2 has emerged as, perhaps, the most relevant player in PD pathogenesis identified to date [60]. One of the consistent pathological features of patients with LRRK2 mutations is α-synuclein-positive LBs pathology [61]. Besides G2019S, there are only a handful of proven pathogenic mutations in LRRK2, which is rather surprising given its large size. Multiple pathogenic mutations (I1371V, R14441C, R1441G, R1441H, Y1699C, Y1699G, G2019S, and I2020T) are located within the GTPase and the kinase domains or within the COR domain. This structural feature can be used as a target in the design of drugs that treat PD [62]. Many of the LRRK2 kinase inhibitors identified to date were discovered by using libraries of defined kinase inhibitors [63]. As with any kinase inhibitor development for human use, issues related to safety will need to be carefully evaluated. This is particularly important for a chronic disease such as PD.

More directly supporting a role of LRRK2 in cancer, chromosomal amplification of the LRRK2 locus is required for oncogenic signaling in papillary renal and thyroid carcinomas [64]. Genetic studies have implicated LRRK2 in the pathogenesis of several human diseases, including cancer and CD [65–67]. In 2011, Liu et al. [68] found that LRRK2 could suppress the activity of the transcription factor Nuclear factor of activated T-cells (NFAT). Overexpression of LRRK2 led to increased retention of NFAT in the cytosol. When *LRRK2* was knocked out, NFAT in the cytosol was translocated to the nucleus and transcriptionally activated the expression of genes encoding cytokines and other key proteins involved in triggering inflammatory responses. It was firstly proposed that LRRK2 might play an important role in the signal pathway that induced CD. Liu and co-workers highlighted the possibility that the M2397T (replacement of methionine 2397 with threonine) polymorphism may alter the steady-state abundance of LRRK2, which is distributed in many tissues and brain regions, generally at low abundance. In addition, the structure of LRRK2 is similar to that of carcinogen B-RAF. Therefore, it can act on the MAPK pathway. G2019S, a common *LRRK2* mutation in PD, can increase the risk of non-skin cancer in Jews by three times [69]. A complex role for LRRK2 in multiple cellular processes is perhaps not surprising, because LRRK2 has multiple domains and is both an active kinase and a GTPase [70]. Binding the different LRRK2 domains and different ligands may have different functions, preventing them from connecting closely with PD, inflammation, or cancer. To understand the roles of LRRK2 in human disease, the best place to start is with examination of the genetics linked to these diseases. Various coding changes in the open reading frame of LRRK2 are linked to disease. In PD, these mutations result in functional changes in LRRK2, although no clear pattern to these changes has emerged. LRRK2 is involved in many diseases result from the distinct influence of genetic mutations. These variants not only change the potential of LRRK2 to interact with upstream regulators or downstream effector, but also can alter the biological functions of LRRK2. The discovery of more LRRK2 functions and a deeper understanding of its pleiotropism should provide the research community with more insight into the pathological functions of the same protein in different diseases. Every protein may have more than one function and may play completely different roles in different diseases. Targeted therapies with minimal side effects may be developed based on the functions of these proteins in different signal pathways.

6. Perspective and conclusion

Increasingly epidemiologic findings demonstrated the correlation between cancer and PD in recent years, but the conclusions were not completely consistent. This is because of the differences of study management. Our understanding of the control of signaling pathways is further advanced in cancer studies compared to neurodegeneration. As a result, many small molecule inhibitors have been approved as anticancer agents or are currently being tested in clinical trials. In 2010, Datamonitor Inc. (USA) estimated that there were over 1.5 million PD patients in the USA, Japan, France, Germany, Italy, Spain, and UK combined, one-third of them in the USA. With the increasing aging of world population, the incidence of PD is increasing yearly [71]. Medication is usually the first option in the treatment of PD. Levodopa is currently the most effective medication, but long-term use can reduce the effectiveness of treatment and cause complications such as motor dysfunction. Thus, discoveries in cancer research are likely to provide a solid base upon which scientists will study the pathophysiology of neurodegenerative diseases, especially PD.

The origins of the association and interplay between cancer and PD are still a matter of debate, but increasing epigenetic modifications such as DNA acetylation, DNA methylation, and miRNA scan conspire with genetic alterations in disease pathogenesis [72]. Recently, Gehrke et al. [73] found that *LRRK2* mutation in Drosophila model could have an antagonist effect on two miRNAs: let-7, a known tumor suppressor, and miR-184, a mediator of neurological development. This led to E2F1/DP over-expression, causing the cells to reenter the cell cycle. These will help us develop an understanding of these two diseases from opposing angles. Although, cancer and PD seem to have little in common, one due to enhanced resistance to cell death and the other due to premature cell death. However, the more we learn about the molecular genetics and cell biology of cancer and PD, the greater the overlap between these disorders appears. Both cancer and PD are thought to be the result of the interaction of genetic and environmental factors. The difference is that different reactions occur based on different cellular backgrounds: cell division and cell death. The inflammation hypothesis is considered one explanation for PD and cancer. The immune factor and ROS released from chronic inflammatory reactions not only promote the occurrence of the disease but also cause cellular DNA to accumulate mutations more easily, forming proteins with aberrant functions. In the end, interactions between genes and the environment cause the diseases. Recently, our group found that P268S in *CARD15* may be a risk factor for PD, and Liu and co-workers provide evidence that *LRRK2* also has a role in a signaling pathway linked with the pathogenesis of Crohn's disease, an inflammatory bowel disease. These findings both implied a correlation between PD and inflammation.

Most degenerative diseases of the brain are incurable and the study of tissue from the brains of people with significant neurodegeneration is difficult, so the postmortem specimen is probably the most valuable research material. However, academic and clinic of cancer research have accumulated a wide range of achievement in the past long time, and these results and experience must be important and beneficial to neurodegeneration study. Understanding the nature of their relationship must help scientist find novel and more efficacious therapeutic approaches for both diseases.

Author details

Zhiming Li[1,2,3] and Chi-Meng Tzeng[1,2,3*]

*Address all correspondence to: cmtzeng@xmu.edu.cn

1 Translational Medicine Research Center, School of Pharmaceutical Sciences, Xiamen University, Xiamen, Fujian, China

2 Key Laboratory for Cancer T-Cell Theranostics and Clinical Translation (CTCTCT), Xiamen, Fujian, China

3 INNOVA Clinics and TRANSLA Health Group University, Xiamen, Fujian, China

References

[1] Farrer MJ. Genetics of Parkinson disease: paradigm shifts and future prospects. Nat Rev Genet. 2006;7:306–318. doi:10.1038/nrg1831

[2] Schapira AH. Molecular and clinical pathways to neuroprotection of dopaminergic drugs in Parkinson disease. Neurology. 2009;72:S44–50. doi:10.1212/WNL.0b013e3181990438

[3] Doshay LJ. Problem situations in the treatment of paralysis agitans. J Am Med Assoc. 1954;156:680–684. doi:10.1001/jama.1954.02950070008003

[4] Hernan MA, Takkouche B, Caamano-Isorna F, Gestal-Otero JJ. A meta-analysis of coffee drinking, cigarette smoking, and the risk of Parkinson's disease. Ann Neurol. 2002;52:276–284. doi:10.1002/ana.10277

[5] D'Amelio M, Ragonese P, Sconzo G, Aridon P, Savettieri G. Parkinson's disease and cancer: insights for pathogenesis from epidemiology. Ann N Y Acad Sci. 2009;1155:324–334. doi:10.1111/j.1749-6632.2008.03681.x

[6] Ong EL, Goldacre R, Goldacre M. Differential risks of cancer types in people with Parkinson's disease: a national record-linkage study. Eur J Cancer. 2014;50:2456–2462. doi:10.1016/j.ejca.2014.06.018

[7] Fiala KH, Whetteckey J, Manyam BV. Malignant melanoma and levodopa in Parkinson's disease: causality or coincidence? Parkinsonism Relat Disord. 2003;9:321–327. doi: 10.1016/S1353-8020(03)00040-3

[8] Zanetti R, Loria D, Rosso S. Melanoma, Parkinson's disease and levodopa: causal or spurious link? A review of the literature. Melanoma Res. 2006;16:201–206. doi: 10.1097/01.cmr.0000215043.61306.d7

[9] Veeriah S, Taylor BS, Meng S, Fang F, Yilmaz E, Vivanco I, et al. Somatic mutations of the Parkinson's disease-associated gene PARK2 in glioblastoma and other human malignancies. Nat Genet. 2010;42:77–82. doi:10.1038/ng.491

[10] Devine MJ, Plun-Favreau H, Wood NW. Parkinson's disease and cancer: two wars, one front. Nat Rev Cancer. 2011;11:812–823. doi:10.1038/nrc3150

[11] Hardy J. Genetic analysis of pathways to Parkinson disease. Neuron. 2010;68:201–206. doi:10.1016/j.neuron.2010.10.014

[12] Tan EK, Skipper LM. Pathogenic mutations in Parkinson disease. Hum Mutat. 2007;28:641–653. doi:10.1002/humu.20507

[13] Balkwill F, Mantovani A. Inflammation and cancer: back to Virchow? Lancet. 2001;357:539–545. doi:10.1016/S0140-6736(00)04046-0

[14] Tansey MG, Goldberg MS. Neuroinflammation in Parkinson's disease: its role in neuronal death and implications for therapeutic intervention. Neurobiol Dis. 2010;37:510–518. doi:10.1016/j.nbd.2009.11.004

[15] Aggarwal BB, Shishodia S, Sandur SK, Pandey MK, Sethi G. Inflammation and cancer: how hot is the link? Biochem Pharmacol. 2006;72:1605–1621. doi:10.1016/j.bcp.2006.06.029

[16] Mantovani A, Allavena P, Sica A, Balkwill F. Cancer-related inflammation. Nature. 2008;454:436–444. doi:10.1038/nature07205

[17] Grivennikov SI, Greten FR, Karin M. Immunity, inflammation, and cancer. Cell. 2010;140:883–899. doi:10.1016/j.cell.2010.01.025

[18] Colotta F, Allavena P, Sica A, Garlanda C, Mantovani A. Cancer-related inflammation, the seventh hallmark of cancer: links to genetic instability. Carcinogenesis. 2009;30:1073–1081. doi:10.1093/carcin/bgp127

[19] Li Z, Lin Q, Huang W, Tzeng CM. Target gene capture sequencing in Chinese population of sporadic Parkinson disease. Medicine (Baltimore). 2015;94:e836. doi: 10.1097/MD.0000000000000836

[20] Block ML, Zecca L, Hong JS. Microglia-mediated neurotoxicity: uncovering the molecular mechanisms. Nat Rev Neurosci. 2007;8:57–69. doi:10.1038/nrn2038

[21] Burguillos MA, Deierborg T, Kavanagh E, Persson A, Hajji N, Garcia-Quintanilla A, et al. Caspase signalling controls microglia activation and neurotoxicity. Nature. 2011;472:319–324. doi:10.1038/nature09788

[22] Mirza B, Hadberg H, Thomsen P, Moos T. The absence of reactive astrocytosis is indicative of a unique inflammatory process in Parkinson's disease. Neuroscience. 2000;95:425–432. doi: 10.1016/S0306-4522(99)00455-8

[23] Orr CF, Rowe DB, Halliday GM. An inflammatory review of Parkinson's disease. Prog Neurobiol. 2002;68:325–340. doi: 10.1016/S0301-0082(02)00127-2

[24] Chen H, Zhang SM, Hernan MA, Schwarzschild MA, Willett WC, Colditz GA, et al. Nonsteroidal anti-inflammatory drugs and the risk of Parkinson disease. Arch Neurol. 2003;60:1059–1064. doi:10.1001/archneur.60.8.1059

[25] Chen H, Jacobs E, Schwarzschild MA, McCullough ML, Calle EE, Thun MJ, et al. Nonsteroidal antiinflammatory drug use and the risk for Parkinson's disease. Ann Neurol. 2005;58:963–967. doi:10.1002/ana.20682

[26] Hugot JP, Chamaillard M, Zouali H, Lesage S, Cezard JP, Belaiche J, et al. Association of NOD2 leucine-rich repeat variants with susceptibility to Crohn's disease. Nature. 2001;411:599–603. doi:10.1038/35079107

[27] Ogura Y, Bonen DK, Inohara N, Nicolae DL, Chen FF, Ramos R, et al. A frameshift mutation in NOD2 associated with susceptibility to Crohn's disease. Nature. 2001;411:603–606. doi:10.1038/35079114

[28] Hampe J, Cuthbert A, Croucher PJ, Mirza MM, Mascheretti S, Fisher S, et al. Association between insertion mutation in NOD2 gene and Crohn's disease in German and British populations. Lancet. 2001;357:1925–1928. doi:10.1016/S0140-6736(00)05063-7

[29] Gao M, Cao Q, Luo LH, Wu ML, Hu WL, Si JM. NOD2/CARD15 gene polymorphisms and susceptibility to Crohn's disease in Chinese Han population. Zhonghua Nei Ke Za Zhi. 2005;44:210–212.

[30] Croucher PJ, Mascheretti S, Hampe J, Huse K, Frenzel H, Stoll M, et al. Haplotype structure and association to Crohn's disease of CARD15 mutations in two ethnically divergent populations. Eur J Hum Genet. 2003;11:6–16. doi:10.1038/sj.ejhg.5200897

[31] Yamazaki K, Takazoe M, Tanaka T, Kazumori T, Nakamura Y. Absence of mutation in the NOD2/CARD15 gene among 483 Japanese patients with Crohn's disease. J Hum Genet. 2002;47:469–472. doi:10.1007/s100380200067

[32] Bialecka M, Kurzawski M, Klodowska-Duda G, Opala G, Juzwiak S, Kurzawski G, et al. CARD15 variants in patients with sporadic Parkinson's disease. Neurosci Res. 2007;57:473–476. doi:10.1016/j.neures.2006.11.012

[33] Crane AM, Bradbury L, van Heel DA, McGovern DP, Brophy S, Rubin L, et al. Role of NOD2 variants in spondylarthritis. Arthritis Rheum. 2002;46:1629–1633. doi:10.1002/art.10329

[34] Proell M, Riedl SJ, Fritz JH, Rojas AM, Schwarzenbacher R. The Nod-like receptor (NLR) family: a tale of similarities and differences. Plos One. 2008;3:e2119. doi:10.1371/journal.pone.0002119

[35] Gasche C, Carethers JM. NOD2 and colorectal cancer: guilt by non-association. Cancer Res. 2004;64:5525; author reply 5525–5526. doi: 10.1158/0008-5472.CAN-03-3791

[36] Papaconstantinou I, Theodoropoulos G, Gazouli M, Panoussopoulos D, Mantzaris GJ, Felekouras E, et al. Association between mutations in the CARD15/NOD2 gene and colorectal cancer in a Greek population. Int J Cancer. 2005;114:433–435. doi:10.1002/ijc.20747

[37] Roberts RL, Gearry RB, Allington MD, Morrin HR, Robinson BA, Frizelle FA. Caspase recruitment domain-containing protein 15 mutations in patients with colorectal cancer. Cancer Res. 2006;66:2532–2535. doi:10.1158/0008-5472.CAN-05-4165

[38] Wyss-Coray T, Mucke L. Inflammation in neurodegenerative disease—a double-edged sword. Neuron. 2002;35:419–432. doi: 10.1016/S0896-6273(02)00794-8

[39] Smith WL, DeWitt DL, Garavito RM. Cyclooxygenases: structural, cellular, and molecular biology. Annu Rev Biochem. 2000;69:145–182. doi:10.1146/annurev.biochem.69.1.145

[40] Feng ZH, Wang TG, Li DD, Fung P, Wilson BC, Liu B, et al. Cyclooxygenase-2-deficient mice are resistant to 1-methyl-4-phenyl1, 2, 3, 6-tetrahydropyridine-induced damage of dopaminergic neurons in the substantia nigra. Neurosci Lett. 2002;329:354–358. doi: 10.1016/S0304-3940(02)00704-8

[41] Sanchez-Pernaute R, Ferree A, Cooper O, Yu M, Brownell AL, Isacson O. Selective COX-2 inhibition prevents progressive dopamine neuron degeneration in a rat model of Parkinson's disease. J Neuroinflammation. 2004;1:6. doi:10.1186/1742-2094-1-6

[42] Gao HM, Liu B, Zhang W, Hong JS. Novel anti-inflammatory therapy for Parkinson's disease. Trends Pharmacol Sci. 2003;24:395–401. doi: 10.1016/S0165-6147(03)00176-7

[43] Prescott SM, Fitzpatrick FA. Cyclooxygenase-2 and carcinogenesis. Biochim Biophys Acta. 2000;1470:M69–78. doi: 10.1034/j.1600-0463.2003.1111001.x

[44] Subbaramaiah K, Dannenberg AJ. Cyclooxygenase 2: a molecular target for cancer prevention and treatment. Trends Pharmacol Sci. 2003;24:96–102. doi:10.1016/S0165-6147(02)00043-3

[45] Hunot S, Vila M, Teismann P, Davis RJ, Hirsch EC, Przedborski S, et al. JNK-mediated induction of cyclooxygenase 2 is required for neurodegeneration in a mouse model of Parkinson's disease. Proc Natl Acad Sci USA. 2004;101:665–670. doi:10.1073/pnas.0307453101

[46] Liu W, Reinmuth N, Stoeltzing O, Parikh AA, Tellez C, Williams S, et al. Cyclooxygenase-2 is up-regulated by interleukin-1 beta in human colorectal cancer cells via multiple signaling pathways. Cancer Res. 2003;63:3632–3636.

[47] Denkert C, Kobel M, Berger S, Siegert A, Leclere A, Trefzer U, et al. Expression of cyclooxygenase 2 in human malignant melanoma. Cancer Res. 2001;61:303–308.

[48] Steinbach G, Lynch PM, Phillips RK, Wallace MH, Hawk E, Gordon GB, et al. The effect of celecoxib, a cyclooxygenase-2 inhibitor, in familial adenomatous polyposis. N Engl J Med. 2000;342:1946–1952. doi:10.1056/NEJM200006293422603

[49] Silverstein FE, Faich G, Goldstein JL, Simon LS, Pincus T, Whelton A, et al. Gastrointestinal toxicity with celecoxib vs nonsteroidal anti-inflammatory drugs for osteoarthritis and rheumatoid arthritis: the CLASS study: a randomized controlled trial. Celecoxib Long-term Arthritis Safety Study. JAMA. 2000;284:1247–1255. doi: 10.1001/jama.284.10.1247.

[50] Zimprich A, Biskup S, Leitner P, Lichtner P, Farrer M, Lincoln S, et al. Mutations in LRRK2 cause autosomal-dominant parkinsonism with pleomorphic pathology. Neuron. 2004;44:601–607. doi:10.1016/j.neuron.2004.11.005

[51] Paisan-Ruiz C, Jain S, Evans EW, Gilks WP, Simon J, van der Brug M, et al. Cloning of the gene containing mutations that cause PARK8-linked Parkinson's disease. Neuron. 2004;44:595–600. doi:10.1016/j.neuron.2004.10.023

[52] Lesage S, Brice A. Parkinson's disease: from monogenic forms to genetic susceptibility factors. Hum Mol Genet. 2009;18:R48–59. doi:10.1093/hmg/ddp012

[53] Berg D, Schweitzer KJ, Leitner P, Zimprich A, Lichtner P, Belcredi P, et al. Type and frequency of mutations in the LRRK2 gene in familial and sporadic Parkinson's disease. Brain. 2005;128:3000–3011. doi:10.1093/brain/awh666

[54] Ohta E, Kawakami F, Kubo M, Obata F. LRRK2 directly phosphorylates Akt1 as a possible physiological substrate: impairment of the kinase activity by Parkinson's disease-associated mutations. FEBS Lett. 2011;585:2165–2170. doi:10.1016/j.febslet.2011.05.044

[55] Bosgraaf L, Van Haastert PJ. Roc, a Ras/GTPase domain in complex proteins. Biochim Biophys Acta. 2003;1643:5–10. doi: 10.1016/j.bbamcr.2003.08.008

[56] Manning G, Whyte DB, Martinez R, Hunter T, Sudarsanam S. The protein kinase complement of the human genome. Science. 2002;298:1912–1934. doi:10.1126/science.1075762

[57] Andrade MA, Perez-Iratxeta C, Ponting CP. Protein repeats: structures, functions, and evolution. J Struct Biol. 2001;134:117–131. doi:10.1006/jsbi.2001.4392

[58] Cookson MR. The role of leucine-rich repeat kinase 2 (LRRK2) in Parkinson's disease. Nat Rev Neurosci. 2010;11:791–797. doi:10.1038/nrn2935

[59] West AB, Moore DJ, Biskup S, Bugayenko A, Smith WW, Ross CA, et al. Parkinson's disease-associated mutations in leucine-rich repeat kinase 2 augment kinase activity. Proc Natl Acad Sci USA. 2005;102:16842–16847. doi:10.1073/pnas.0507360102

[60] Aasly JO, Toft M, Fernandez-Mata I, Kachergus J, Hulihan M, White LR, et al. Clinical features of LRRK2-associated Parkinson's disease in central Norway. Ann Neurol. 2005;57:762–765. doi:10.1002/ana.20456

[61] Simon-Sanchez J, Schulte C, Bras JM, Sharma M, Gibbs JR, Berg D, et al. Genome-wide association study reveals genetic risk underlying Parkinson's disease. Nat Genet. 2009;41:1308–1312. doi:10.1038/ng.487

[62] Mata IF, Wedemeyer WJ, Farrer MJ, Taylor JP, Gallo KA. LRRK2 in Parkinson's disease: protein domains and functional insights. Trends Neurosci. 2006;29:286–293. doi:10.1016/j.tins.2006.03.006

[63] Lee BD, Dawson VL, Dawson TM. Leucine-rich repeat kinase 2 (LRRK2) as a potential therapeutic target in Parkinson's disease. Trends Pharmacol Sci. 2012;33:365–373. doi:10.1016/j.tips.2012.04.001

[64] Looyenga BD, Furge KA, Dykema KJ, Koeman J, Swiatek PJ, Giordano TJ, et al. Chromosomal amplification of leucine-rich repeat kinase-2 (LRRK2) is required for

oncogenic MET signaling in papillary renal and thyroid carcinomas. Proc Natl Acad Sci USA. 2011;108:1439–1444. doi:10.1073/pnas.1012500108

[65] Zhang J, Baran J, Cros A, Guberman JM, Haider S, Hsu J, et al. International Cancer Genome Consortium Data Portal—a one-stop shop for cancer genomics data. Database (Oxford). 2011;2011:bar026. doi:10.1093/database/bar026

[66] Franke A, McGovern DP, Barrett JC, Wang K, Radford-Smith GL, Ahmad T, et al. Genome-wide meta-analysis increases to 71 the number of confirmed Crohn's disease susceptibility loci. Nat Genet. 2010;42:1118–1125. doi:10.1038/ng.717

[67] Greenman C, Stephens P, Smith R, Dalgliesh GL, Hunter C, Bignell G, et al. Patterns of somatic mutation in human cancer genomes. Nature. 2007;446:153–158. doi:10.1038/nature05610

[68] Liu Z, Lee J, Krummey S, Lu W, Cai H, Lenardo MJ. The kinase LRRK2 is a regulator of the transcription factor NFAT that modulates the severity of inflammatory bowel disease. Nat Immunol. 2011;12:1063–1070. doi:10.1038/ni.2113

[69] Inzelberg R, Cohen OS, Aharon-Peretz J, Schlesinger I, Gershoni-Baruch R, Djaldetti R, et al. The LRRK2 G2019S mutation is associated with Parkinson disease and concomitant non-skin cancers. Neurology. 2012. doi:10.1212/WNL.0b013e318249f673

[70] Lewis PA, Manzoni C. LRRK2 and human disease: a complicated question or a question of complexes? Sci Signal. 2012;5:pe2. doi:10.1126/scisignal.2002680

[71] Huynh T. The Parkinson's disease market. Nat Rev Drug Discov. 2011;10:571–572. doi:10.1038/nrd3515

[72] Jones PA, Baylin SB. The epigenomics of cancer. Cell. 2007;128:683–692. doi:10.1016/j.cell.2007.01.029

[73] Gehrke S, Imai Y, Sokol N, Lu B. Pathogenic LRRK2 negatively regulates microRNA-mediated translational repression. Nature. 2010;466:637–641. doi:10.1038/nature09191

[74] Kawashima M, Suzuki SO, Doh-ura K, Iwaki T. Alpha-synuclein is expressed in a variety of brain tumors showing neuronal differentiation. Acta Neuropathol. 2000;99:154–160. doi: 10.1007/PL00007419

[75] Matsuo Y, Kamitani T. Parkinson's disease-related protein, alpha-synuclein, in malignant melanoma. Plos One. 2010;5:e10481. doi:10.1371/journal.pone.0010481

[76] Bruening W, Giasson BI, Klein-Szanto AJ, Lee VM, Trojanowski JQ, Godwin AK. Synucleins are expressed in the majority of breast and ovarian carcinomas and in preneoplastic lesions of the ovary. Cancer. 2000;88:2154–2163. doi:10.1002/(SICI)1097-0142(20000501)88:9<2154::AID-CNCR23>3.0.CO;2-9

[77] Li L, Tao Q, Jin H, van Hasselt A, Poon FF, Wang X, et al. The tumor suppressor UCHL1 forms a complex with p53/MDM2/ARF to promote p53 signaling and is frequently

silenced in nasopharyngeal carcinoma. Clin Cancer Res. 2010;16:2949–2958. doi: 10.1158/1078-0432.CCR-09-3178

[78] Okochi-Takada E, Nakazawa K, Wakabayashi M, Mori A, Ichimura S, Yasugi T, et al. Silencing of the UCHL1 gene in human colorectal and ovarian cancers. Int J Cancer. 2006;119:1338–1344. doi:10.1002/ijc.22025

[79] Berthier A, Navarro S, Jimenez-Sainz J, Rogla I, Ripoll F, Cervera J, et al. PINK1 displays tissue-specific subcellular location and regulates apoptosis and cell growth in breast cancer cells. Hum Pathol. 2011;42:75–87. doi:10.1016/j.humpath.2010.05.016

[80] MacKeigan JP, Clements CM, Lich JD, Pope RM, Hod Y, Ting JP. Proteomic profiling drug-induced apoptosis in non-small cell lung carcinoma: identification of RS/DJ-1 and RhoGDIalpha. Cancer Res. 2003;63:6928–6934.

Chapter 6

Is Chronic Systemic Inflammation a Determinant Factor in Developing Parkinson's Disease?

Perla Ugalde-Muñiz, Jesús Pérez-H and
Anahí Chavarría

Additional information is available at the end of the chapter

http://dx.doi.org/10.5772/62955

Abstract

The etiology of Parkinson's disease (PD) is complex and involves numerous risk factors as environmental and hereditary. Nevertheless, recent studies have established that systemic inflammation and neuroinflammation are both present in the prodromal phase and sustained during the progression of the disease. Evidence suggests that the activation of the peripheral immune system exacerbates the brain inflammatory response, which may initiate or enhance neurodegenerative processes. Understanding the impact of chronic systemic inflammation in the neuroinflammation and the progression of the disease will provide a broader view of the etiology and pathology of PD. In this chapter, we review the role of the chronic systemic inflammation in neuroinflammation and its effect on PD, considering cell types, molecular, and inflammatory mediators that predispose to the development of the disease.

Keywords: Parkinson's disease, chronic systemic inflammation, neuroinflammation, microglial activation, pro-inflammatory cytokines

1. Introduction

The contribution of systemic inflammation in the progression of several neurodegenerative diseases slightly has been studied. Inflammatory processes and activation of microglia are both important components in the pathogenesis of many neurodegenerative diseases such as Parkinson's disease (PD). Data support that microglial age-related cell changes induce cytotoxicity; this may contribute to the onset of neurodegenerative changes.

Indeed, low levels of chronic inflammation are associated with age-related diseases, including atherosclerosis, cardiovascular diseases, diabetes, and PD [1]. This phenomenon is caused by a persistent antigenic response and oxidative stress accompanied by reduced ability to counteract with a variety of stress factors, as well as a progressive increase in the pro-inflammatory state [2].

The etiology of PD is complex and involves numerous risk factors as environmental and hereditary. Nevertheless, recent studies have established that systemic inflammation and neuroinflammation are both present in the prodromal phase and sustained during the progression of the disease. Evidence suggests that the activation of the peripheral immune system exacerbates the brain inflammatory response, which may initiate or enhance neurodegenerative processes. Understanding the impact of chronic systemic inflammation in the neuroinflammation and the progression of the disease will provide a broader view of the etiology and pathology of PD. In this chapter, we discuss the role of the chronic systemic inflammation in neuroinflammation and its effect on PD, considering cell types, molecular, and inflammatory mediators that predispose to the development of the disease.

2. Neuroinflammation

A few decades ago the central nervous system (CNS) was considered an immunologically privileged site, a feature that has been attributed mainly to the presence of the blood-brain barrier (BBB), the low expression of major histocompatibility complex class II (MHCII), and the lack of brain lymphatic vessels [3].

Under systemic or endogenous pathological conditions, brain immune and glial cells start local inflammatory events, a situation named neuroinflammation, which is a mechanism of host defense that aims to restore the structure, recover normal functions, and insult neutralization [4].

Several hypotheses have been postulated on the possible causes of neurodegeneration in PD patients, which include genetic factors, environmental toxins, mitochondrial dysfunction, and cell death associated with free radicals [4, 5]. However, now research has focused on neuroinflammation as possible neurodegeneration activator in PD as epidemiological data indicate that is present even during the asymptomatic phase of the disease [6].

The main neuroinflammatory characteristics present in PD are the presence of activated microglia and reactive astrocytes; participation of the adaptive immune system; increased immune molecules such as cytokines, chemokines, among others; and increased oxygen and nitrogen reactive species concentration (ROS/RNS). These features can lead to the impairment of the BBB [7].

3. The blood-brain barrier

The BBB is a cellular barrier that regulates the environment of the CNS of vertebrates. It represents the border between CNS capillaries and extracellular fluid of neurons and glial cells, and ensures specific brain homeostasis, allowing proper function of neurons [8]. Although the BBB becomes more permeable during systemic inflammation [9], the total area of the microvasculature that composes the BBB in the adult human brain is 12–18 m^2 [10] and is the primary interface for the brain-blood exchange.

The primary function of the BBB is to provide a stable microenvironment for neural function. At first, it provides optimal concentrations of ions for neural communication, due to the functional combination of channels and transporters specific ions. For example, in mammals, the plasma concentration of potassium is 4.5 mM; however, in the cerebrospinal fluid (CSF) and the interstitial fluid, the levels range between 2.5 and 2.9 mM [11, 12]. Also, brain calcium and magnesium levels, and the pH are actively regulated by the BBB [13–15].

Moreover, although the peripheral nervous system and CNS use the same neurotransmitters, the BBB impedes the free flow and maintains the concentrations to avoid phenomena such as excitotoxicity [16, 17]. Similarly, the CSF protein content is lower than that of blood plasma. High levels of proteins such as albumin, prothrombin, and plasminogen can activate apoptotic cascades, therefore, be locally harmful to the nervous tissue [18–20].

The main elements that conform the BBB are endothelial cells, pericytes, astrocytes (specifically astrocytic foots), neurons, microglia cells, and the extracellular matrix. The close interactions between these components form the neurovascular unit [21] (**Figure 1**).

The endothelial cells of the BBB differ from the rest of the endothelial cells because they present tight junctions, low vesicular transport, and multiple transporters, restricting and selecting molecule flow [22]. Transmembrane tight junctions proteins (occludins, claudins 1–20 and JAMs) seal the intercellular space of endothelial cells and interact intracellularly with scaffold proteins (ZO-1, ZO-2, and ZO-3), and other cytoskeletal proteins. In adherens junctions, cadherins stabilize the adhesion between endothelial cells and catenin binds the cadherin to the cytoskeleton [23].

Through analysis of the microvasculature of the brain, it showed that astrocytic foot forms a thin film on the outer surface of the endothelium, suggesting that the astroglia is responsible for the development and specialization of brain endothelial phenotype [16]. An example that illustrates this point is the transforming growth factor-β (TGF-β) and angiopoietin-1 produced by astrocytes, which increases the expression of tight junction proteins and decreases the permeability of H3-Sucrose [8].

On the other hand, pericytes share the basement membrane with the endothelial cells of capillaries, venules, and arterioles, stabilizing the blood vessel wall. Also, pericytes present receptors for catecholamines, angiotensin II, vasoactive intestinal peptide, vasopressin, and endothelin-1 that prevent pericyte apoptosis rates in coculture of endothelial cells with astrocytes [22].

Multiple CNS pathologies such as hypoxia, ischemia [24], edema [25], and neurodegenerative diseases such as Alzheimer's, PD and multiple sclerosis [26–28] involve some degree of BBB dysfunction. An increased BBB permeability facilitates entry of macromolecules such as albumin into the CNS [29] and changes in blood vessels [30] in patients with PD. These changes of BBB permeability contribute to neuronal death in MPTP-intoxicated animal models of PD [31, 32].

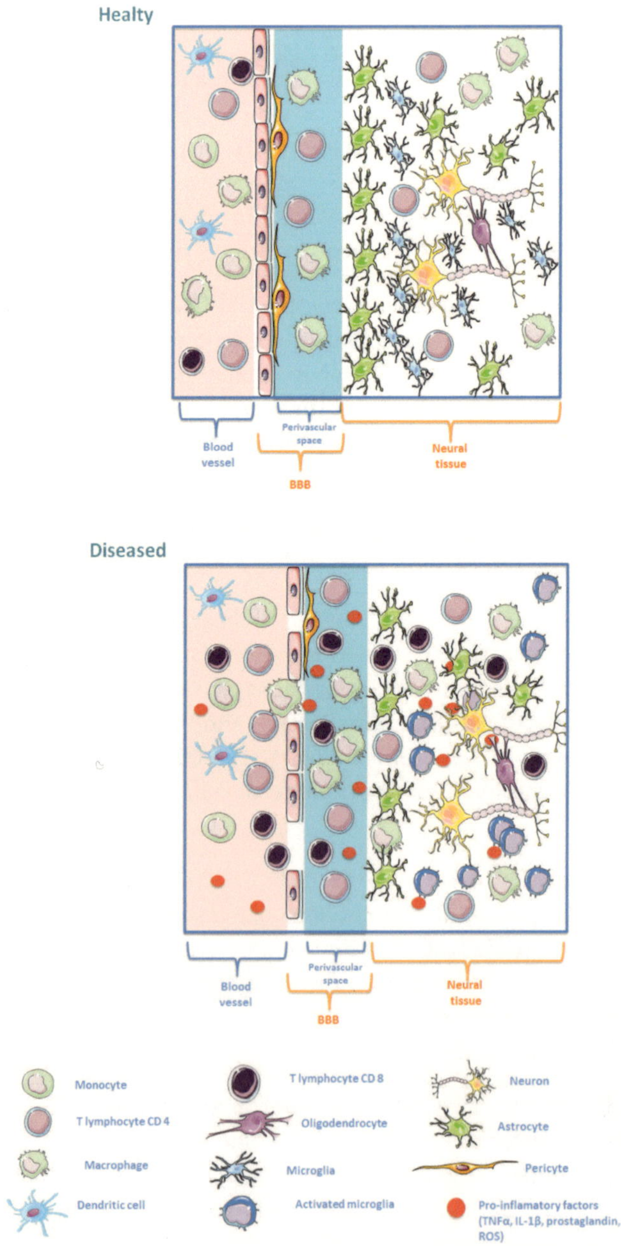

Figure 1. Under physiological conditions, astrocytes and neurons modulate the activation of the microglia. Peripheral immune cells maintain immune surveillance of brain parenchyma and perivascular space, and CD4+ T cell and macrophages could enter across of intact BBB into the CNS. But under systemic inflammation conditions, peripheral immune cells can penetrate the BBB and contribute to neuroinflammation.

One of the main evidence that involves BBB changes in patients with PD stems from a study of positron emission tomography (PET) that showed an increase of the [11C] verapamil capture in the midbrain of PD patients suggesting a decrease of P-glycoprotein [33]. Also, it has been proposed that in these individuals developing changes in the BBB permeability, increased traffic of iron and magnesium, both involved in the PD pathogenesis [34].

There is growing interest in the study of inflammation as a pathogenic mechanism of PD, which involves BBB properties alterations as shown in several experimental models [35]. These events facilitate the establishment of neuroinflammatory phenomena (**Figure 1**). Regardless of whether these developments are cause or consequence of neuronal death in PD, the attention of researchers focuses on identifying new therapeutic targets for alternative therapies in the treatment of this disease.

4. Brain-immune cells response in Parkinson's disease

4.1. Microglia: the major surveillance cell in the CNS

Microglial cells are vital in maintaining an immune homeostasis in the CNS; these cells are the first defenders against infectious agents and injury-related products in the CNS. Similar to tissue macrophages, microglia survey the brain for pathogens and support CNS homeostasis and plasticity, by guarding and remodeling synapses [36].

Under physiological conditions, astrocytes and neurons maintain the microglia in a quiescent or non-activated state [37, 38]. Non-activated microglia constitutively expresses low levels of HLA-DR in the healthy human brain [39] and MHCII in the rodent brain [40]. In this state, microglia mainly maintain brain homeostasis with astrocytes. Nevertheless, activated microglia display more molecular markers of an antigen presentation cell such as MHCII, CD80, CD86, CD40, CD11a, CD54, and CD58 [41, 42]. These properties show the capability for antigen presentation of this cell and thus its function of immune surveillance of the brain. Microglia have all the machinery necessary to detect any foreign molecule that accesses the CNS parenchyma and can rapidly mount a potent inflammatory response. After immune stimuli, such as a viral infection or brain injury, microglia cells quickly activate [43, 44] and acquire a compact phenotype. They upregulate several surface receptors such as receptors for neurotransmitters, cytokines, and chemokines, as well as pattern-recognition receptors [45–47]. Several TLRs are expressed on the microglial surface, including TLR2, TLR4, and TLR6 [48, 49].

Microglia also respond and propagate inflammatory signals initiated at the periphery, by activating and producing pro-inflammatory cytokines such as IL-1β, IL-6, and tumor necrosis factor alpha (TNFα) [50, 51](**Figure 2**). These cytokines are indispensable for the induction and maintenance of the CNS inflammatory state. They also promote the release of secondary inflammatory mediators including prostaglandins and nitric oxide (NO) [52–54]. Also, they facilitate the production of reactive oxygen species (ROS) through the induction or activation of NADPH and NO release [55, 56]. Though the activation of microglia and the production of cytokines are transient, once the immune insult is resolved, the microglia return to a surveying state.

Similar to peripheral macrophages, microglial exposure to IFNγ or TNFα, or stimulation by microbial agents such as LPS, or other TLR-agonistic compounds or pathogen-associated molecular patterns, would establish in microglia a "classical" macrophagic activation with an M1 phenotype. These cells are defense-oriented, release pro-inflammatory and cytotoxic factors. Cytokines, such as IL-4 or IL-13, instead facilitate an "alternative" activation of macrophages, also known as M2 phenotype [57]. Recent studies proved that brain microglia display a distinct profile that is not present in microglial cell lines and differ from M1 or M2 polarized microglia, but rather implicate genes associated with nervous system development [58].

During aging or in some pathologies such as Alzheimer's disease, microglia display a heterogeneity analogous to systemic tissue-resident populations [59, 60]. These studies showed that early in disease progression, microglia develop an altered inducible "activated" state, which functionally differs from steady state microglia. This activation state is further subdivided into classical M1 and alternative M2 state [61, 62].

More interestingly is that in neurodegenerative diseases, microglia can get overactivated resulting in reactive microgliosis, and this might induce neurotoxicity, perturbation of the neuronal network, maladaptive plasticity, and leading to tissue damage [63]. In PD, microglia can release pro-inflammatory cytokines, such as IFNγ, IL-1β, TNFα, IL-2, and IL-6 [64], increases the levels of TNFα receptor R1 (p55), bcl-2, soluble Fas, caspase-1 and caspase-3, which may contribute to the dopaminergic neurons degeneration [65, 66]. In turn, dopaminergic neuronal death may trigger microglial activation through the loss of the neural inhibitory CD200 signaling, exposure to α-synuclein, through binding of neuron-bound complement or antibodies, etc. [67, 68].

4.2. Astrocytes

Astrocytes are the most abundant glial cells of neuroectodermal origin that preserve brain homeostasis and neuronal functions, participate in maintaining and inducing the BBB, as well as in nervous tissue repair. Also, they significantly regulate the immune response and express a set of pattern-recognition receptors involved in innate immune response such as TLRs, mannose receptors, scavenger receptors, and some components of the complement system [69]. Astrocytes have a strategic location close to other glial cells and blood vessels and form a connection between the blood vessels and the brain parenchyma. Moreover, astroglia can be activated by pattern-recognition receptors ligands or exposure to IFNγ; increasing the expression of the glial fibrillary acidic protein (GFAP), MHCII, costimulatory molecules (CD80, CD86, CD40), and adhesion molecules [69]. They possess the ability to secrete cytokines such as IL 12 and chemokines (CCL2, CCL19, CCL20, and CXCL10) that promote changes in BBB permeability and favor thus an inflammatory-type response TH1 [69–72]. However, its role as antigen presenting cell is controversial, and it is thought that their participation is secondary [3].

Most findings indicate that microglial cells are the main mediators of neuroinflammation in the PD, but the presence of reactive astrocytes in the substantia nigra of PD patients is a constant pathological feature [73]. The increased GFAP expression observed suggests not only a morphological change but also a functional shift in this type of cell [74]. This phenomenon is consistent with the decreased production of trophic factors as derived neurotrophic factor glia and ciliary neurotrophic factor, both substances generated by astrocytes under normal physiological conditions [74, 75], and this reactivity is proportional to damage dopaminergic neurons [76].

Astrocytes can detect neurons with α-synuclein accumulation (the main component of Lewy bodies) and can be activated as a measure of neural protection. A recent study showed that neural α-synuclein is transferred and accumulated in astrocytes and induces activation of genes associated with the immune response. In these conditions, astrocytes express cytokines such as IL-1α, IL-1β, IL-6, IL-18, and colony stimulating factor 1, 2, and 3 [6], chemokines type CC, CXC, and type CX3C [69].

Also, intercellular adhesion molecule 1 (ICAM-1) positive astrocytes are present in the substantia nigra of PD patients; it is possible that they attract reactive microglia to the site of injury since microglial cells expressing the LFA-receptor 1 in the same place are found [77]. The action of α-synuclein on astrocytes is thought to occur via receptors, but the identity of these receptors is currently unknown [5].

5. Peripheral immune cells participation in Parkinson's disease

5.1. Macrophages and dendritic cells

The phagocytic cells such as macrophages are restricted to the perivascular space, leptomeninges, and choroid plexus. Macrophages constitutively express MHCII, CD11b, and CD45, which can help distinguish the microglia since it has a low expression of CD45 in the inactivated state [70]. In the healthy brain, the primary function is immune surveillance, antigen capture, and presentation locally and in the cervical lymph nodes. In the case of a lesion, macrophages participate as antigen presenting cells, in phagocytosis and secretion of pro-inflammatory cytokines (IFNγ, TNFα, IL-12) and chemokines (CCL2, CCL3) favoring chemotaxis and inflammation [78, 79]. Also, peripheral macrophages and brain microglia can secrete inflammasome components (caspase-1, IL-1β, and IL-18) that can induce neurotoxicity [78, 79]. In contrast, macrophages also have a regulatory role since they can produce anti-inflammatory and neurotrophic factors as nerve growth factor [80].

Dendritic cells (DCs) can be found primarily in the choroid plexus and meninges [81]. However, they have also been identified in regions lacking BBB such as the circumventricular organs, in sites of postnatal neurogenesis, in the perivascular space and even forming part of the glia limitans of the BBB [82, 83]. They are classified into two main groups (lymphoid and myeloid) and are assorted into several subpopulations due to cell expressing markers. The main attributed function in the CNS is immune surveillance, antigen capture, and delivery to the cervical lymph nodes, and antigen presentation [84]. However, they also have an important role in inflammation by producing cytokines such as IL-23, IL-1β, IL-12, TNFα, and IFNγ also IL-10 [81].

After recognizing molecules associated with inflammation, damaged tissue, or autoantigens, the DCs migrate to sites of inflammation and to lymph nodes to activate T cells and thus connect the innate immune response and the adaptive immune response. There is little evidence of the involvement of the DCs in the pathogenesis of PD, but they are recruited from the blood to the brain where they prime T cells and contribute to the neuroinflammation. A decrease in the number of peripheral DCs, mainly myeloid, associated with the increased severity of cognitive and motor symptoms of the disease [85]. Additionally, it has been reported that DCs treated with neuromelanin (the pigment present in dopaminergic neurons) acquire a mature phenotype, produce IL-6 and TNFα, and can stimulate T cell proliferation [86].

5.2. Lymphocytes

Leukocyte trafficking into the CNS is a highly regulated process, which protects the brain from a generalized inflammatory phenomenon that could significantly compromise the homeostasis required for neural functions [87, 88].

Interestingly, the cellular immune surveillance in the healthy human brain differs among CNS regions and the greatest numbers of immune cells are located in brain regions where the tight junction barrier of the BBB is reduced, such as the circumventricular organs and the ventrorostral areas of the medulla oblongata [89].

In healthy humans, predominantly activated central memory T cells that expressed high levels of CCR7, CXCR3, and L-selectin are found in the choroid plexus, the subarachnoid space, and the CSF [90]. Also, P-selectin facilitates migration of T cells into the CSF of mice and healthy humans. Furthermore, P-selectin, E-selectin, and ICAM-1 have been detected in vessels of the choroid plexus and subarachnoid space in humans [91].

Under physiological conditions, the immune surveillance in the perivascular space, with the participation of T cells that cross the vessel wall of postcapillary venules, however, progress towards the brain parenchyma dependent antigen presentation by perivascular macrophages or DCs [3, 83]. Questions have been raised whether the antigen specificity of T cells is a prerequisite for easy transit to the CNS. Still, several studies have transferred reactive T cells against neural antigens or irrelevant antigens to animals, and both types infiltrate the perivascular space similarly, though antigen specificity is required for final access to the brain [87, 92].

Given the evidence of the role of T cells in the maintenance of brain homeostasis, these could be implicated in the initiation and progression of PD. In this regard, PD patients and animal models of PD present infiltrating T CD4+ and CD8+ cells in the substantia nigra [93, 94] and decreased blood naive T lymphocytes [64, 95, 96]. Similarly, patients with PD have a cytotoxic response by T cell due to a change in the proportion of markers CD4:CD8 and the increase in the secreted IFNγ production versus IL-4 by lymphocytes [95, 97].

Other changes in peripheral blood lymphocytes of patients with PD have been reported, and lymphocytes from patients with PD have a higher incidence of micronuclei, DNA breaks, and oxidized purine bases [98]. Interestingly, levodopa treatment appears to reduce DNA damage in lymphocytes of these patients [99]. Furthermore, apoptotic markers, caspase-3, and the activity of Cu/Zn superoxide dismutase are increased in lymphocytes from patients with PD [100]. The increased levels of apoptosis and DNA damage could be indicative of a fundamental process pathogenic that involves oxidative stress, specific immune responses, and/or intrinsic factors such as genetic.

B cells are antibody-secreting cells of the immune system and the key mediators of the humoral response [101].

Patients with PD display antibodies against α-synuclein as well as against other epitopes from the CNS [102, 103]. Nevertheless, the presence of antibody producing B cells in the CNS of PD patients has not been reported [93, 94] despite the decrease in peripheral B lymphocytes [95, 96]. Deletion of the B cell counts in autoimmune diseases and other inflammatory diseases are secondary to reduced circulating memory B cells, which can be related to an inflammatory process or cellular activation [104, 105]. These events can occur in the substantia nigra in PD and that could explain the B cell decrease in the periphery of these patients.

6. Main cytokines and chemokines involved

Cytokines are proteins with pleiotropic actions that mediate many of the functions of immune cells and are mainly secreted by immune cells but also parenchyma brain cells. Multiple cytokines (IFNγ TNFα, IL-1β, IL-6, IL-18, IL-4, IL-10, IL-11, IL-13, TGF-β, IL-17, and IL-23) are found in the CNS, even under physiological conditions [106, 107].

It has been shown that PD patients present increased plasma cytokines such as IL-2, IL-4, IL-6, IL-10, TNFα, and IFNγ [108, 109]. Also, high levels of these cytokines and other inflammation markers are related to the risk of idiopathic PD [110]. Postmortem studies have found over-expression of pro-inflammatory cytokines (IL-1β TGF-α, IFNγ, and IL-6) in CSF and nigrostriatal regions of PD patients [111, 112]. Also, proteins of the complement system are found associated with extra-neuronal Lewy bodies [113]. As mentioned earlier, genetic factors are strongly related to the PD, polymorphisms of IL-8, IL-17, and IL-10 genes are associated with the risk of developing sporadic PD [114]. The findings suggest that activation of the immune response occurs in association with or in response to the Lewy bodies' formation [115].

Chemokines, which play important roles in neuroinflammation as mediators of leukocyte infiltration, are among the most important inflammatory factors [116]. They are proteins mediating the response and traffic of leukocytes and are classified into four subfamilies: C, CC, CXC, and CX 3. In the CNS, chemokines are mainly produced by glial cells and its primary function is chemotaxis or attraction of leukocytes to the damaged area promoting inflammation. The main CNS chemokines are monocyte (CCL2, CCL3, CCL4), lymphocyte (CCL5) chemoattractant, IFNγ-induced (CXCL10), among others [117, 118].

A prominent member of the chemokine family is CXCL12 or stromal-derived factor-1 alpha (SDF-1a) and its receptor CXCR4. Both CXCL12 and CXCR4 are constitutively expressed and modulate a variety of CNS functions, including neurogenesis [119], axonal growth [120], pain [121], and neurotransmission [122]. High expression of CXCL12 and CXCR4 is present in the rodent substantia nigra [123] and modulate dopamine transmission [124]. In the human substantia nigra, CXCR4 immunoreactivity was high in dopaminergic neurons [125].

Regarding PD, patients show elevated levels of CCL5 in the serum, and its concentrations are higher in patients with greater severity of symptoms [109]. Interestingly, the substantia nigra of patients with PD exhibited higher expression of CXCR4 and CXCL12 than control subjects despite the loss of dopaminergic neurons. This effect was accompanied by an increase in activated microglia [125].

We can finally say that levels of CCL2 expressed by peripheral blood mononuclear cells were higher in PD patients than in healthy control. CCL2 levels are also correlated with the Unified Parkinson's Disease Rating Scale (UPDRS)-III and Hoehn-Yahr stage [109]. Moreover, a recent study showed that elevated CCL2 CSF levels were associated with more severe symptoms of depression in PD patients [126].

7. Contribution of systemic and neuroinflammation in Parkinson's disease development

The contribution of systemic inflammation in the progression of several neurodegenerative diseases has been slightly studied. Inflammatory processes and activation of microglia are both important components in the pathogenesis of many neurodegenerative disorders such as PD; epidemiological evidence suggests an association between neuroinflammation and PD [35].

The PD, such as other neurodegenerative diseases, is associated with aging, which is related to increased formation of ROS predisposing the cell to damage and dysfunction. The evidence points to a relationship between oxidative stress and inflammation in the excessive production of free radicals that can induce an inflammatory response [1].

7.1. Cytokines contribution

Several studies have reported increases and decreases in the levels of pro-inflammatory cytokines and neurotrophins in the brain of PD patients [127], suggesting that neurons could be more susceptible to neuroinflammation and apoptosis, thus contributing to the pathogenesis of PD.

High levels of TNFα, IL-1β, IL-2, IL-4, IL-6, TGF-α, TGF-β1, and β2 have been detected in the brain parenchyma or CSF of PD patients [94, 128–130]. In accordance, the activated microglia can be a source of pro-inflammatory cytokines since in the substantia nigra of PD patients microglial overactivity was observed [46, 131–135]. An additional source of pro-inflammatory cytokines is the presence of CD8+ T lymphocytes in the vicinity of degenerating neurons

[94]. Cytotoxic T CD8+ is directly neurotoxic in autoimmune and aging-associated neurodegenerative disorders of the CNS [136]. This observation suggests that an infiltration of immune cells through the BBB may also contribute to the pathophysiology of PD. In this regard, peripheral blood mononuclear cells from PD patients express significantly higher levels of CCL2, CCL3, CCL5, IL-8, IFNγ, IL-1β, and TNFα after LPS stimulation than in healthy subjects [109].

It is possible that as well local as peripheral pro-inflammatory cytokines contribute to the loss of the BBB integrity facilitating the entrance of peripheral immune cells into the CNS. The role of peripheral immune cell traffic into the brain and its relevance in PD have not been extensively explored, but some studies show the implication of CD4+ T cells since mice lacking CD4+ cells are protected from MPTP-induced nigrostriatal neurons degeneration [93].

7.2. Microglia priming

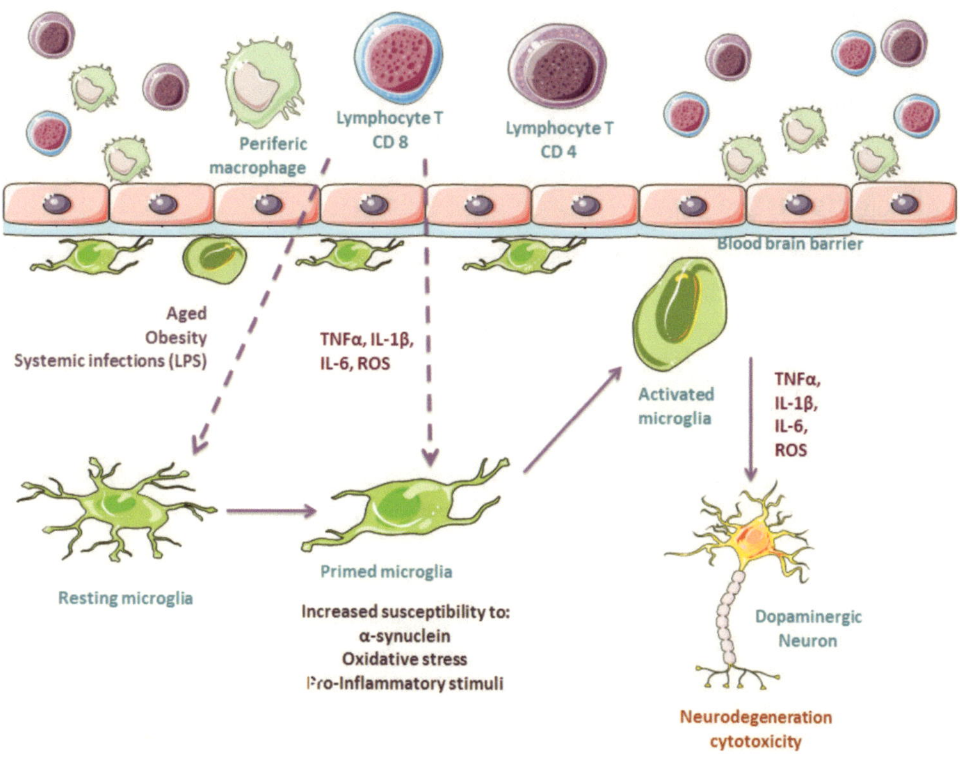

Figure 2. The relationship between peripheral inflammation and neuronal loss in PD. Neurodegenerative diseases present microglial activation as the chief hallmark, which can change its morphology from resting towards an activated or primed shape. The intermediate stage, "primed microglia," describes the atypical microglial stage, which precedes a further neurotoxic microglial activation as a consequence of a secondary pro-inflammatory stimulus. This intermediate stage could be a consequence of pro-inflammatory stimuli evoked by obesity, aged, or a systemic infection. Activated microglia releases pro-inflammatory cytokines which can act on dopaminergic neuronal integrity.

Primed microglia is the state when microglia respond to a secondary inflammatory stimulus with an exaggerated inflammatory response; this form of microglia contributes significantly to neuroinflammation and death of dopaminergic neurons (**Figure 2**). A recent study reported that a single paraquat exposure induced microglia activation with induction of the NADPH oxidase. If this activation was blocked with the anti-inflammatory drug minocycline, subsequent exposures to the paraquat failed to cause oxidative stress and neurodegeneration [137]. Also, systemic LPS administration resulted in rapid brain TNFα increase that remained elevated for 10 months activating microglia and secondarily increasing the expression of brain pro-inflammatory factors (i.e., TNFα, CCL2, IL-1β, and NF-κB). Further, tyrosine hydroxylase-immunoreactive neurons in the substantia nigra are reduced after LPS exposure and these data demonstrate that peripheral inflammation can activate brain microglia to produce chronically elevated pro-inflammatory factors, favoring a progressive loss of dopaminergic neurons of the substantia nigra [138].

Other works showed that priming of microglia with LPS predisposes susceptibility of dopaminergic neurons to neural toxins such as paraquat and 6-hydroxydopamine (6-OHDA), favoring the secretion of IL-1β, triggering the loss of these neurons, and suggesting a close relationship between neurodegeneration and inflammation [139, 140].

Therefore, microglial priming may in part regulate microglial phenotype and shift microglial activities from neuroprotective to neurotoxic (i.e., from trophic factor synthesis to production of ROS/RNS, among others), leading to hasten the death of vulnerable neuronal populations [141, 142].

Increased susceptibility to inflammation-induced nigral degeneration was shown in Parkin-deficient mice treated chronically with intraperitoneal low-dose of LPS, mice developed neuroinflammation and selective loss of dopaminergic neurons of substantia nigra [143].

Also, the systemic co-administration in mice of LPS and α-synuclein significantly increased IL-1β, IL-6, and TGF-β mRNA when compared with animals treated with α-synuclein alone. These observations suggest that any activator of the innate immune system, such as a peripheral pathogen, will alter the pathogenesis of PD by generating a transient pro-inflammatory environment that is likely to accelerate neurodegeneration [144].

7.3. What role plays aging?

Many age-related changes affect the CNS, contributing to both oxidative stress and inflammation deterioration of certain functions; thus, these processes singly and collectively affect neuronal viability and increase vulnerability. Data support that microglial age-related cell changes induce cytotoxicity, and this may provide to the onset of neurodegenerative changes. It has been observed that basal mRNA expression of markers of activated microglia such as CD11b and Iba-1 was higher in the aged hippocampus when compared to the adult [145]. Moreover, aging increased macrophage infiltration in the brain, with increased expression of IFNγ and the TLR4 agonists, high-mobility group protein B1 (HMGB1) [146].

Microglia seem to be activated at baseline in the elderly [94]. Furthermore, microglial cells obtained from aged mice developed lipofuscin granules, reduced the complexity of processes ramification, and increased mRNA levels of several pro-inflammatory cytokines (TNFα, IL-1β, and IL-6) as well as several anti-inflammatory cytokines (IL-10 and TGF-β) when compared with young mice. Also, when a pro-inflammatory stimulus is performed by a single dose of LPS, expression of TNFα IL-1β, IL-6, and IL-10 is increased but not of TGF-β [147]. These elevated cytokine levels may modify the microglial function and predispose microglial cells to become cytotoxic and cause neurodegenerative changes [148].

Upon aging, there are hormonal, immunological, and fatty changes that lead to a chronic inflammatory state [149]. These changes promote cognitive, cardiac, neuronal deterioration, and the occurrence of vascular events. However, if pro-inflammatory molecules outgrow anti-inflammatory responses, an imbalance occurs establishing a chronic inflammatory state [1, 150]. Therefore, this apparent imbalance in innate immune responses and pro-inflammatory molecules present in aging leads to a low-grade chronic inflammatory condition commonly present in elderly [150].

In this context, obesity results in a chronic inflammatory environment and may be associated with increased systemic oxidative stress. Levels of pro-inflammatory cytokines, such as IL-6 and TNFα, are significantly higher in obese subjects than in lean subjects [151, 152]. It becomes relevant since mortality was higher in obese animals than in control mice in the MPTP mice model, suggesting that obesity may increase the vulnerability of dopaminergic neurons to MPTP via increased levels of ROS and pro-inflammatory cytokines [153].

8. Conclusions

In recent decades, has deepened in the study of neuroinflammation as an important factor in etiology and development of PD, finding enough evidence to affirm that neuroinflammation is an adverse process for neuronal survival and function of individuals with this disease.

The immune system continues to undergo changes throughout life. The evidence shows that chronic inflammatory conditions caused by infectious, degenerative diseases or conditions such as aging and obesity, contribute to the establishment of neuroinflammation and the development of neurodegenerative phenomena, mainly in microglia rich brain regions, as the substantia nigra.

The full impact of systemic inflammation on brain immune changes remain poorly understood. The existence of a close association between systemic inflammation and neuroinflammation is evident in the progression of neurodegenerative disorders.

The cross-talk between immune cells and nervous system, especially microglia, is of particular importance in damage processes that precede PD. Based on current evidence, blocking microglia-derived inflammatory mediators or modulating the peripheral immune cells may be potentially useful therapies. However, it is important to explore in parallel the cellular, molecular and functional changes occurring during systemic inflammation, and thus, it may be possible to analyze the implications of this inflammation in recent Parkinson development.

Although research has been extensive, it is necessary to deepen this area of knowledge, especially in countries with a high number of individuals with obesity or metabolic syndrome, to assess and reduce the risks of increasing prevalence of PD and other neurodegenerative diseases.

Acknowledgements

Perla Ugalde-Muñiz and Jesús Pérez-H contributed equally to this paper. Funding for this research was provided by the Medical School and grants from Dirección General de Asuntos del Personal Académico (DGAPA; IN222215), National Autonomous University of Mexico (UNAM). Perla Ugalde-Muñiz is recipient of a fellowship sponsored by the Consejo Nacional de Ciencia y Tecnología (CONACyT) and Jesús Pérez-Hernández is recipient of a postdoctoral fellowship sponsored by CONACYT.

Author details

Perla Ugalde-Muñiz[1,2], Jesús Pérez-H[1,3] and Anahí Chavarría[1*]

*Address all correspondence to: anahi.chavarria@gmail.com

1 Unidad de Medicina Experimental, Facultad de Medicina, Universidad Nacional Autónoma de México, Mexico City, Mexico

2 Posgrado de Ciencias Biológicas, Universidad Nacional Autónoma de México, Mexico City, Mexico

3 Programa de Estancias Posdoctorales del Consejo Nacional de Ciencia y Tecnología, Mexico City, Mexico

References

[1] de la Fuente M, Miquel J. An update of the oxidation-inflammation theory of aging: the involvement of the immune system in oxi-inflamm-aging. Curr Pharm Des. 2009;15:3003–26. doi:10.2174/138161209789058110

[2] Franceschi C, Bonafè M, Valensin S, Olivieri F, De Luca M, Ottaviani E, De Benedictis G. Inflamm-aging. An evolutionary perspective on immunosenescence. Ann N Y Acad Sci. 2000;908:244–54. doi:10.1111/j.1749-6632.2000.tb06651.x

[3] Becher B, Bechmann I, Creter M. Antigen presentation in autoimmune and CNS inflammation: how T limphocytes recognize the brain. J Mol Med. 2006;84:532–43. doi:10.1007/s00109-006-0065-1

[4] More SV, Kumar H, Kim IS, Song SY, Choi DK. Cellular and molecular mediators of neuroinflammation in the pathogenesis of Parkinson's disease. Mediat Inflamm. 2013;2013:952375. doi:10.1155/2013/952375

[5] McGeer PL, McGeer EG. Glial reactions in Parkinson's disease. Mov Disord. 2008;23:474–83. doi:10.1089/rej.2010.1134

[6] Lee J, Tran T, Tansey MG. Neuroinflammation in Parkinson's disease. J Neuroimmune Pharmacol. 2009;4:419–29. doi:10.1007/s11481-009-9176-0

[7] Ransohoff RM, Perry VH. Microglial physiology: unique stimuli, specialized responses. Annu Rev Immunol. 2009;27:119–45. doi:10.1146/annurev.immunol.021908.132528

[8] Haseloff RF, Blasig IE, Bauer HC, Bauer H. In search of the astrocytic factor(s) modulating blood-brain barrier functions in brain capillary endothelial cells in vitro. Cell Mol Neurobiol. 2005;25:25–39. doi:10.1007/s 10571-004-1375-x

[9] Weiss N, Miller F, Cazaubon S, Couraud PO. The blood-brain barrier in brain homeostasis and neurological diseases. Biochim Biophys Acta. 2009;1788:842–57. doi:10.1016/j.bbamem.2008.10.022

[10] Nag S, Begley DJ. Blood-brain barrier, exchange of metabolites and gases. In: Kalimo H, editor. Pathology and Genetics. Cerebrovascular Diseases. Basel: Neuropath Press. 2005; pp. 22–29.

[11] Bradbury MW, Stubbs J, Hughes IE, Parker P. The distribution of potassium, sodium, chloride and urea between lumbar cerebrospinal fluid and blood serum in human subjects. Clin Sci. 1963;25:97–105.

[12] Hansen AJ. Effect of anoxia on ion distribution in the brain. Physiol Rev. 1985;65:101–148.

[13] Somjen GG. Ions in the brain: normal function, seizures. Neurology. 2006;66:618–618. doi:10.1212/01.wnl.0000176392.40778.f2

[14] Jeong SM, Hahm KD, Shin JW, Leem JG, Lee C, Han SM. Changes in magnesium concentration in the serum and cerebrospinal fluid of neuropathic rats. Acta Anaesthesiol Scand. 2006;50:211–216. doi:10.1111/j.1399-6576.2006.00925.x

[15] Nischwitz V, Berthele A, Michalke B. Speciation analysis of selected metals and determination of their total contents in paired serum and cerebrospinal fluid samples: an approach to investigate the permeability of the human blood-cerebrospinal fluid-barrier. Anal Chim Acta. 2008;627:258–69. doi:10.1016/j.aca.2008.08.018

[16] Abbott N, Rönnbäck L, Hansson E. Astrocyte-endothelial interactions at the blood-brain barrier. Nat Rev Neurosci. 2006;7:41–53. doi:10.1038/nrn1824

[17] Bernacki J, Dobrowolska A, Nierwińska K, Małecki A. Physiology and pharmacological role of the blood-brain barrier. Pharmacol Rep. 2008;60:600–622.

[18] Nadal A, Fuentes E, Pastor J, McNaughton PA. Plasma albumin is a potent trigger of calcium signals and DNA synthesis in astrocytes. Proc Natl Acad Sci USA 1995;92:1426–30. doi:10.1073/pnas.92.5.1426

[19] Gingrich MB, Junge CE, Lyuboslavsky P, Traynellis SF. Potentiation of NMDA receptor function by the serine protease thrombin. J Neurosci. 2000;20:4582–4595.

[20] Gingrich MB, Traynelis SF. Serine proteases and brain damage: is there a link? Trends Neurosci. 2000;23:399–407. doi:10.1016/S0166-2236(00)01617-9

[21] Alvarez JI, Katayama T, Prat A. Glial influence on the blood brain barrier. Glia 2013;61:1939–58. doi:10.1002/glia.22575

[22] Ballabh P, Braun A, Nedergaard M. The blood-brain barrier: an overview structure, regulation, and clinical implications. Neurobiol Dis. 2004;16:1–13. doi:10.1016/j.nbd.2003.12.016

[23] Gloor SM, Wachtela M, Bolligera MF, Ishiharab H, Landmannc R, Freib K. Molecular and cellular permeability control at the blood-brain barrier. Brain Res Brain Res Rev. 2001;36:258–264. doi:10.1016/S0165-0173(01)00102-3

[24] Kaur C, Ling EA. Blood brain barrier in hypoxic-ischemic conditions. Curr Neurovasc Res. 2008;5:71–81. doi:10.2174/156720208783565645

[25] Rosenberg GA, Yang Y. Vasogenic edema due to tight junction disruption by matrix metalloproteinases in cerebral ischemia. Neurosurg Focus. 2007;22:E4.

[26] Zlokovic BV. The blood-brain barrier in health and chronic neurodegenerative disorders. Neuron. 2008;57:178–201. doi:10.1016/j.neuron.2008.01.003

[27] Desai BS, Monahan AJ, Carvey PM, Hendey B. Blood-brain barrier pathology in Alzheimer's and Parkinson's disease: implications for drug therapy. Cell Trans. 2007;16:285–299. doi:10.3727/000000007783464731

[28] Correale J, Villa A. The blood-brain-barrier in multiple sclerosis: functional roles and therapeutic targeting. Autoimmunity. 2007;40:148–160. doi:10.1080/08916930601183522

[29] Pisani V, Stefani A, Pierantozzi M, Natoli S, Stanzione P, Franciotta D, Pisani A. Increased blood cerebrospinal fluid transfer of albumin in advanced Parkinson's disease. J Neuroinflamm. 2012;9:188. doi:10.1186/1742-2094-9-188

[30] Faucheux BA, Bonnet AM, Agid Y, Hirsch EC. Blood vessels change in the mesencephalon of patients with Parkinson's disease. Lancet. 1999;353:981–82. doi:10.1016/S0140-6736(99)00641-8

[31] Chao YX, He BP, Tay SSW. Mesenchymal stem cell transplantation attenuates blood brain barrier damage and neuroinflammation and protects dopaminergic neurons

against MPTP toxicity in the substantia nigra in a model of Parkinson's disease. J Neuroimmunol. 2009;30:39–50. doi:10.1016/j.jneuroim.2009.09.003

[32] Zhao C, Ling Z, Newman MB, Bhatia A, Carvey PM. TNF-α knockout and minocycline treatment attenuates blood brain barrier leakage in MPTP-treated mice. Neurobiol Dis. 2007;26:36–46. doi:10.1016/j.nbd.2006.11.012

[33] Kortekaas R, Leenders KL, van Oostrom JC, VaalburgW, Bart J, Willemsen AT, Hendrikse NH. Blood-brain barrier dysfunction in parkinsonian midbrain in vivo. Ann Neurol. 2006;57:176–9. doi:10.1002/ana.20369

[34] Yokel RA. Blood-brain barrier flux of aluminum, manganese, iron and other metals suspected to contribute to metal-induced neurodegeneration. J Alzheimers Dis. 2006;10:223–53.

[35] Whitton PS. Inflammation as a causative factor in the aetiology of Parkinson's disease. Br J Pharmacol. 2007;150:963–76. doi:10.1038/sj.bjp.0707167

[36] Parkhurst CN, Yang G, Ninan I, Savas JN, Yates JR, Lafaille JJ, Hempstead BL, Littman DR, Gan WB. Microglia promote learning-dependent synapse formation through brain-derived neurotrophic factor. Cell 2013;155:1596–609. doi:10.1016/j.cell.2013.11.030

[37] Neumann H. Control of glial immune function by neurons. Glia 2001;36:191–9. doi:10.1002/glia.1108

[38] Tian L, Ma L, Kaarela T, Li Z. Neuroimmune crosstalk in the central nervous system and its significance for neurological diseases. J Neuroinflamm. 2012;9:155. doi:10.1186/1742-2094-9-155.

[39] Hayes GM, Woodroofe MN, Cuzner ML. Microglia are the major cell type expressing MHC class II in human white matter. J Neurol Sci. 1987;80:25–37. doi:10.1016/0022-510X(87)90218-8

[40] Akiyama H, Itagaki S, McGeer P. Major histocompatibility complex antigen expression on rat microglia following epidural kainic acid lesions. J Neurosci Res. 1988;20:147–57.

[41] Akiyama H, McGeer P. Brain microglia constitutively express β-2 integrins. J Neuroimmunol. 1990;30:81–93. doi:10.1016/0165-5728(90)90055-R

[42] Shrikant P, Benveniste EN. The central nervous system as an immunocompetent organ: role of glial cells in antigen presentation. J Immunol. 1996;157:1819–22.

[43] Davalos D, Grutzendler J, Yang G, Kim J V, Zuo Y, Jung S, Littman DR, Dustin ML, Gan WB. ATP mediates rapid microglial response to local brain injury in vivo. Nat Neurosci. 2005;8:752–8. doi:10.1038/nn1472

[44] Nimmerjahn A, Kirchhoff F, Helmchen F. Resting microglial cells are highly dynamic surveillants of brain parenchyma in vivo. Science. 2005;308:1314–18. doi:10.1126/science.1110647

[45] Rock RB, Gekker G, Hu S, Sheng WS, Cheeran M, Lokensgard JR, Peterson PK. Role of microglia in central nervous system infections. Clin Microbiol Rev. 2004;17:942–64. doi:10.1128/CMR.17.4.942-964.2004

[46] Block M, Zecca L, Hong J. Microglia-mediated neurotoxicity: uncovering the molecular mechanisms. Nat Rev Neurosci. 2007;8:57–69. doi:10.1038/nrn2038

[47] Block M, Hong J. Chronic microglial activation and progressive dopaminergic neurotoxicity. Biochem Soc Trans. 2007;35:1127–32. doi:10.1042/BST0351127

[48] Stewart CR, Stuart LM, Wilkinson K, van Gils JM, Deng J, Halle A, Rayner KJ, Boyer L, Zhong R, Frazier WA, Lacy-Hulbert A, El Khoury J, Golenbock DT, Moore KJ. CD36 ligands promote sterile inflammation through assembly of a Toll-like receptor 4 and 6 heterodimer. Nat Immunol. 2010;11:155–61. doi:10.1038/ni.1836

[49] Fellner L, Irschick R, Schanda K, Reindl M, Klimaschewski L, Poewe W, Wenning GK, Stefanova N. Toll-like receptor 4 is required for [alpha]-synuclein dependent activation of microglia and astroglia. Glia 2013;61:349–60. doi:10.1002/glia.22437

[50] Lee SC, Liu W, Dickson DW, Brosnan CF, Berman JW. Cytokine production by human fetal microglia and astrocytes. Differential induction by lipopolysaccharide and IL-1 beta. J Immunol. 1993;150:2659–67.

[51] Hanisch UK, Kettenmann H. Microglia: active sensor and versatile effector cells in the normal and pathologic brain. Nat Neurosci. 2007;10:1387–94. doi:10.1038/nn1997

[52] Ericsson A, Arias C, Sawchenko PE. Evidence for an intramedullary prostaglandin-dependent mechanism in the activation of stress-related neuroendocrine circuitry by intravenous interleukin-1. J Neurosci. 1997;17:7166–79.

[53] Marty V, El Hachmane M, Amedee T. Dual modulation of synaptic transmission in the nucleus tractus solitarius by prostaglandin E2 synthesized downstream of IL-1beta. Eur J Neurosci. 2008;27:3132–50. doi:10.1111/j.1460-9568.2008.06296.x

[54] Konsman JP, Kelley K, Dantzer R. Temporal and spatial relationships between lipopolysaccharideinduced expression of Fos, interleukin-1beta and inducible nitric oxide synthase in rat brain. Neuroscience. 1999;89:535–48. doi:10.1016/S0306-4522(98)00368-6

[55] Shimohama S, Tanino H, Kawakami N, Okamura N, Kodama H, Yamaguchi T, Hayakawa T, Nunomura A, Chiba S, Perry G, Smith MA, Fujimoto S. Activation of NADPH oxidase in Alzheimer's disease brains. Biochem Biophys Res Commun. 2000;273:5–9. doi:10.1006/bbrc.2000.2897

[56] Heneka MT, Wiesinger H, Dumitrescu-Ozimek L, Riederer P, Feinstein DL, Klockgether T. Neuronal and glial coexpression of argininosuccinate synthetase and

inducible nitric oxide synthase in Alzheimer disease. J Neuropathol Exp Neurol. 2001;60:906–16. doi:10.1093/jnen/60.9.906

[57] Hanisch UK. Functional diversity of microglia: how heterogeneous are they to begin with? Front Cell Neurosci. 2013;7:65. doi:10.3389/fncel.2013.00065

[58] Butovsky O, Bukshpan S, Kunis G, Jung S, Schwartza M. Microglia can be induced by IFN-γ or IL-4 to express neural or dendritic-like markers. Mol Cell Neurosci. 2007;35:490–500. doi:10.1016/j.mcn.2007.04.009

[59] Varnum MM, Ikezu T. The classification of microglial activation phenotypes on neurodegeneration and regeneration in Alzheimer's disease brain. Arch Immunol Ther Exp. 2012;60:251–66. doi:10.1007/s00005-012-0181-2

[60] Amor S, Peferoen L, Vogel D, Breur M, van der Valk P, Baker D, van Noort J. Inflammation in neurodegenerative diseases: an update. Immunology 2014;142:151–66. doi:10.1111/imm.12233

[61] Perry VH, Teeling J. Microglia and macrophages of the central nervous system: the contribution of microglia priming and systemic inflammation to chronic neurodegeneration. Semin Immunopathol. 2013;35:601–12. doi:10.1007/s00281-013-0382-8

[62] Eggen BJL, Raj D, Hanisch U-K, Boddeke HWGM. Microglial phenotype and adaptation. J Neuroimmune Pharmacol. 2013;8:807–23. doi:10.1007/s11481-013-9490-4

[63] Papa M, De Luca C, Petta F, Alberghina L, Cirillo G. Astrocyte-neuron interplay in maladaptive plasticity. Neurosci Biobehav Rev. 2014;42:35–54. doi:10.1016/j.neubiorev.2014.01.010

[64] Fiszer U, Mix E, Fredrikson S, Kostulas V, Link H. Parkinson's disease and immunological abnormalities: increase of HLA-DR expression on monocytes in cerebrospinal fluid and of CD45RO+ T cells in peripheral blood. Acta Neurol Scand. 1994;90:160–6. doi:10.1111/j.1600-0404.1994.tb02699.x

[65] Botta-Orfila T, Sanchez-Pla A, Fernandez M, Carmona F, Ezquerra M, Tolosa E. Brain transcriptomic profiling in idiopathic and LRRK2-associated Parkinson's disease. Brain Res. 2012;1466:152–7. doi:10.1016/j.brainres.2012.05.036

[66] Bialecka M, Kurzawski M, Klodowska-Duda G, Opala G, Juzwiak S, Kurzawski G, Tan EK, Drozdzik M. CARD15 variants in patients with sporadic Parkinson's disease. Neurosci Res. 2007;57:473–6. doi:10.1016/j.neures.2006.11.012

[67] Aloisi F. Immune function of microglia. Glia 2001;36:165–79. doi:10.1002/glia.1106

[68] Kim SU, de Vellis J. Microglia in health and disease. J Neurosci Res. 2005;81:302–313. doi:10.1002/jnr.20562

[69] Farina C, Aloisi F, Meinl E. Astrocytes are active players in cerebral innate immunity. Trends Immunol. 2007;28:138–45. doi:10.1016/j.it.2007.01.005

[70] Hauwel M, Furon E, Canova C, Griffiths M, Neal J, Gasque P. Innate (inherent) control of brain infection, brain inflammation and brain repair: the rol of microglía, astrocytes, "protective" glial stem cells and stromal ependymal cells. Brain Res Brain Res Rev. 2005;48:220–33. doi:10.1016/j.brainresrev.2004.12.012

[71] Nikcevich KM, Gordon KB, Tan L, Hurst SD, Kroepfl JF, Gardinier M, Barrett TA, Miller SD. IFN-gamma-activated primary murine astrocytes express B7 costimulatory molecules and prime naive antigen-specific T cells. J Immunol. 1997;158:614–21.

[72] Park C, Lee S, Cho IH, Lee HK, Kim D, Choi SY, Oh SB, Park K, Kim JS, Lee SJ. TLR3-mediated signal induces proinflammatory cytokine and chemokine gene expression in astrocytes: differential signaling mechanisms of TLR3-induced IP-10 and IL-8 gene expression. Glia 2006;53:248–56. doi:10.1002/glia.20278

[73] Hirsch EC, Hunot S. Neuroinflammation in Parkinson's disease: a target for neuroprotection? Lancet Neurol. 2009;8:382–97. doi:10.1016/S1474-4422(09)70062-6

[74] Wu DC, Tieu K, Cohen O, Choi DK, Vila M, Jackson-Lewis V, Teismann P, Przedborski S. Glial cell response: a pathogenic factor in Parkinson's disease. J Neurovirol. 2002;8:551–8. doi:10.1080/13550280290100905

[75] Sellers RS, Antman M, Phillips J, Khan KN, Furst SM. Effects of Miglyol 812 on rats after 4 weeks of gavage as compared with methylcellulose/Tween 80. Drug Chem Toxicol. 2005;28:423–32. doi:10.1080/01480540500262839

[76] Damier P, Hirsch EC, Zhang P, Agid Y, Javoy-Agid F. Glutathione peroxidase, glial cells and Parkinson's disease. Neuroscience 1993;52:1–6.

[77] Miklossy J, Doudet DD, Schwab C, Yu S, McGeer EG, McGeer PL. Role of ICAM-1 in persisting inflammation in Parkinson disease and MPTP monkeys. Exp Neurol. 2006;197:275–83. doi:10.1016/j.expneurol.2005.10.034

[78] Sarkar A, Mitra S, Mehta S, Raices R, Wewers MD. Monocyte derived microvesicles deliver a cell death message via encapsulated caspase-1. PLoS One. 2009;4:e7140. doi: 10.1371/journal.pone.0007140

[79] Gulinelli S, Salaro E, Vuerich M, Bozzato D, Pizzirani C, Bolognesi G, Idzko M, Di Virgilio F, Ferrari D. IL-18 associates to microvesicles shed from human macrophages by a LPS/TLR-4 independent mechanism in response to P2X receptor stimulation. Eur J Immunol. 2012;42:3334–45. doi:10.1002/eji.201142268

[80] Yamate J, Ishimine S, Izawa T, Kumagai D, Kuwamura M. Macrophage populations and expressions of regulatory proinflammatory factors in the rat meninx under lipopolysaccharide treatment in vivo and in vitro. Histol Histopathol. 2009;24:13–24.

[81] McMahon EJ, Bailey SL, Miller SD. CNS dendritic cells: critical participants in CNS inflammation? Neurochem Int. 2007;49:195–203. doi:10.1016/j.neuint.2006.04.004

[82] Bulloch K, Miller MM, Gal-Toth J, Milner TA, Gottfried-Blackmore A, Waters EM, Kaunzner UW, Liu K, Lindquist R, Nussenzweig MC, Steinman RM, McEwen BS.

CD11c/EYFP transgene illuminates a discrete network of dendritic cells within the embryonic, neonatal, adult, and injured mouse brain. J Comp Neurol. 2008;508:687–710. doi:10.1002/cne.21668

[83] Prodinger C, Bunse J, Krüger M, Schiefenhövel F, Brandt C, Laman JD, Greter M, Immig K, Heppner F, Becher B, Bechmann I. CD11c-expressing cells reside in the juxtavascular parenchyma and extend processes into the glia limitans of the mouse nervous system. Acta Neuropathol. 2011;121:445–58. doi:10.1007/s00401-010-0774-y

[84] Colton CA. Immune heterogeneity in neuroinflammation: dendritic cells in the brain. J Neuroimmune Pharmacol. 2013;8(1):145–62. doi:10.1007/s11481-012-9414-8

[85] Ciaramella A, Salani F, Bizzoni F, Pontieri FE, Stefani A, Pierantozzi M, Assogna F, Caltagirone C, Spalletta G, Bossù P. Blood dendritic cell frequency declines in idiopathic Parkinson's disease and is associated with motor symptom severity. PLoS One. 2013;11:e65352. doi:10.1371/journal.pone.0065352

[86] Oberländer U, Pletinckx K, Dohler A, Muller N, Lutz MB, Arzberger T, Riederer P, Gerlach M, Koutsilieri E, Scheller C. Neuromelanin is an immune stimulator for dendritic cells in vitro. BMC Neurosci. 2011;12:116. doi:10.1186/1471-2202-12-116

[87] Galea I, Palin K, Newman TA, Van Rooijen N, Perry VH, Boche D. Mannose receptor expression specifically reveals perivascular macrophages in normal, injured, and diseased mouse brain. Glia 2005;49:375–84. doi:10.1002/glia.20124

[88] Ousman SS, Kubes P. Immune surveillance in the central nervous system. Nat Neurosci. 2012;15:1096–101. doi:10.1038/nn.3161

[89] Loeffler C, Dietz K, Schleich A, Schlaszus H, Stoll M, Meyermann R, Mittelbronn M. Immune surveillance of the normal human CNS takes place in dependence of the locoregional blood-brain barrier configur and is mainly performed by CD^{3+}/CD^{8+} lymphocytes. Neuropathology 201;31:230–8. doi:10.1111/j.1440-1789.2010.01167.x

[90] Carrithers MD, Visintin I, Viret C, Janeway CS. Role of genetic background in P selectin-dependent immune surveillance of the central nervous system. J Neuroimmunol. 2002;129:51–57. doi:10.1016/S0165-5728(02)00172-8

[91] Kivisäkk P, Mahad DJ, Callahan MK, Trebst C, Tucky B, Wei T, Wu L, Baekkevold ES, Lassmann H, Staugaitis SM, Campbell JJ, Ransohoff RM. Human cerebrospinal fluid central memory CD4+ T cells: evidence for trafficking through choroid plexus and meninges via P-selectin. Proc Natl Acad Sci USA 2003;100:8389–94. doi:10.1073/pnas.1433000100

[92] Archambault AS, Sim J, Gimenez MA, Russell JH. Defining antigen-dependent stages of T cell migration from the blood to the central nervous system parenchyma. Eur J Immunol. 2005;35:1076–85. doi:10.1002/eji.200425864

[93] Brochard V, Combadiere B, Prigent A, Laouar Y, Perrin A, Beray-Berthat V, Bonduelle O, Alvarez-Fischer D, Callebert J, Launay JM, Duyckaerts C, Flavell RA, Hirsch

EC, Hunot S. Infiltration of CD4+ lymphocytes into the brain contributes to neurodegeneration in a mouse model of Parkinson disease. J Clin Invest. 2009;119:182–92. doi: 10.1172/JCI36470

[94] McGeer PL, Itagaki S, Boyes BE, McGeer EG. Reactive microglia are positive for HLA-DR in the substantia nigra of Parkinson's and Alzheimer's disease brains. Neurology 1988;38:1285–91.

[95] Bas J, Calopa M, Mestre M, Mollevi G, Cutillas B, Ambrosio S, Buendia E. Lymphocyte populations in Parkinson's disease and in rat models of parkinsonism. J Neuroimmunol. 2001;113:146–52. doi:10.1016/S0165-5728(00)00422-7

[96] Stevens CH, Rowe D, Morel-Kopp MC, Orr C, Russell T, Ranola M, Ward C, Halliday GM. Reduced T helper and B lymphocytes in Parkinson's disease. J Neuroimmunol. 2012;252:95–9. doi:10.1016/j.jneuroim.2012.07.015

[97] Baba Y, Kuroiwa A, Uitti RJ, Wszolek ZK, Yamada T. Alterations of T-lymphocyte populations in Parkinson disease. Parkinsonism Relat Disord. 2005;11:493–8. doi: 10.1016/j.parkreldis.2005.07.005

[98] Migliore L, Petrozzi L, Lucetti C, Gambaccini G, Bernardini S, Scarpato R, Trippi F, Barale R, Frenzilli G, Rodilla V, Bonuccelli U. Oxidative damage and cytogenetic analysis in leukocytes of Parkinson's disease patients. Neurology 2002;58:1809–15. doi:10.1212/WNL.58.12.1809

[99] Cornetta T, Palma S, Aprile I, Padua L, Tonali P, Testa A, Cozzi R. Levodopa therapy reduces DNA damage in peripheral blood cells of patients with Parkinson's disease. Cell Biol Toxicol. 2009;25:321–30. doi:10.1007/s10565-008-9086-6

[100] Blandini F, Mangiagalli A, Cosentino M, Marino F, Samuele A, Rasini E, Fancellu R, Martignoni E, Riboldazzi G, Calandrella D, Frigo GM, Nappi G. Peripheral markers of apoptosis in Parkinson's disease: the effect of dopaminergic drugs. Ann N Y Acad Sci. 2003;1010:675–8. doi:10.1196/annals.1299.123

[101] Shlomchik MJ, Weisel F. Germinal center selection and the development of memory B and plasma cells. Immunol Rev. 2012;247:52–63. doi:10.1111/j.1600-065X.2012.01124.x.

[102] Besong-Agbo D, Wolf E, Jessen F, Oechsner M, Hametner E, Poewe W, Reindl M, Oertel WH, Noelker C, Bacher M, Dodel R. Naturally occurring α-synuclein autoantibody levels are lower in patients with Parkinson disease. Neurology 2013;80:169–75. doi: 10.1212/WNL.0b013e31827b90d1

[103] Han M, Nagele E, DeMarshall C, Acharya N, Nagele R. Diagnosis of Parkinson's disease based on disease-specific autoantibody profiles in human sera. PLoS One 2012;7:e32383. doi:10.1371/journal.pone.0032383

[104] Hansen A, Odendahl M, Reiter K, Jacobi AM, Feist E, Scholze J, Burmester GR, Lipsky PE, Dorner T. Diminished peripheral blood memory B cells and accumulation of

memory B cells in the salivary glands of patients with Sjogren's syndrome. Arthritis Rheum. 2002;46:2160–71. doi:10.1002/art.10445

[105] Souto-Carneiro MM, Mahadevan V, Takada K, Fritsch-Stork R, Nanki T, Brown M, Fleisher TA, Wilson M, Goldbach-Mansky R, Lipsky PE. Alterations in peripheral blood memory B cells in patients with active rheumatoid arthritis are dependent on the action of tumour necrosis factor. Arthritis Res Ther. 2009;11:R84. doi:10.1186/ar2718

[106] Dammann O, O'Shea TM. Cytokines and perinatal brain damage. Clin Perinatol. 2008;35:643–63. doi:10.1016/j.clp.2008.07.011.

[107] Churchill L, Taishi P, Wang M, Brandt J, Cearley C, Rehman A, Krueger J. Brain distribution of cytokine mRNA induced by systemic administration of interleukin-1β or tumor necrosis factor α. Brain Res. 2006;1120:64–73. doi:10.1016/j.brainres. 2006.08.083

[108] Brodacki B, Staszewski J, Toczyłowska B, Kozłowska E, Drela N, Chalimoniuk M, Stepien A. Serum interleukin (IL-2, IL-10, IL-6, IL-4), TNFα, and INFγ concentrations are elevated in patients with atypical and idiopathic parkinsonism. Neurosci Lett. 2008;441:158–62. doi:10.1016/j.neulet.2008.06.040

[109] Reale M, Iarlori C, Thomas A, Gambi D, Perfetti B, Di Nicola M, Onofrj M. Peripheral cytokines profile in Parkinson's disease. Brain Behav Immun. 2009;23:55–63. doi: 10.1016/j.bbi.2008.07.003

[110] Song IU, Kim JS, Chung SW, Lee KS. Is there an association between the level of high-sensitivity C-reactive protein and idiopathic Parkinson's disease? A comparison of Parkinson's disease patients, disease controls and healthy individuals. Eur Neurol. 2009;62:99–104. doi:10.1159/000222780.

[111] Mogi M, Harada M, Kondo T, Riederer P, Inagaki H, Minami M, Nagatsu T. Interleukin-1β, interleukin-6, epidermal growth factor and transforming growth factor-α are elevated in the brain from parkinsonian patients. Neurosci Lett. 1994;180:147–50.

[112] Mount MP, Lira A, Grimes D, Smith PD, Faucher S, Slack R, Anisman H, Hayley S, Park DS. Involvement of interferon-γ in microglial-mediated loss of dopaminergic neurons. J Neurosci. 2007;27:3328–37. doi:10.1523/JNEUROSCI.5321-06.2007

[113] Chao Y, Wong SC, Tan EK. Evidence of inflammatory system involvement in Parkinson'sdisease. Biomed Res Int. 2014;2014:308654. doi:10.1155/2014/308654.

[114] Nie K, Zhang Y, Gan R, Wang L, Zhao J, Huang Z, Tang H, Wang L. Polymorphisms in immune/inflammatory cytokine genes are related to Parkinson's disease with cognitive impairment in the Han Chinese population. Neurosci Lett. 2013;541:111–5. doi:10.1016/j.neulet.2013.02.024

[115] Yamada T, McGeer PL, McGeer EG. Lewy bodies in Parkinson's disease are recognized by antibodies to complement proteins. Acta Neuropathol. 1992;84:100–4.

[116] Kannarkat GT, Boss JM, Tansey MG. The role of innate and adaptive immunity in Parkinson's disease. J Parkinsons Dis. 2013;3:493–514. doi:10.3233/JPD-130250

[117] Babcock A, Kuziel W, Rivest S, Owens T: Chemokine Expression by glial cells directs leukocytes to sites of axonal injury in the CNS. J Neurosci. 2003;23:7922–30.

[118] Baggiolini M. Chemokines in pathology and medicine. J Intern Med. 2001;250:91–104. doi:10.1046/j.1365-2796.2001.00867

[119] Tran PB, Miller RJ. HIV-1, chemokines and neurogenesis. Neurotox Res. 2005;8:149–58.

[120] Lieberam I, Agalliu D, Nagasawa T, Ericson J, Jessell TM. A Cxcl12-CXCR4 chemokine signaling pathway defines the initial trajectory of mammalian motor axons. Neuron. 2005;47:667–79. doi:10.1016/j.neuron.2005.08.011

[121] Szabo I, Chen XH, Xin L, Adler MW, Howard OM, Oppenheim JJ, Rogers TJ. Heterologous desensitization of opioid receptors by chemokines inhibits chemotaxis and enhances the perception of pain. Proc Natl Acad Sci USA 2002;99:10276–81. doi: 10.1073/pnas.102327699

[122] Limatola C, Giovannelli A, Maggi L, Ragozzino D, Castellani L, Ciotti MT, Vacca F, Mercanti D, Santoni A, Eusebi F. SDF-1alpha-mediated modulation of synaptic transmission in rat cerebellum. Eur J Neurosci. 2000;12:2497–504. doi:10.1046/j.1460-9568.2000.00139.x

[123] Skrzydelski D, Guyon A, Daugé V, Rovère C, Apartis E, Kitabgi P, Nahon JL, Rostène W, Mélik Parsadaniantz M. The chemokine stromal cell-derived factor-1/CXCL12 activates the nigrostriatal dopamine system. J Neurochem. 2007;102:1175–83. doi: 10.1111/j.1471-4159.2007.04639.x

[124] Guyon A, Skrzydelski D, Rovère C, Apartis E, Rostène W, Kitabgi P, Mélik Parsadaniantz S, Nahon JL. Stromal-cell-derived factor alpha/CXCL12 modulates high-threshold calcium currents in rat substantia nigra. Eur J Neurosci. 2008;28:862–70. doi: 10.1111/j.1460-9568.2008.06367.x

[125] Shimoji M, Pagan F, Healton EB, Mocchetti I. CXCR4 and CXCL12 expression is increased in the nigro-striatal system of Parkinson's disease. Neurotox Res. 2009;16:318–28. doi:10.1007/s12640-009-9076-3

[126] Lindqvist D, Hall S, Surova Y, Nielsen HM, Janelidze S, Brundin L, Hansson O. Cerebrospinal fluid inflammatory markers in Parkinson's disease-associations with depression, fatigue, and cognitive impairment. Brain Behav Immun. 2013;33:183–189. doi:10.1016/j.bbi.2013.07.007

[127] Mogi M, Togari A, Kondo T, Mizuno Y, Komure O, Kuno S, Ichinose H, Nagatsu T. Brain-derived growth factor and nerve growth factor concentrations are decreased in the substantia nigra in Parkinson's disease. Neurosci Lett. 1999;270:45–8. doi:10.1016/S0304-3940(99)00463-2

[128] Nagatsu T, Sawada M. Inflammatory process in Parkinson's disease: role for cytokines. Curr Pharm Des. 2005;11:999–1016. doi:10.2174/1381612053381620

[129] Sawada M, Imamura K, Nagatsu T. Role of cytokines in inflammatory process in Parkinson's disease. J Neural Transm Suppl. 2006;70:373–81

[130] McGeer PL, McGeer EG. Inflammation and neurodegeneration in Parkinson's disease. Parkinsonism Relat Disord. 2004;10:S3–S7. doi:10.1016/j.parkreldis.2004.01.005

[131] Lawson L, Perry V, Dri P, Gordon S. Heterogeneity in the distribution and morphology of microglia in the normal adult mouse brain. Neuroscience 1990;39:151–70. doi: 10.1016/0306-4522(90)90229-W

[132] Czlonkowska A, Kohutnicka M, Kurkowska-Jastrzebska I, Czlonkowski A. Microglial reaction in MPTP (1-methyl-4-phenyl-1,2,3,6-tetrahydropyridine) induced Parkinson's disease mice model. Neurodegen 1996;5:137–43.

[133] Gao H, Jiang J, Wilson B, Zhang W, Hong J, Liu B. Microglial activation-mediated delayed and progressive degeneration of rat nigral dopaminergic neurons: relevance to Parkinson's disease. J Neurochem. 2002;81:1285–97. doi:10.1046/j.1471-4159.2002.00928.x

[134] Imamura K, Hishikawa N, Sawada M, Nagatsu T, Yoshida M, Hashizume Y. Distribution of major histocompatibility complex class II-positive microglia and cytokine profile of Parkinson's disease brains. Acta Neuropathol. 2003;106:518–26. doi:10.1007/s00401-003-0766-2

[135] Barcia C, Sánchez-Bahillo A, Fernández-Villalba E, Bautista V, Poza Y, Fernández-Barreiro A, Hirsch E, Herrero M. Evidence of active microglia in substantia nigra pars compacta of parkinsonian monkeys 1 year after MPTP exposure. Glia 2004;46:402–9. doi:10.1002/glia.20015

[136] Neumann H, Medana IM, Bauer J, Lassmann H. Cytotoxic T lymphocytes in autoimmune and degenerative CNS diseases. Trends Neurosci. 2002;25:313–9.

[137] Purisai MG, McCormack AL, Cumine S, Li J, Isla MZ, Di Monte DA. Microglial activation as a priming event leading to paraquat-induced dopaminergic cell degeneration. Neurobiol Dis. 2007;25:392–400.

[138] Qin L, Wu X, Block ML, Liu Y, Breese GR, Hong JS, Knapp DJ, Crews FT. Systemic LPS causes chronic neuroinflammation and progressive neurodegeneration. Glia 2007;55:453–62. doi:10.1002/glia.20467

[139] Koprich JB, Reske-Nielsen C, Mithal P, Isacson O. Neuroinflammation mediated by IL-1 beta increases susceptibility of dopamine neurons to degeneration in an animal model of Parkinson's disease. J Neuroinflamm. 2008;27:5–8. doi:10.1186/1742-2094-5-8

[140] Mangano EN, Hayley S. Inflammatory priming of the substantia nigra influences the impact of later paraquat exposure: neuroimmune sensitization of neurodegeneration. Neurobiol Aging. 2009;30:1361–78. doi:10.1016/j.neurobiolaging.2007.11.020

[141] Block ML, Hong JS. Microglia and inflammation-mediated neurodegeneration: multiple triggers with a common mechanism. Prog Neurobiol. 2005;76:77–98. doi: 10.1016/j.pneurobio.2005.06.004

[142] Kim YS, Joh TH. Microglia, major player in the brain inflammation: their roles in the pathogenesis of Parkinson's disease. Exp Mol Med. 2006;38:333–47. doi:10.1038/emm. 2006.40

[143] Frank-Cannon TC, Tran T, Ruhn KA, Martinez TN, Hong J, Marvin M, Hartley M, Trevino I, O'Brien DE, Casey B, Goldberg MS, Tansey MG. Parkin deficiency increases vulnerability to inflammation-related nigral degeneration. J Neurosci. 2008;28:10825–34. doi:10.1523/JNEUROSCI.3001-08.2008

[144] Couch Y, Alvarez-Erviti L, Sibson NR, Wood MJ, Anthony DC. The acute inflammatory response to intranigral α-synuclein differs significantly from intranigral lipopolysaccharide and is exacerbated by peripheral inflammation. J Neuroinflamm. 2011;8:166. doi:10.1186/1742-2094-8-166

[145] Sandhir R, Onyszchuk G, Berman NE. Exacerbated glial response in the aged mouse hippocampus following controlled cortical impact injury. Exp Neurol. 2008;213:372–80. doi:10.1016/j.expneurol.2008.06.013

[146] Barrett JP, Costello DA, O'Sullivan J, Cowley TR, Lynch MA. Bone marrow-derived macrophages from aged rats are more responsive to inflammatory stimuli. J Neuroinflamm. 2015;12:67. doi:10.1186/s12974-015-0287-7

[147] Sierra A, Gottfried-Blackmore AC, McEwen BS, Bulloch K. Microglia derived from aging mice exhibit an altered inflammatory profile. Glia 2007;55:412–24. doi:10.1002/glia.20468

[148] Fiala M, Lin J, Ringman J, Kermani-Arab V, Tsao G, Patel A, Lossinsky AS, Graves MC, Gustavson A, Sayre J, Sofroni E, Suarez T, Chiappelli F, Bernard G. Ineffective phagocytosis of amyloid-beta by macrophages of Alzheimer's disease patients. J Alzheimers Dis. 2005;7:221–32.

[149] Wu J, Xia S, Kalionis B, Wan W, Sun T. The role of oxidative stress and inflammation in cardiovascular aging. Biomed Res Int. 2014;2014:615312. doi:10.1155/2014/615312

[150] Douziech N, Seres I, Larbi A, Szikszay E, Roy PM, Arcand M, Dupuis G, Fulop T Jr. Modulation of human lymphocyte proliferative response with aging. Exp Gerontol. 2002;37:369–87. doi:10.1016/S0531-5565(01)00204-2

[151] Zahorska-Markiewicz B, Janowska J, Olszanecka-Glinianowicz M, Zurakowski A. Serum concentrations of TNF-alpha and soluble TNF-alpha receptors in obesity. Int J Obes Relat Metab Disord. 2000;24:1392–5.

[152] Fried SK, Bunkin DA, Greenberg AS. Omental and subcutaneous adipose tissues of obese subjects release interleukin-6: depot difference and regulation by glucocorticoid. J Clin Endocrinol Metab. 1998;83:847–50.

[153] Choi JY, Jang EH, Park CS, Kang JH. Enhanced susceptibility to 1-methyl-4-phenyl-1,2,3,6-tetrahydropyridine neurotoxicity in high-fat diet-induced obesity. Free Radic Biol Med. 2005;38:806–16. doi:10.1016/j.freeradbiomed.2004.12.008

Chapter 7

Disorders of Sleep and Motor Control During the Impaired Cholinergic Innervation in Rat – Relevance to Parkinson's Disease

Jasna Saponjic, Jelena Petrovic, Jelena Ciric and
Katarina Lazic

Additional information is available at the end of the chapter

http://dx.doi.org/10.5772/62949

Abstract

The medical profession has been generally very slow to acknowledge the importance of sleep medicine and sleep research. Disorders of sleep are related to anxiety, many mental and neurodegenerative diseases, cardiovascular and respiratory disorders, and obesity.

Our knowledge of the neural substrates of sleep/wake states and sleep-related behavior disorders regulation in health and the diseases, over more than 50 years of sleep research, is based on the experiments in animal models, pharmacotherapy, and the neuropathological studies in humans. But, we still need further work in fundamental multidisciplinary and clinical research between sleep and neurodegenerative disease investigators to understand normal and abnormal sleep, and to provide new insights into preventive or disease-altering approaches for therapy.

Our aim is to give an overview of our recent results related to the importance of thalamocortical cholinergic brain system in the disorders of sleep and motor control during sleep, with particular relevance to Parkinson's disease.

Keywords: sleep, motor control, the pedunculopontine tegmental nucleus (PPT), excitotoxic lesion, rat

1. Introduction

1.1. Importance of sleep research

The medical profession has been generally very slow to acknowledge the importance of sleep medicine and sleep research. The tendency to sleep less — perhaps 20% less in industrialized countries than a century ago — has serious consequences for economy and public safety. According to US National Science Foundation data, 75% of patients report sleep problems, but less than one-third were asked by their doctors about it, and one-third of American drivers admit to having nodded off behind the wheel [1]. Furthermore, the mounting body of evidence links lack of sleep to anxiety, many mental and neurodegenerative diseases [2–4], cardiovascular and respiratory disorders [5, 6], and obesity [7–9].

On the other hand, our knowledge of the neural substrates for sleep/wake states and sleep-related behavior disorders regulation in health and the diseases, over more than 50 years of sleep research, is based on the experiments in animal models, pharmacotherapy, central nervous system lesions, and the neuropathological studies in humans [2].

But, we still do not know why we sleep [10], and only further work in fundamental multidisciplinary and clinical research between sleep and neurodegenerative disease investigators is promising to enable us understand normal and abnormal sleep, and to provide new insights into preventive or disease-altering approaches for therapy.

1.2. Sleep and neurodegenerative diseases

Sleep is a complex, global and reversible behavioral state of all mammals, that is homeostatically regulated [11, 12]. It is also defined as a rapidly reversible state of immobility and reduced sensory responsiveness [12]. Still, there is no definition that has succeded in satisfying all aspects of sleep. The failure to define sleep as a single behavior lies in several facts [11, 13]: (1) sleep is not a homogenous state, but continuum of a number of mixed states; (2) the control mechanisms of sleep are manifested at all levels of biological organization - from genes and intracellular mechanisms to the networks of neuronal populations within the central nervous system that control movement, arousal, autonomic functions, behavior and cognition; (3) the activity and interactions of these neurochemically greatly heterogenous neuronal populations are dependent on two nested biological rhythms — the circadian rhythm of wake/sleep and about 90 minutes long periodic cycles of non-rapid-eye-movement (NREM)/ rapid-eye-movement (REM) sleep as two main sleep states [11–13].

Brain neurodegenerative diseases, like Alzheimer's (AD), and Parkinson's (PD) diseases, are devastating and rather common diseases. According to Nussbaum and Ellis [14] their prevalence is 0.5–1%; increasing to 1–3% for PD, and up to 50% for AD in ages over 69. In spite of a long knowledge of their clinical description and brain pathology (lesions of the cholinergic neurons in basal forebrain, lesions of the dopaminergic neurons in substantia nigra, etc.), they remain incurable with only limited success in temporal amelioration of their symptoms. Their symptoms are either cognitive (dementia in AD), or motor (tremor and bradykinesia in PD) or eventually both, and with age they progress to affective and cognitive deterioration as well as autonomic and sleep related behavioral disturbances. Clinical symptoms first appear at 65–69 years on average, but there are indications that subclinical features may start many years earlier. Namely, the patients with REM sleep behavior disorder (RBD) face close to a 20% 5-year risk of developing PD or dementia, and that risk rises to more than 40% after 10 years, and exceeds 50% after 12 years.

It is well known that human development, maturation, healthy aging [15, 16], and many neurological diseases [2] are associated with profound changes in sleep/wake states distribution and with variety of the sleep-related behavioral disorders. Neurodegenerative diseases such as AD and PD involve the selective loss of specific neuronal populations within the brain. Human studies evidenced that sleep/wake cycle disturbance, as no cognitive symptom of dementia, precedes on average 3 years before the clinical diagnosis of the AD [17], and that RBD, reflecting an underlying synucleinopathy neurodegeneration, precedes as a symptom the onset of motor and cognitive disturbances by years or decades, with presence of the α – synuclein protein pathology within the REM sleep-related regulatory structures of the dorsal midbrain and pons at the onset of disease, with ascending pattern of neurodegeneration progression from brainstem to basal areas of the brain [3].

1.3. Sleep and the brain cholinergic systems

Generally, the activation state of mammalian neocortex is regulated by a complex interplay of cortical and subcortical neuronal networks. Slow EEG oscillations are present in isolated neocortical tissue, while high-frequency oscillations (β and γ frequency oscillations) are not, suggesting a dependence on subcortical impulse flow [18]. The cholinergic afferent fibers system originating in the basal forebrain plays a critical role in switching cortical activity from deactivated slow to high-frequency, activated EEG patterns. Inputs to the cortex originated in the thalamus constitute the second major system involved in regulation of the cortical activity, and the pedunculopontine tegmental nucleus (PPT - the cholinergic nucleus within the pons; the main thalamo-cortical cholinergic source of innervation) efferent fibers exert, through the thalamus, widespread control over neocortical EEG activation during waking and REM sleep. Because direct projections from the PPT reach both the basal forebrain and thalamus, this nucleus is an ideal candidate to study the integrated contributions of these two systems to regulating activation of the neocortex [18]. PPT is postulated to have important functions relevant to the regulation of REM sleep [19, 20], arousal [21–29], and various motor control systems [30–32], including breathing control [33–38]. In addition, the PPT has a central role in the REM sleep phenomenon control [39–41], and each individual REM-sleep-sign generating nucleus receives afferent inputs from PPT [28].

Degeneration of the PPT thalamo-cortical cholinergic neurons was related to RBD [42], and to the motor control impairment, including falls in PD [43, 44.] Recent PET imaging [45] and neuropathological studies [44] suggested that the neurodegeneration of thalamic cholinergic afferent projections may contribute to the PD specific motor and cognitive abnormalities [45]. Clinical studies also evidenced the beneficial effect of AChE inhibitor donepezil in 50% reduction of falls in PD patients [46], and suggested that PD is a neurodegeneration of different CNS systems [44].

Obviously, counseling and prevention of AD or PD would be highly enriched by the development of a practical, sensitive and reliable methodology for detecting those patients with RBD, or other sleep disorders who are at risk for developing AD or PD.

In this chapter we will give an overview of our results in the animal studies related to the importance of thalamo-cortical cholinergic brain system (the PPT cholinergic neurons) in the disorders of sleep and motor control during sleep, which is of particular relevance to PD.

2. Experimental procedure in the animal studies of the impaired PPT cholinergic control

2.1. The rat model of impaired PPT cholinergic innervation

In our studies we used the bilateral PPT lesioned rats as the *"in vivo"* model of the severe thalamo-cortical cholinergic neuropathology. We followed the sleep/wake states architecture and transition structure, the EEG microstructure and motor control across sleep, and all the sleep state episodes dynamics. Adult, male, Wistar rats were chronically implanted for sleep recording [47, 48]. During operative procedure for the stereotaxic implantation of the EEG and EMG electrodes the bilateral PPT lesions were performed by the stereotaxically guided microinfusion of 100 nl of 0.1 M ibotenic acid/ 0.1 M phosphate buffered saline into the PPT of each brain side [49–53].

The animals were maintained on a 12-hour light-dark cycle, and were housed at 25°C with free access to food and water, and all experimental procedures were in accordance with the EEC Directive (86/609/EEC) on the protection of animals used for experimental and other scientific purposes, and were approved by the Ethical Committee for the Use of Laboratory Animals of the Institute for Biological Research "Sinisa Stankovic", University of Belgrade (Approval N° 2-21/10).

2.2. Surgical procedure of the chronic electrodes implantation for sleep recording in rat

We implanted under ketamine/diazepam anesthesia (Zoletil 50, VIRBAC, France, 50 mg/kg; i.p.), in 2.5 months old rats, 4 epidural parietal stainless-steel screw electrodes for electroencephalographic (EEG) cortical activity recording: 2 in the motor (MCx; A/P: +1.0 mm from bregma; R/L: 2.0 mm from sagittal suture), and 2 in the sensorimotor (SMCx; A/P: -3.0 mm from bregma; R/L: 2.0 mm from sagittal suture) cortex [54]. Bilateral electromyogram (EMG) stainless steel teflon coated wire electrodes (Medwire, NY, USA) were implanted into the dorsal nuchal musculature to assess skeletal muscle activity, and a stainless-steel screw electrode was implanted in the nasal bone. All the electrode leads were soldered to a miniature connector plug (39F1401, Newark Electronics, Schaumburg, IL, USA), and the assembly was fixed to the screw electrodes and skull using acrylic dental cement (Biocryl-RN, Galenika a.d. Beograd, Serbia).

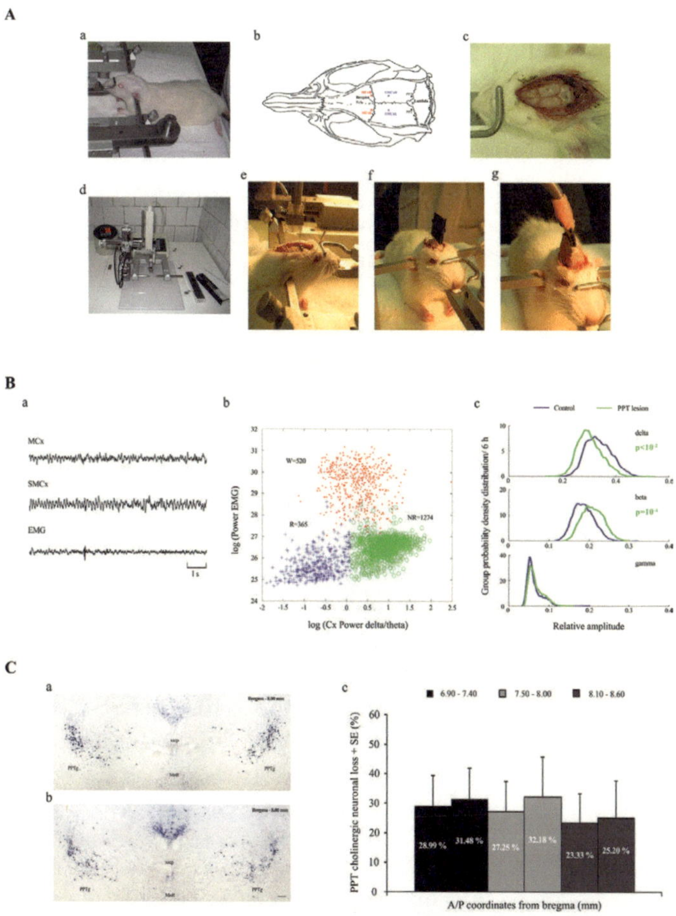

Figure 1. Schematic illustration of the experimental procedure in the animal studies of the impaired PPT cholinergic control. Operative procedure for the stereotaxic implantation of the chronic EEG and EMG electrodes for sleep recording and the stereotaxically guided microinfusion for the PPT excitotoxic lesion (**Aa-g**) with the illustrations of stereotaxic positions on the rat scull for the EEG electrodes implantation and the PPT lesions (**Ab**); Sleep recording, sleep states differentiation and analysis (**Ba-c**): the analog signals (10 s) recorded from the sensorimotor (SMCx) and motor (MCx) cortex, and EMG from dorsal nuchal muscle (**Ba**); an individual example of the final scattergram for Wake/NREM/REM differentiation during the 6 h of sleep recording. Each symbol corresponds to one 10 s epoch. W cluster – Wake 10 s epochs, dots; NR cluster – NREM 10 s epochs, circles; R cluster – REM 10 s epochs, crosses (**Bb**); and an example of the group probability density distributions of the sleep/wake state-related EEG frequency band relative amplitudes/6 h in bilateral PPT lesion vs. control, representing the EEG microstructure during NREM, with statistically significant attenuation (the left shifted green delta amplitude group distribution) and augmentation (the right shifted green beta amplitude group distribution) of the corresponding EEG relative amplitudes (**Bc**). Typical examples of the control PPT (**Ca**) and the bilateral PPT lesion (**Cb**), histologically identified by NADPH-diaphorase staining and quantified throughout the overall PPT rostro-caudal dimension (6.90 – 8.60 mm caudal from bregma), with the cholinergic neuronal loss expressed as the group mean percent difference of the NADPH-diaphorase positive cells with respect to control, taken as 100% for each stereotaxic range, and also per each brain side (**Cc**). PPTg – pedunculopontine tegmental nucleus; xscp – decussation of the superior cerebellar peduncle; MnR – median raphe nucleus. Scale bar is 200 μm.

2.3. Excitotoxic lesion of the PPT

During surgical procedure for the EEG and EMG electrodes implantations we performed the bilateral PPT lesions (**Figure 1A**). These excitotoxic lesions were induced by the stereotaxically guided microinfusion of 0.1 M ibotenic acid (IBO)/ 0.1 M phosphate buffered saline (PBS) bilaterally into the PPT (A/P: –7.8 mm from bregma; R/L: 1.9 mm from sagittal suture; D/V: 7.0 mm from the brain surface), using a Digital Lab Standard Stereotaxic Instrument with a Hamilton syringe (1 μl). The IBO (Sigma; pH = 7.4) concentration was chosen on the basis of previous studies [49–53, 55]. The microinfusions were introduced at a volume of 100 nl, using a single, 60 s pulse.

2.4. Sleep recording

At the end of surgical procedure, the scalp wounds were sutured and the rats were allowed to recover 13 days before their adaptation to the recording cable and plexiglass chamber (30 cm x 30 cm x 30 cm) for one day. The EEG and EMG activities were carried from the connector plug on the rat head by cable, passed through a sealed port on the recording box, and differentially recorded. Differential mode consisted of 6 inputs (left MCx, right MCx, left SMCx, right SMCx, left EMG, right EMG), each with a (+) on the left and a (–) on the right side and all with the same ground (a screw electrode implanted in the nasal bone). The activities were displayed on a computer monitor, and stored on disk for further off-line analysis (**Figure 1Ba**). After conventional amplification and filtering (0.3–100 Hz band pass; A-M System Inc. Model 3600, Carlborg, WA, USA), the analog data were digitized (sampling frequency 256/s), and recorded for 6 h, during the normal inactive circadian phase for rats (from 9 a.m. to 3 p.m.), using DataWave SciWorks Experimenter Version 8.0 (Datawave Technologies, Longmont, CO, USA).

Additionally, we have followed the impact of different anesthetized states of surgical level in all the experimental groups, during 20 min of ketamine/diazepam or pentobarbital anesthesia [52], and we recorded EEG and respiratory movements using the piezo electric strain gauge (Infant-Ped Sleepmate Technologies, Midlothain, VA).

The stability of the anesthesia was estimated on the bases of the observed loss of consciousness, muscle atonia, absence of tail-pinch, ear-pinch (analgesia) and corneal reflexes before the onset of each 20 min recording of the stable anesthetized state, and on the bases of polygraphic recording during the experimental procedure, including regular breathing pattern [52]. In all acute experiments, the anesthesia was administered at 9 a.m.

2.5. Identification and quantification of the PPT lesion

We identified the PPT lesions by NADPH - diaphorase histochemistry [56], and we quantified the PPT cholinergic cell loss using Image J 1.46 software. NADPH - diaphorase positive cells were counted in three 40 μm thick coronal sections per each brain within an overall rostro-caudal PPT dimension [49–53]. The number of NADPH - diaphorase positively stained cells was intended to provide an estimate of the lesion damage or the cholinergic neuronal numbers, rather than an attempt to determine the absolute numbers of cholinergic neurons within the PPT. The cholinergic neuronal loss was expressed per each brain side, and per each defined stereotaxic range, within the overall PPT rostro-caudal dimension, as the percent difference of NADPH - diaphorase positive cells versus the controls. Namely, all percent differences were expressed with respect to the mean control absolute numbers per each stereotaxic range taken as 100%. All statistical analyses for the PPT cholinergic cells number changes were done using nonparametric Mann-Whitney U two-tailed tests [49–53]. We have shown that by using a 100 nl microinfusion of 0.1 M IBO for the excitotoxic PPT lesion we induced the partial bilateral lesions of the PPT pars compacta (as dominantly cholinergic part of the PPT), and we achieved the selectivity of the lesions within the PPT limits (**Figure 1Ca,b**). We have demonstrated (**Figure 1Ca,b,c**) that the cholinergic neuronal loss induced by our methodological approach was > 20% throughout the overall rosto-caudal dimension within the each brain side [49–53].

2.6. Data analysis

Analysis of the recorded signals was conducted using original software we developed [48–53] using MATLAB 6.5 (**Figure 1Bb,c**). We applied Fourier analysis to the signals acquired throughout each 6 h recording (2160 10 s Fourier epochs), and each 10 s epoch was differentiated as Wake, NREM or REM state (**Figure 1Bb**) for further analysis of the Wake, NREM and REM related EEG relative amplitudes of all the conventional frequency bands (δ = 0.3–4 Hz; θ = 4.1–8 Hz; σ = 10.1–15 Hz; β = 15.1–30 Hz; γ = 30.1–50 Hz).

We particularly analyzed two distinct REM clusters that emerged within the scattergrams, and each REM 10 s epoch was differentiated, based on the EMG power, as REM with higher muscles tone (REM1) or REM with atonia (REM2). Differentiation of the Wake epochs from sleep epochs, and further differentiation of the NREM and REM/REM1/REM2 epochs was achieved using the two clusters K means algorithm (**Figure 1Bb; Figure 2A**). We improved these differentiation results by using the logarithmic values of quantities on both axes [48–53].

To analyze the sleep/wake state related EEG amplitude changes we calculated group probability density distributions of all the Wake, NREM and REM/REM1/REM2 conventional EEG frequency bands relative amplitudes over 6 h, using the Probability Density Estimate (PDE) routine supplied with MATLAB 6.5 (**Figure 1Bc; Figure 2B**). In order to eliminate any influence from absolute signal amplitude variations on the recordings, we computed the relative Fourier amplitudes [48–53, 57]:

$$(RA)_b = \frac{\sum_b \mathrm{Amp}}{\sum_{tot} \mathrm{Amp}}, \quad b = \{\delta, \theta, \sigma, \beta, \gamma\}. \tag{1}$$

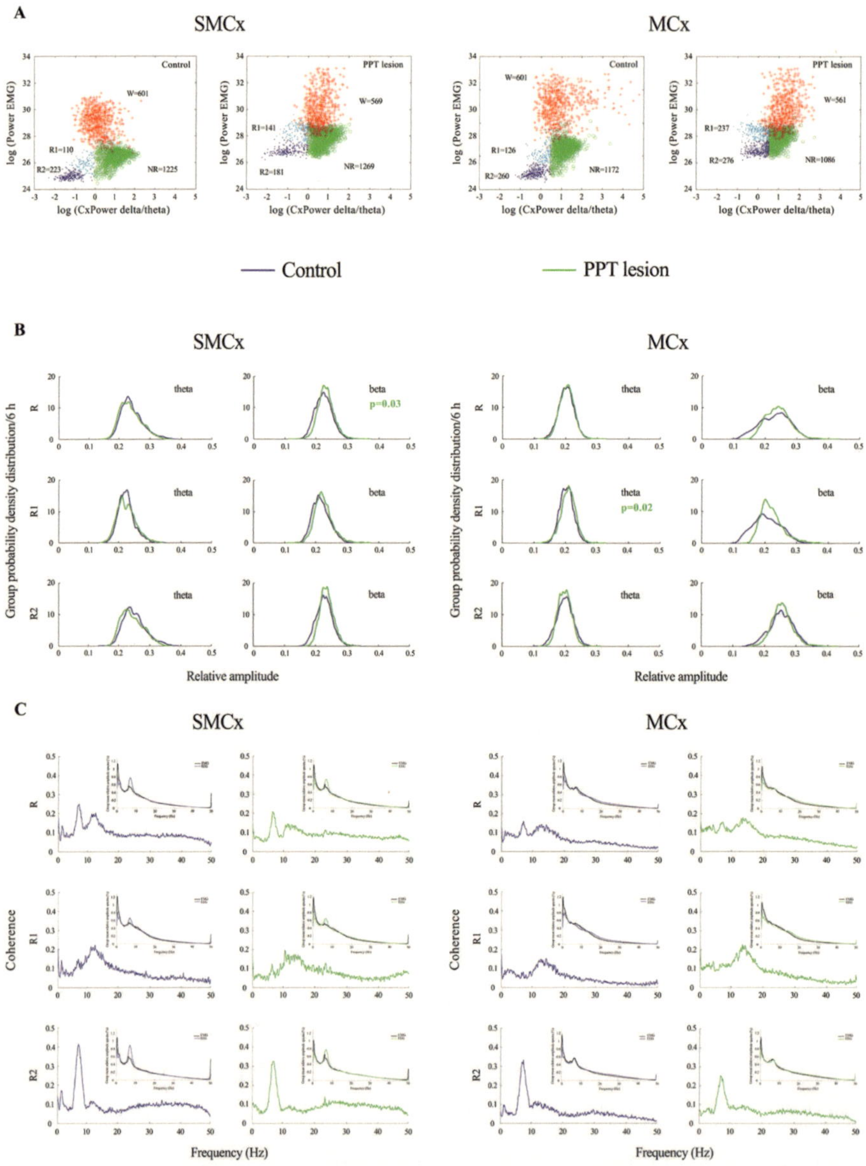

Figure 2. Topography of the REM sleep alterations following the PPT lesion. Examples of the final scattergrams for the Wake/NREM/REM/REM1/REM2 differentiation within the sensorimotor (SMCx) and motor (MCx) cortex during 6 h of sleep recordings (**A**) of the control (Control) and bilaterally PPT lesioned rat (PPT lesion). In all scattergrams the Wake 10 s epochs (W cluster, crosses) are transferred to these final scattergrams from the preceding Wake/Sleep differentiations. NR cluster, circles – NREM 10 s epoch; R1, R2, clusters, dots – REM1, REM2 10 s epochs (**A**); REM/REM1/REM2 EEG microstructure within the SMCx and MCx cortex of the control (Control, blue line) and bilaterally PPT lesioned rat (PPT lesion, green line); p values correspond to the statistically significant Mann-Whitney U two-tailed comparisons (**B**); REM/REM1/REM2 group coherence spectra between the SMCx or MCx EEGs and the dorsal nuchal muscle EMGs of the control (Control, blue line) and bilaterally PPT lesioned rat (PPT lesion, green line) with the inserts of their corresponding group mean relative amplitude EEG and EMG spectra used for the corticomuscular coherence analysis (**C**).

For each sleep/wake state and each frequency band, PDE analysis was performed on the ensembles of relative amplitudes by pooling measured values $(RA)_b$ from all animals belonging to a specific experimental group (**Figure 1Bc; Figure 2B; Figure 3A; Figure 4Ac; Figure 4Bc**).

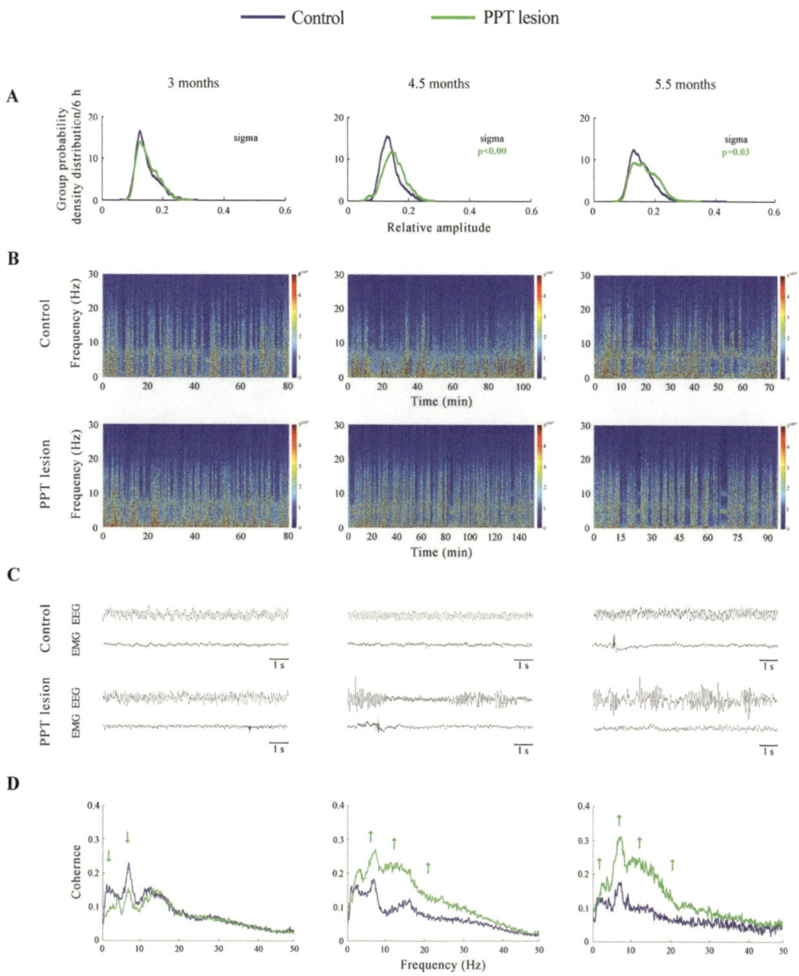

Figure 3. Differing impact of aging on the EEG microstructure during REM sleep in the PPT lesioned rats vs. control rats at the onset (3 months), and at two last (4.5 months and 5.5 months) aging follow-up periods. The group probability density distributions of the EEG sigma relative amplitude/6 h during REM sleep depict the age related augmentation of the REM sigma amplitude within the motor cortex (MCx) in the PPT lesioned rats vs. control rats (the right shifted green distributions) - p values correspond to the obtained significant results of Mann-Whitney U two-tailed tests (**A**). Individual examples of the MCx REM spectrograms across the overall aging follow up period during the bilateral PPT lesions vs. controls (**B**), with their typical 10 s analog EEG and EMG signals during REM (**C**) used for the construction of REM spectrograms as well as for the corticomuscular coherence analysis during REM. For all REM spectrograms the EEG 10 s epochs during REM were extracted and concatenated in the same order as they occurred in a real-time domain during the whole 6 h sleep of each rat, and at each time during aging follow up period. The group mean coherence spectra between the MCx EEG and the dorsal nuchal muscle EMG during REM in the bilateral PPT lesions vs. controls (**D**). Aging consistently increased the MCx delta, theta, sigma and beta drives during the bilateral PPT lesion (green arrows).

Additionally, we have analyzed the Wake, NREM and REM/REM1/REM2 corticomuscular coherences (CMCs) separately for each experimental group, each state, and for all the conventional EEG frequency bands (**Figure 2C**; **Figure 3D**), using the SMCx or MCx EEG, and the EMG of the dorsal nuchal muscles [51, 53, 57]. CMC values were calculated using the "cohere" routine of the MATLAB 6.5 Signal Processing Toolbox. It actually computes the magnitude squared coherence between signals x(EEG) and y(EMG) as:

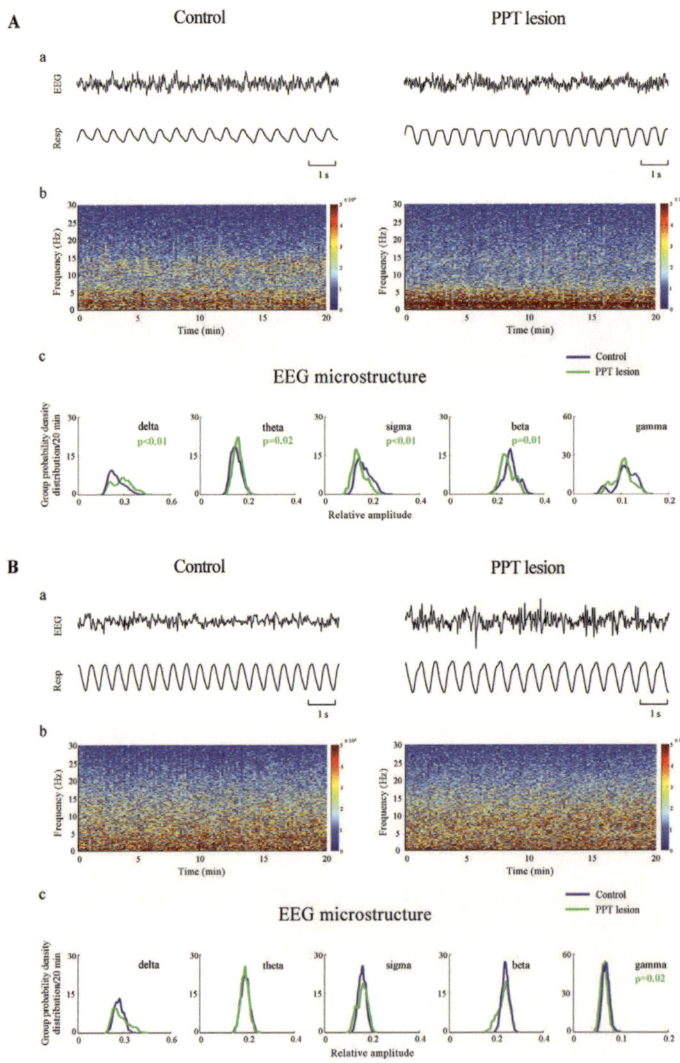

Figure 4. Impact of ketamin/diazepam (A) and pentobarbital (B) anesthetic regimens at surgical level on EEG microstructure and respiratory pattern in the bilaterally PPT lesioned rat vs. control rat. Individual examples of the analog 10 s EEG and respiratory signals (**a**), as well as their EEG spectrograms (**b**) and the group EEG microstructure during 20 min of stable anesthetized state (**c**) in the bilaterally PPT lesioned vs. control rats. The p values correspond to the statistically significant Mann-Whitney U two-tailed comparisons.

$$C_{xy}(f) = \frac{\left|P_{xy}(f)\right|^2}{P_{xx}(f)P_{yy}(f)} \tag{2}$$

where $P_{xy}(f)$ stands for the cross spectrum of x and y, while $P_{xx}(f)$ and $P_{yy}(f)$ denote the power spectra of the two signals. All P_{xy}, P_{xx}, and P_{yy} values were determined for every 10 s of each 6 h recording, and for each frequency within the overall 0.3 - 50 Hz range, with 0.1 Hz resolution.

Namely, previously identified Wake/NREM/REM/REM1/REM2 EEG and EMG 10 s epochs were concatenated and pooled within each experimental group of rats. Then, the CMC spectra were calculated for every 60 min of Wake and NREM, and for every 30 min of REM/REM1/REM2, using 10 s FFT epochs for the MATLAB "cohere" routine, resulting in 0.1 Hz frequency resolution. Then, the CMC values within each conventional frequency band (δ, θ, σ, β, γ) were averaged for each spectrum, and finally their means were calculated from the collection of all available CMC spectra, for each state.

We have also drawn the REM sleep EEG spectrograms (Figure 3B) or the EEG spectrograms of distinct anesthetized states at surgical level (**Figure 4Ab**, **Figure 4Bb**) using the same Fourier analysis parameters: a 10 s Fourier epoch, resulting in 0.1 Hz y-axis frequency resolution; a 10 s moving Fourier epoch step, yielding the same x-axis time resolution.

For the respiratory pattern time-domain analysis during anesthesia, the respiratory signal was passed through a 0.5–5 Hz band pass filter to remove baseline drift and attenuate the high frequency noise and we used our originally developed analysis for breath detection, differentiation, and the quantification of the eupnea, bradypnea/apnea and sigh breath-to-breath intervals within the respiratory pattern. All the details for the respiratory pattern analysis are explained elsewhere [52].

For the statistical analysis of PDE/6 h and CMC/6 h we calculated the relative amplitude means for Wake and NREM per each 60 min, and for REM/REM1/REM2 per each 30 min. Further, we employed the Kruskal-Wallis ANOVA and Mann-Whitney U two-tailed tests for the statistical analysis of all group means over 6 h: the group mean durations of Wake, NREM, and REM/REM1/REM2; the group mean number and group mean duration of Wake, NREM and REM/REM1/REM2 episodes; the group means of Wake, NREM and REM/REM1/REM2 EEG relative amplitudes for all frequency bands; and the group CMC means of Wake, NREM and REM/REM1/REM2. In all cases the differences were considered statistically significant for $p \leq 0.05$.

3. Disorders of sleep and motor control in the rat model of Parkinson's disease cholinergic neuropathology

Our studies in the rat model *"in vivo"* demonstrated that the severe PPT cholinergic neuronal loss (the severe thalamo-cortical cholinergic control impairment) did not change the sleep/wake states architecture, but disturbed the sleep/wake state transitions structure and augmented cortical activation during all sleep/wake states [49]. Beside the "tonically" increased

Wake/REM and REM/Wake transitions, the bilateral PPT lesion was expressed from the onset (14 days following lesion) as a generalized Wake, NREM and REM beta amplitude augmentation, which was sustainable for 5 weeks. This effect was followed from the onset by the NREM delta attenuation and REM gamma augmentation. In addition, there was the Wake delta attenuation from 21 days after the PPT lesion [49].

Furthermore, our studies have shown for the first time that the bilateral PPT cholinergic neuronal loss in rat was differently expressed in sensorimotor vs. motor cortex (**Figure 2A, B**), and the differing EEG microstructure and transition structure, particularly within the motor cortex and during NREM and REM sleep are the hallmarks of lesion [50]. Moreover, the bilateral PPT lesion increased a likelihood of the emergence of two REM sleep states [51], particularly within the motor cortex (**Figure 2A**): REM1 (REM without atonia, or "sigma coherent REM"), and REM2 (REM with atonia, or "theta coherent REM"). Namely, aside from the differential total EMG power of the dorsal nuchal musculature (**Figure 2A**), REM1 and REM2 have the topographically distinct EEG microstructures (**Figure 2B**) and cortical locomotor drives (**Figure 2C**) from the sensorimotor and motor cortices to dorsal nuchal muscles. These PPT lesion induced alteration of the cortical drives are commonly expressed as the impaired theta and sigma cortico-muscular coherences [51]. Although the bilateral PPT lesion altered both cortical drives during both REM states [51], its impact was more severe during REM2 state (healthy REM, REM with atonia), and more severely through the sensorimotor cortical drive (there were the impaired theta, sigma, beta and gamma coritco-muscular coherences). These results indicate the simultaneous breakdown of the PPT cholinergic direct ascending thalamo-coritcal control, and the indirect descending control of the REM sleep atonia regulatory circuitry, for the emergence of two differential REM states following the bilateral PPT lesion in rats [51].

We have also demonstrated the age-related and topographically specific EEGs and cortical drives alterations during sleep in the PPT lesioned rats (**Figure 3**). The hallmark of earlier aging onset in the PPT lesioned rats vs. physiological controls was the augmented EEG sigma amplitude within the motor cortex during REM (**Figure 3A, B, C**), as the unique pathological phenomenon [53]. Beside this EEG microstructure disorder during REM sleep, we have evidenced for the first time the altered cortical drives as the hallmarks of the earlier aging onset during severely impaired PPT cholinergic control (**Figure 3D**). This compensatory and aging induced plasticity was differently expressed through the sensorimotor cortical drive alterations, but it was broadly and commonly expressed through the motor cortical drive alterations during all the sleep/wake states [53]. Namely, during severely impaired PPT thalamocortical innervation aging consistently increased the motor cortical delta, theta, sigma and beta drives during NREM and REM sleep (**Figure 3D**).

Furthermore, we have shown that distinct anesthetic regimens at surgical level were expressed differently in the bilaterally PPT lesioned rats (the rat model of cholinergic PD neuropathology) vs. physiological controls (**Figure 4A, B**) in terms of the EEG microstructure, respiratory pattern, and post-anesthesia sleep [52]. Namely, the ketamine/diazepam anesthesia induced more alterations in the EEG microstructure and respiratory pattern (**Figure 4A**) than did the pentobarbital anesthesia (**Figure 4B**) in the PPT lesioned rats vs. physiological controls [52]. Although the ketamine/diazepam anesthesia at surgical level induced the apneustic breathing pattern in the PPT lesioned rats, the equal time to establish an anesthetized state in the PPT lesioned rats vs. control rats, and the long-term post-anesthesia suppressive effect on the augmented cortical activation during NREM (the augmented beta and theta amplitudes during NREM as a hallmarks of the PPT lesion), suggested the ketamine/diazepam anesthesia as potentially more beneficial both for anesthesia induction and post-anesthesia sleep in the surgical procedures of elderly, Parkinson's and Alzheimer's patients.

4. Discussion

Our studies have shown that the sleep/wake states related disturbances were topographically differently expressed within the sensorimotor and motor cortex in terms of their EEG microstructure and transitions structure, particularly during NREM and REM sleep, in the rat model of severely impaired PPT cholinergic thalamo-cortical innervation [49, 50]. Moreover, we have evidenced the emergence of two REM sleep states in the bilateral PPT lesioned rats, differential with regard to the total EMG power, the topographically distinct EEG microstructures and the sensorimotor and motor cortical drives to the dorsal nuchal muscles. These altered cortical drives were commonly expressed during both REM states, as the impaired beta oscillation drive [51]. In addition, the sensorimotor cortical drive was altered more severely during "healthy" REM (REM with atonia, theta REM) than during the emerged pathological REM (REM without atonia, sigma REM).

It is well known that the output of the basal ganglia (the efferents from globus palidus internus and substantia nigra pars reticulata) is sent primarily to thalamus and from there to the frontal cortex, forming the partially closed cortico-basal ganglia loop. PPT, as the main source of thalamo-cortical cholinergic innervation, monosynaptically innervates the substantia nigra and to less extent the globus palidus internus [58], but through its descending cholinergic efferents indirectly promotes REM sleep atonia [59–61]. Therefore, the degeneration of PPT cholinergic neurons could underlie the motor symptoms in patients with PD and RBD [59]. Since the PPT may be severely affected by PD pathology, it is regarded as a promising target for therapeutic deep-brain stimulation [59].

However, our understanding of the PPT role in PD pathogenesis is limited by the lack of a suitable model of PPT cholinergic neuronal degeneration. All animal models [62–65], the toxic and transgenic animal models, have their own specificities and limitations that must be carefully taken into consideration when choosing the model to be used, and when interpreting the results. For example, recent studies [66, 67] demonstrated different results within the PPT, as a consequence of the substantia nigra dopaminergic neuronal loss caused by 6-OHDA or Lactacystin: mostly non-cholinergic PPT neuronal loss [67] vs. mostly PPT cholinergic loss [66]. We have overviewed our results in the animal model of severe PPT cholinergic neuropathology (the rat model of PD cholinergic neuropathology) to provide new insights into the importance and relevance of thalamo-cortical cholinergic system regulatory role in sleep and motor control in PD.

Acknowledgements

This work was supported by Serbian Ministry of Education, Science and Technological Development Grant OI 173022.

Author details

Jasna Saponjic*, Jelena Petrovic, Jelena Ciric and Katarina Lazic

*Address all correspondence to: jasnasap@ibiss.bg.ac.rs; jasnasaponjic@yahoo.com

University of Belgrade, Department of Neurobiology, Institute for Biological Research - Sinisa Stankovic, Belgrade, Serbia

References

[1] Nature Editorial. Waking up to the importance of sleep. Nature. 2005;437:1207. DOI: 10.1038/4371207a

[2] Boeve BF, Silber MH, Saper CB, Ferman TJ, Dickson DW, Parisi JE, Benarroch EE, Ahlskog JE, Smith GE, Caselli RC, Tippman-Peikert M, Olson EJ, Lin SC, Young T, Wszolek Z, Schenck CH, Mahowald MW, Castillo PR, Del Tredici K, Braak H. Pathophysiology of REM sleep behaviour disorder and relevance to neurodegenerative disease. Brain. 2007;130:2770–2788. DOI: 10.1093/brain/awm056

[3] Whitwell JL, Weigand SD, Shiung MM, Boeve BF, Ferman TJ, Smith GE, Knopman DS, Petersen RC, Benarroch EE, Josephs KA, Jack CRJr. Focal atrophy in dementia with Lewy bodies on MRI: a distinct pattern from Alzheimer's disease. Brain. 2007;130:708–719. DOI: 10.1093/brain/awl388

[4] Raggi A, Ferri R. Sleep disorders in neurodegenerative diseases. Eur J Neurol. 2010; 17:1326–1338. DOI: 10.1111/j.1468-1331.2010.03034.x.

[5] Maria B, Sophia S, Michalis M, Charalampos L, Andreas P, John ME, Nikolaos SM. Sleep breathing disorders in patients with idiopathic Parkinson's disease. Respir Med. 2003;97:1151–1157. DOI: 10.1016/S0954-6111(03)00188-4

[6] McKay LC, Janczewski WA, Feldman JL. Sleep-disordered breathing after targeted ablation of preBötzinger complex neurons. Nat Neurosci. 2005;8:1142–1144. DOI: 10.1038/nn1517

[7] Kok SW, Overeem S, Visscher TLS, Lammers GJ, Seidell JC, Pijl H, Meinders AE. Hypocretin deficiency in narcoleptic humans is associated with abdominal obesity. Obes Res. 2003;11:1147–1154. DOI: 10.1038/oby.2003.156

[8] Resta O, Foschino Barbaro MP, Bonfitto P, Giliberti T, Depalo A, Pannacciulli N, de Pergola G. Low sleep quality and daytime sleepiness in obese patients without obstructive sleep apnoea syndrome. J Intern Med. 2003;253:536–543. DOI: 10.1046/j.1365-2796.2003.01133.x

[9] Sakurai T. Roles of orexin/hypocretin in regulation of sleep/wakefulness and energy homeostasis. Sleep Med Rev. 2005;9:231–241. DOI: 10.1016/j.smrv.2004.07.007

[10] White DP. The pathogenesis of obstructive sleep apnea - Advances in the past 100 years. Am J Respir Cell Mol Biol. 2006;34:1–6. DOI: 10.1165/rcmb.2005-0317OE

[11] Pace-Schott EF, Hobson JA. The neurobiology of sleep: genetics, cellular physiology and subcortical networks. Nat Rev Neurosci. 2002;3:591–605. DOI: 10.1038/nrn895

[12] Siegel JM. Do all animals sleep? Trends Neurosci. 2008;31:208–213. DOI: 10.1016/j.tins.2008.02.001

[13] Hobson JA, Pace-Schott EF. The cognitive neuroscience of sleep: neuronal systems, consciousness and learning. Nat Rev Neurosci. 2002;3:679–693. DOI: 10.1038/nrn915

[14] Nussbaum RL, Ellis CE. Alzheimer's Disease and Parkinson's Disease. N Engl J Med. 2003;348:1356–1364. DOI: 10.1056/NEJM2003ra020003

[15] Garcia-Rill E, Charlesworth A, Heister D, Ye M, Hayar A. The developmental decrease in REM sleep: the role of transmitters and electrical coupling. Sleep. 2008;31:673–690. DOI:

[16] Dijk DJ, Groeger JA, Stanley N, Deacon S. Age-related reduction in daytime sleep propensity and nocturnal slow wave sleep. Sleep. 2010;33:211–223. DOI:

[17] Simic G, Stanic G, Mladinov M, Jovanov-Milosevic N, Kostovic I, Hof PR. Does Alzheimer's disease begin in the brainstem? Neuropathol App Neurobiol. 2009; 35:532–554. DOI: 10.1111/j.1365-2990.2009.01038.x

[18] Dringenberg HC, Olmstead MC. Integrated contributions of basal forebrain and thalamus to neocortical activation elicited by pedunculopontine tegmental stimulation in urethane-anesthetized rats. Neuroscience. 2003;119:839–853. DOI: 10.1016/S0306-4522(03)00197-0

[19] Lu J, Sherman D, Devor M, Saper CB. A putative flip-flop switch for control of REM sleep. Nature. 2006;441:589–594. DOI: 10.1038/nature04767

[20] McCarley RW, Hobson JA. Neuronal excitability modulation over the sleep cycle: a structural and mathematical model. Science. 1975;189:58–60. DOI: 10.1126/science.1135627

[21] Bringmann A. Different functions of rat's pedunculopontine tegmental nucleus are reflected in cortical EEG. Neuroreport. 1995;6:2065–2068. DOI:

[22] Bringmann A. Nicotine affects the occipital theta rhythm after lesion of the pedunculopontine tegmental nucleus in rats. Neuropsychobiology. 1997;35:102–107. DOI: 10.1159/000119399

[23] Datta S. Evidence that REM sleep is controlled by the activation of brain stem pedunculopontine tegmental kainate receptor. J Neurophysiol. 2002;87:1790–1798. DOI: 10.1152/jn.00763.2001

[24] Datta S, Spoley EE, Patterson EH. Microinjection of glutamate into the pedunculopontine tegmentum induces REM sleep and wakefulness in the rat. Am J Physiol Regul Integr Comp Physiol. 2001;280:R752–R759. DOI:

[25] Datta S, MacLean RR. Neurobiological mechanisms for the regulation of mammalian sleep-wake behavior: reinterpretation of historical evidence and inclusion of contemporary cellular and molecular evidence. Neurosci Biobehav Rev. 2007;31:775–824. DOI: 10.1016/j.neubiorev.2007.02.004

[26] Datta S, Siwek DF. Excitation of the brain stem pedunculopontine tegmentum cholinergic cells induces wakefulness and REM sleep. J Neurophysiol. 1997;77:2975–2988. DOI:

[27] Kleiner S, Bringmann A. Nucleus basalis magnocellularis and pedunculopontine tegmental nucleus: control of slow EEG waves in rats. Arch Ital Biol. 1996;134:153–167. DOI:

[28] Rye DB. Contributions of the pedunculopontine region to normal and altered REM sleep. Sleep. 1997;20:757–788. DOI:

[29] Vertes RP. Brainstem control of the events of REM sleep. Prog Neurobiol. 1984;22:241–288. DOI: 10.1016/0301-0082(84)90020-0

[30] Inglis WL, Allen LF, Whitelaw RB, Latimer MP, Brace HM, Winn P. An investigation into the role of the pedunculopontine tegmental nucleus in the mediation of locomotion and orofacial stereotypy induced by D-amphetamine and apomorphine in the rat. Neuroscience. 1994;58:817–833. DOI: 10.1016/0306-4522(94)90459-6

[31] Saper CB, Loewy AD. Projections of the pedunculopontine tegmental nucleus in the rat: evidence for additional extrapyramidal circuitry. Brain Res. 1982;252:367–372. DOI: 10.1016/0006-8993(82)90404-8

[32] Takakusaki K, Habaguchi T, Saitoh K, Kohyama J. Changes in the excitability of hindlimb motoneurons during muscular atonia induced by stimulating the pedunculopontine tegmental nucleus in cats. Neuroscience. 2004;124:467–480. DOI: 10.1016/j.neuroscience.2003.12.016

[33] Lydic R, Baghdoyan HA. Pedunculopontine stimulation alters respiration and increases Ach release in the pontine reticular formation. Am J Physiol. 1993;264:R544–R554. DOI:

[34] Radulovacki M, Pavlovic S, Saponjic J, Carley DW. Modulation of reflex and sleep related apnea by pedunculopontine tegmental and intertrigeminal neurons. Respir Physiol Neurobiol. 2004;143:293–306. DOI: 10.1016/j.resp.2004.02.012

[35] Saponjic J, Radulovacki M, Carley DW. Respiratory pattern modulation by the pedunculopontine tegmental nucleus. Respir Physiol Neurobiol. 2003;138:223–237. DOI: 10.1016/j.resp.2003.08.002

[36] Saponjic J, Cvorovic J, Radulovacki M, Carley DW. 2005. Serotonin and noradrenaline modulate respiratory pattern disturbances evoked by glutamate injection into pedunculopontine tegmentum of anesthetized rats. Sleep. 2005;28:560–570. DOI:

[37] Saponjic J, Radulovacki M, Carley DW. Injection of glutamate into the pedunculopontine tegmental nuclei of anesthetized rat causes respiratory dysrhythmia and alters EEG and EMG power. Sleep Breath. 2005;9:82–91. DOI: 10.1007/s11325-005-0010-5

[38] Saponjic J, Radulovacki M, Carley DW. Modulation of respiratory pattern and upper airway muscle activity by the pedunculopontine tegmentum: Role of NMDA receptors. Sleep Breath. 2006;10:195–202. DOI 10.1007/s11325-006-0075-9

[39] Datta S. Neuronal activity in the peribrachial area: relationship to behavioral state control. Neurosci Biobehav Rev. 1995;19:67–84. DOI: 10.1016/0149-7634(94)00043-Z

[40] Datta S. Cellular basis of pontine ponto-geniculo-occipital wave generation and modulation. Cell Mol Neurobiol. 1997;17:341–365. DOI:

[41] Garcia-Rill E. 1991. The pedunculopontine nucleus. Prog Neurobiol. 1991;36:363–389. DOI: 10.1016/0301-0082(91)90016-T

[42] Kotagal V, Albin RL, Müller MLTM, Koeppe RA, Chervin RD, Frey KA, Bohnen NI. Symptoms of rapid eye movement sleep behavior disorder are associated with cholinergic denervation in Parkinson disease. Ann Neurol. 2012;7:560–568. DOI: 10.1002/ana.22691

[43] Bohnen NI, Müller MI, Koeppe RA, Studenski SA, Kilbourn MA, Fey KA, Albin RL. History of falls in Parkinson disease is associated with reduced cholinergic activity. Neurology. 2009;73:1670–1676. DOI: 10.1212/WNL.0b013e3181c1ded6

[44] Bohnen NI, Albin RL. The cholinergic system and Parkinson disease. Behav Brain Res. 2011;221:564–573. DOI: 10.1016/j.bbr.2009.12.048

[45] Kotagal V, Müller MLTM, Kaufer DI, Koeppe RA, Bohnen NI. Thalamic cholinergic innervation is spared in Alzheimer disease compared to parkinsonian disorders. Neurosci Lett. 2012;514:169–172. DOI: 10.1016/j.neulet.2012.02.083

[46] Chung KA, Lobb BM, Nutt JG, Horak F. Cholinergic augmentation in frequently falling subjects with Parkinson's disease. Mov Disord. 2009; 24(Suppl 1):S259. DOI:

[47] Saponjic J, Radulovacki M, Carley DW. Monoaminergic system lesions increase post-sigh respiratory pattern disturbance during sleep in rats. Physiol Behav. 2007;90:1–10. DOI: 10.1016/j.physbeh.2006.08.019

[48] Saponjic J, Petrovic J, Kalauzi A, Ciric J, Lazic K, Radulovacki M, Carley DW. Sleep-state related EEG amplitude distribution in the rat model of cortical cholinergic innervation disorder. Sleep Biol Rhythms. 2013;11:105–115. DOI: 10.1111/sbr.12011

[49] Petrovic J, Ciric J, Lazic K, Kalauzi A, Saponjic J. Lesion of the pedunculopontine tegmental nucleus in rat augments cortical activation and disturbs sleep/wake state transitions structure. Exp Neurol. 2013;247:562–571. DOI: 10.1016/j.expneurol.2013.02.007

[50] Petrovic J, Lazic K, Ciric J, Kalauzi A, Saponjic J. Topography of the sleep/wake states related EEG microstructure and transitions structure differentiates the functionally distinct cholinergic innervation disorders in rat. Behav Brain Res. 2013;256:108–118. DOI: 10.1016/j.bbr.2013.07.047

[51] Petrovic J, Lazic K, Kalauzi A, Saponjic J. REM sleep diversity following the pedunculopontine tegmental nucleus lesion in rat. Behav Brain Res. 2014;271:258–268. DOI: 10.1016/j.bbr.2014.06.026

[52] Lazic K, Petrovic J, Ciric J, Kalauzi A, Saponjic J. Impact of anesthetic regimen on the respiratory pattern, EEG microstructure and sleep in the rat model of cholinergic Parkinson's disease neuropathology. Neuroscience. 2015;304:1–13. DOI: 10.1016/j.neuroscience.2015.07.020

[53] Ciric J, Lazic K, Petrovic J, Kalauzi A, Saponjic J. Age-related disorders of sleep and motor control in the rat models of functionally distinct cholinergic neuropathology. Behav Brain Res. 2016;301:273–286. DOI: 10.1016/j.bbr.2015.12.046

[54] Paxinos G, Watson C. The Rat Brain in Stereotaxic Coordinates, 5th ed., Elsevier Academic Press, San Diego, USA; 2005. DOI:

[55] Inglis WL, Semba K. Discriminable excitotoxic effects of ibotenic acid, AMPA, NMDA and quinolinic acid in the rat laterodorsal tegmental nucleus. Brain Res. 1997;755:17-27. DOI: 10.1016/S0006-8993(97)00101-7

[56] Paxinos G, Watson C, Carrive P, Kirkcaldie M, Ashwell KWS. Chemoarchitectonic Atlas of The Rat Brain, 2nd ed. Academic Press, London, UK; 2009. DOI:

[57] Ciric J, Lazic K, Petrovic J, Kalauzi A, Saponjic J. Aging induced cortical drive alterations during sleep in rats. Mech Ageing Dev. 2015;146–148:12-22. DOI: 10.1016/j.mad.2015.03.002

[58] Krause V, Wach C, Sudmeyer M, Ferrea S, Schnitzler A, Pollok B. Cortico-muscular coupling and motor performance are modulated by 20 Hz transcranial alternating

current stimulation (tACS) in Parkinson's disease. Front Hum Neurosci. 2014;7:1–10. DOI: 10.3389/fnhum.2013.00928

[59] Peever J, Luppi PH, Montplaisir J. Breakdown in REM sleep circuitry underlies REM sleep behavior disorder. Trends Neurosci. 2014;37:279–288. DOI: 10.1016/j.tins.2014.02.009

[60] Kristeva R, Patino L, Omlor W. Beta-range cortical motor spectral power and corticomuscular coherence as a mechanism for effective corticospinal interaction during steady-state motor output. NeuroImage. 2007;36:785–792. DOI: 10.1016/j.neuroimage.2007.03.025

[61] Salenius S, Avikainen S, Kaakkola S, Hari R, Brown P. Defective cortical drive to muscle in Parkinson's disease and its improvement with levodopa. Brain. 2002;125:491–500. DOI: 10.1093/brain/awf042

[62] Bezard E, Przedborski S. A tale on animal models of Parkinson's disease. Mov Disord. 2011;26:993–1002. DOI: 10.1002/mds.23696

[63] Blandini F, Armentero MT, Martignoni E. The 6-hidroxydopamine model: news from the past. Parkinsonism Relat Disord. 2008;14 Suppl 2:S124–129. DOI: 10.1016/j.parkreldis.2008.04.015

[64] Blandini F, Armentero MT. Animal models of Parkinson's disease. FEBS J. 2012;279:1156–1166. DOI: 10.1111/j.1742-4658.2012.08491.x

[65] Duty S, Jenner P. Animal models of Parkinson's disease: a source of novel treatments and clues to the cause of the disease. Br J Pharmacol. 2011;164:1357–1391. DOI: 10.1111/j.1476-5381.2011.01426.x

[66] Pienaar IS, Harrison IF, Elson JL, Bury A, Woll P, Simon AK, Dexter DT. An animal model mimicking pedunculopontine nucleus cholinergic degeneration in Parkinson's disease. Brain Struct Funct. 2015;220:479–500. DOI: 10.1007/s00429-013-0669-5

[67] Pienaar IS, van de Berg W. A non-cholinergic neuronal loss in the pedunculopontine nucleus of toxin-evoked parkinsonian rats. Exp Neurol. 2013;248:213–223. DOI: 10.1016/j.expneurol.2013.06.008

Chapter 8

Cognitive Impairment in Parkinson's Disease: Historical Review, Past, and Present

Ivan Galtier, Antonieta Nieto and Jose Barroso

Additional information is available at the end of the chapter

http://dx.doi.org/10.5772/62888

Abstract

Parkinson's disease (PD) is a neurodegenerative disorder of unknown etiology, not only characterized by motor signs but also by non-motor symptoms, including neuropsychiatric and cognitive dysfunction. The results obtained in the last decades show that the cognitive changes in PD are heterogeneous; impairment in different cognitive domains such as attention, executive, language, memory, and visuospatial functions can be present even in the early stages of the disease. Mild cognitive impairment is frequent in non-demented PD patients and is considered as a risk factor for the development of dementia. As a response to the heterogeneity of cognitive impairment associated with PD, the Movement Disorders Society has recently developed formal diagnostic criteria for mild cognitive impairment and dementia associated with PD. In the present chapter, the authors have conducted a revision of cognitive impairment in PD, describing the results obtained in numerous investigations, from the first studies in the1970s to the advances of the last few years.

Keywords: Parkinson's disease, review, mild cognitive impairment, dementia, predictors variables

1. Introduction

Parkinson's disease (PD) is a neurodegenerative disorder of unknown etiology, characterized by tremor, rigidity, bradykinesia, and impairment of balance that are usually of an asymmetric course. The neuropathology of PD affects several structures that are implicated in movement control. The main neuropathologic feature of PD is the loss of dopaminergic neurons in the substantia nigra pars compacta, leading to a dysfunction of the frontostriatal system.

Ever since James Parkinson published his best known medical study, entitled "an essay on the shaking palsy" in 1817, this pathology has awakened scientific interest. Initially, most research effort focused on the understanding of motor symptoms and the search for effective treatment options. Levodopa, a precursor of dopamine, was discovered in the 1960s, and years later would be used as an effective treatment for the motor symptoms of PD. Coinciding with this historic landmark, a significant increase in interest in the non-motor symptoms associated with PD began to be observed, with special attention being paid to the cognitive symptoms, because of their impact on the quality of life of patients.

This chapter focuses on cognitive impairment in PD, from the first studies that paid attention to cognitive deficits to the present day concept of dementia associated to PD (PDD). There is a description of the neuropsychological profile classically associated with PD, going into the concept of mild cognitive impairment in PD (PD-MCI) in greater depth, which has given rise to numerous investigations in recent years. There is also a summary of the most relevant clinical and demographic variables associated with cognitive impairment in PD.

2. Cognitive impairment in PD: a historical review

2.1. First studies

PD is a neurodegenerative disorder described for the first time in 1817 by James Parkinson [1]. In the monographic entitled "an essay on the shaking palsy," the author described the clinical characteristics of a limited series of PD patients (Paralysis agitans). He defined the pathology as *"Involuntary tremulous motion, with lessened muscular power, in parts not in action and even when supported; with a propensity to bend the trunk forwards, and to pass from a walking to a running pace"* and affirmed that *"the senses and intellects being uninjured"*. However, subsequent studies showed that the last statement is not correct.

Charcot [2], is among the first authors to describe changes in mental functioning in PD. The author stated that in PD patients *"…the mind becomes clouded and the memory is lost"*. However, it was not until the 1960s and 1970s, coinciding with the first levodopa treatments, that scientific interest of the cognitive disorders associated with this pathology increased significantly. Over the following years, and even during 1980s, investigations were carried out without excessive control over the clinical variables (cause of Parkinsonism, stage of disease, duration of illness, etc.). An example is the study of Reitan and Boll [3]. These authors selected a group of 25 PD patients and twenty five controls matched on sex, age, and education, which were evaluated with a battery of psychological tests. The results showed that PD patients suffered deterioration in general cognition, memory, problem-solving, abstract reasoning, and organizing abilities. This was a pioneer study in the use of a wide assessment of cognitive functions. However, information about the clinical features of the patients was not provided (disease stage, duration, motor symptoms, etc.).

The study of cognitive deficits associated with PD and other neurological diseases characterized by basal ganglia pathology, such as Huntington's disease and progressive supranuclear palsy, gave rise to the concept of subcortical dementia, as opposed to predominantly cortical dementia characteristic of Alzheimer's disease [4, 5]. In this period, the concept of subcortical dementia is frequently associated in the literature with descriptions of cognitive impairment in PD. However, different authors consider that this label is often inaccurate and misleading because its application is not always suitable when referring to the cognitive impairment in PD; patients with PD may have cognitive deficits, without significantly affecting their daily lives [6, 7].

The discussions generated by the association between PD and the concept of subcortical dementia led to the development of numerous investigations with an increase in the interest in the control of clinical variables (disease stage, duration, motor symptoms, depression, etc.) and with more exhaustive neuropsychological evaluations [8–11]. The investigation conducted by Lees and Smith [12] is among the first studies to consider these characteristics. The authors conducted a careful sample selection according to the different variables related to the disease; they selected a sample of PD patients, in early-mid-stage of the disease (Hoehn and Yahr stage I–II), under 65 years of old, without depression and without antiparkinsonian drugs. The instruments administered included measures of general intelligence, executive functions, and memory. The PD patients only showed deficits in executive functions. Various investigations, such as the study of Lees and Smith [12], were performed in the 1980s and 1990s, and they led to the establishment of the neuropsychological profile classically associated with PD.

2.2. Neuropsychological profile of PD

Cognitive deficits in PD have traditionally been seen as an executive dysfunction secondary to frontostriatal system impairment. In this schema, this executive dysfunction is responsible for other cognitive disturbances that can appear in this pathology. However, the recently obtained results, in the last few decades, show that the cognitive changes in PD are more heterogeneous than initially thought. PD patients can have deficits in multiple cognitive domains including the executive functions but also in processing speed, attention, visuospatial functions, memory, and language. As will be seen below, the heterogeneity of cognitive impairment associated with PD cannot be explained exclusively as a consequence of dysexecutive syndrome.

PD is associated with cognitive slowing (bradyphrenia). Numerous studies have used reaction time tasks to evaluate processing speed and found that PD patients have deficits in simple and choice reaction time tests [13–18]. However, other investigations show that PD patients only present an altered execution in the choice reaction time task [19, 20]. The results of a meta-analysis conducted by Gauntlett-Gilbert and Brown [21] showed that patients exhibit an altered performance in simple and choice reaction time tasks, but the magnitude of the deficits was associated with the test complexity. This result has been explained in terms of a limitation of resources in tasks with more cognitive demands. Processing speed was also measured by Symbol Digit test and similar instruments; PD patients showed an altered execution with this type of test [22].

As regards attention and working memory, PD patients tend to perform normally in verbal tasks, such as digit span [22, 23], while their execution in visuospatial tasks is altered (visual span) [23, 24]. Siegert et al. [25] conducted a meta-analysis including 56 studies. They differentiated the working memory tests according to the stimuli characteristic (verbal, visual) and difficulty level (direct, inverse). The results showed that PD patients performed poorly in all the working memory tasks. However, in the verbal tests, the difficulty was more significant in the more complex tasks (inverse), while patients showed significant difference in simple and complex tasks in visual tests. Other authors studied working memory based on the n-back paradigm and found that patients had deficits, compared to controls, unrelated to the level of demand or the nature of the stimuli [26].

Visuospatial functions tend to be altered in PD, even in the early stage of the disease. Different authors reported an altered performance in judgment of line orientation [23, 27], facial recognition test [28, 29], and visuospatial reasoning such as Raven's test [8, 10]. Block design [27–30] and the copy of Rey Complex figure test [27, 29] were other instruments in which PD patients showed poor execution. It should be noted that the motor component involving this type of tasks was not controlled in most of these investigations.

Executive functions include a complex set of processes that has been defined as wide and diverse. Lezak [31] define the executive functions as those skills to respond adaptively to novel situations: *"The executive functions can be conceptualized as having four components: (1) volition; (2) planning; (3) purposive action; and (4) effective performance. Each involves a distinctive set of activity-related behaviors. All are necessary for appropriate, socially responsible, and effectively self-serving adult conduct" (page 650).*

The Wisconsin Cart Shorting Test (WCST) is one of the most widely used instruments for the assessment of executive functions; it measures the ability to form abstract concepts, develop strategies and use feedback to maintain or change the mental set on the objective. Numerous authors found that PD patients show an altered performance in this test, including less categories and a greater number of errors (e.g., see [32, 33]). Verbal fluency (VF) tests were also used to evaluate executive functions, as they are considered measures of cognitive flexibility and search strategy. Henry and Crawford [34] propose that phonetic fluency has more validity and specificity as a frontal impairment measure, compared with the WCST. The results obtained in PD with measures of VF are highly heterogeneous, both with phonetic and semantic fluency tests; different studies found an altered execution in PD patients [35–37], whereas other authors do not report the same results [38–40]. Henry and Crawford [41] studied the VF in PD by a meta-analysis that included 68 investigations and a total of 4644 participants. They found that PD is associated with a deficit in VF, with a greater involvement of semantic fluency in comparison with the phonetic fluency test. The difficulties are greater when versions of these tasks in which alternate consigns are used. According to the authors, the performance in VF in PD patients is not exclusively attributable to a deficit of executive functions (according to scores on the WCST); the relationship between the deficit of denomination task and VF performance suggests that PD is associated with a deficit in the recovery of information from semantic memory. Furthermore, the action fluency test has been considered an alternative VF measure of executive functions, since verb generation is strongly associated with the prefrontal cortex. PD patients show a poor performance with this task compared to controls [42].

Other instruments used to evaluate the executive functions in PD are the Trail Making Test (part B) and the Stroop test. As for the Trail Making Test, PD patients often have an altered performance [13, 19, 27]. However, with respect to the Stroop test, the results are heterogeneous: some authors report an altered performance in PD patients [15, 37, 43], whereas other research studies do not describe the same results [20, 22].

Regarding memory deficits in PD, classical descriptions consider that the alterations are confined to new information acquisition and spontaneous retrieval; the patients would show a normal performance in cued recall and recognition tasks. However, the results obtained in different investigations confirm that the affectation of memory functions in PD is more complex. PD patients often show an altered performance in different memory tests (Verbal Paired Associates, Logical Memory) [6, 44, 45], with a normal execution in recognition [44]. However, patients can perform poorly, compared to controls, even in recognition memory tasks [6]. Using tasks that allowed a more precise examination of different memory components (e.g., the Auditory Verbal Learning Test and the California Verbal Learning Test), some authors reported deficits in learning and spontaneous recall, without alteration in recognition [27, 37, 46]. However, this impairment pattern was not confirmed by other authors who found alterations in cued recall and recognition [47–50]. Whittington et al. [51] conducted a meta-analysis and concluded that PD patients have recognition deficits. Therefore, alteration of the verbal memory in PD is not exclusively limited to a deficit of information retrieval.

In regard to visual memory, there are fewer studies than those which are focused on verbal memory. The results obtained are diverse, probably as a consequence of the wide range of instruments used (Visual Retention Test, Visual Paired Associates, Face Memory Test, Complex Figure Test, etc.) [27, 45, 46, 52]. Visuospatial learning has been evaluated by Pillon et al. [53, 54] who found that PD patients present an altered execution. This result was confirmed in a more recent research study [23].

The first research studies into language functions in PD considered that the linguistic deficits observed in patients were a consequence of motor symptoms. Speech disorders were associated to alterations of phonation, facial musculature, reflections, articulation, and prosody [55–57]. However, in addition to the deficits described above, other alterations related to language production and comprehension are common in PD patients. The results of different studies show alterations in speech related to a lower proportion of sentences which are grammatically less complex [58–60]. On the other hand, the results obtained with the Boston naming test are not conclusive: some authors show an altered execution [8, 61], whereas other studies do not observe the same results [6, 44, 62]. Other investigations have been focused on the differentiation between the naming of actions and objects, based on the association of action generation with the frontal cortex. PD patients showed an altered performance in both naming tasks (naming and action), but the execution in the action naming was poorer than the naming of objects [63–65].

As for language comprehension in PD, it is worth mentioning the research line developed by the Grossman group. They reported the following results in a series of publications: patients had a normal performance in simple sentences and a deficient execution in complex sentences, with greater difficulty in those with subordinate clauses; patients show more difficulty when analyzing sentences with subordinate clauses, when the semantic information does not allow their understanding; patients make more mistakes in tasks requiring the matching of a sentence with a picture and patients show deficits when identifying phonetic errors in grammatical morphemes, such as pronouns. Taking all the results together, the authors concluded that PD patients show deficit in language comprehension, related to the limitation of cognitive resources including, attention, cognitive slowing and working memory [66–70]. However, other results do not confirm the conclusions of Grossman [66]. Skeel et al. [62] showed that the alterations of comprehension can be present even in simple sentences and that this deficit was not associated with the status of working memory. Other authors have recently described similar results to Skeel et al. [62]; Galtier et al. [47] reported deficits in language comprehension that cannot be exclusively explained by a limitation of cognitive resources.

In summary, the results obtained in a large number of research studies over the last 40 years confirm that the cognitive deficits associated with PD are heterogeneous, including alterations in different cognitive domains such as attention, memory, executive functions, language, and visuospatial functioning. In addition, these data also confirm that the cognitive alterations in PD patients cannot be exclusively reduced to an executive dysfunction, as has traditionally been thought.

3. Mild cognitive impairment in PD

3.1. Concept of PD-MCI

Reisberg et al. [71] published the Global Deterioration Scale (GDS) in 1982 describing seven stages from normal to severe dementia associated with Alzheimer's disease. The GDS differentiates between stage 2 in which persons complain of memory deficits (without objective evidence in clinical interview, in employment or social situations) and stage 3 which was initially termed "mild cognitive decline". Clinical deficits appear in stage 3 although the objective evidence of memory deficit is only obtained by means of an intensive interview conducted by a clinician. In addition, decreased performance becomes manifest in demanding employment and social situations. Stage 3 is different to a GDS 4 stage which is considered as the earliest stage of dementia. Deficits are manifest in many areas in stage 4 and patients can no longer perform complex tasks accurately and efficiently. A cross-sectional study in 1988 used the terminology "mild cognitive impairment" (MCI) for the first time to refer the GDS stage 3 [72]. The results showed that MCI patients performed poorly in different cognitive measures, compared to GDS stage 2 subjects group (subjective deficits only). In addition, the group with mild dementia (GDS stage 4) performed significantly more poorly than the MCI group in the Mini-Mental State Examination and other cognitive measurements.

The concept of MCI was developed and popularized years later by Petersen et al. [73] who proposed the following diagnostic criteria: (1) memory complaint, preferably corroborated by an informant; (2) objective memory impairment; (3) normal general cognitive function; (4) intact activities of daily living; (5) not demented. The International Working group on Mild

Cognitive Impairment statement in 2004 recommended the criteria which are currently accepted [74] (**Table 1**).

Inclusion criteria

- Not normal, not demented [does not meet criteria (DSM IV, ICD 10) for a dementia syndrome]
- Cognitive decline:

  -Self and/or informant report and impairment on objective cognitive tasks

  And/or

  -Evidence of decline over time on objective cognitive tasks

- Preserved basic activities of daily living and minimal impairment in complex instrumental functions

Adapted with permission from Winblad et al. [74]. © 2004 Blackwell Publishing Ltd.

Table 1. General criteria for MCI.

The construct of MCI in PD (PD-MCI) is a more recent concept, as a result of the gradual increase of interest in non-motor symptoms, the heterogeneity of cognitive deficits, and their impact on the quality of life of PD patients. The investigation of Janvin et al. [75] was the first study that focused on PD-MCI; it included 76 PD patients who were evaluated with a limited selection of neuropsychological tests (Benton Visual Retention Test, Judgment of Line Orientation test, Stroop Word Test). Forty-two patients had PD-MCI (55%), defined as scoring −2 standard deviations below the mean of the control group in at least one of the tests. In the PD-MCI group, 57% of the patients had an altered performance in one neuropsychological test, 33% in two tests while the remaining 10% had an altered execution in all the three tests.

In a recent review conducted by Litvan et al. [76], the authors reported that between 18.9% and 38.2% of PD patients met MCI criteria. However, the study of Janvin et al. [75], described above, and other investigations have reported results with higher percentages (51–55%) [77, 78]. These discrepancies can be explained by differences in the PD-MCI diagnostic criteria, number of cognitive domains explored or selection and number of neuropsychological tests used. Several studies used a less restrictive level (−1 standard deviation) to determine cognitive impairment, while other authors opted for a −1.5 standard deviation or −2 standard deviation cut-off. For example, Foltynie et al. [79] evaluated a group of 159 PD patients with different cognitive tests, including a pattern recognition memory, spatial recognition memory and the Tower of London task from the CANTAB battery. The results showed that 36% of PD patients were considered cognitively impaired, defined as scoring ≥1 standard deviation below the normative mean of at least one of the tests. Janvin et al. [80] conducted a study of cognitive function in a sample of 145 PD patients. Subjects with Mini-Mental State Examination score <25 were considered demented and excluded. Of the total sample, 72 PD patients without dementia were studied and compared to 38 normal controls. Of the nondemented PD patients, 52.8% were diagnosed with MCI, defined as impaired performance [−1.5 standard deviation or more below the mean of the control group) in one, two, or all three of the given neuropsychological tests (Benton Visual Retention Test, Judgment of Line Orientation test, Stroop Word Test). In the study of Muslimovic et al. [81], the authors opted for a −2 standard deviation cut-off. They assessed a sample of 115 nondemented newly diagnosed PD patients with neuropsychological tests which examined the following six cognitive domains: psychomotor speed, attention, language, memory, executive functions, and visuospatial. Cognitive dysfunction was considered to be present whether performance in three or more neuropsychological tests was impaired. The results showed that 27 PD patients (23.5%) had cognitive dysfunction.

As one can see, there has been no consensus on the number of tests that need to be considered as altered to establish a diagnosis of MCI; alteration in one or more tests was taken as a criterion for the diagnosis of MCI [80], while other authors consider that impairment should be present in at least three tests (either within a single cognitive domain or across different cognitive domains) [81]. Moreover, most of the studies used brief batteries or a set of neuropsychological tests that do not allow the evaluation of all cognitive domains with a sufficient level of accuracy. Some authors described cognitive impairment as defined by poor performance in a selection of tests from the CANTAB battery (pattern recognition memory, spatial recognition memory and the Tower of London task) [82]. Other research only evaluated four cognitive domains, including memory, executive, attention, and visuospatial. Only one test was used for the case of memory and attention. Moreover, visuospatial function was examined by one item of the Montreal Cognitive Assessment test, which is a screening instrument [83]. Muslimovic et al. [81] selected a wide range of neuropsychological tests to examine cognitive functions in the following six domains: psychomotor speed, attention, language, memory, executive functions, and visuospatial/constructive skills. However, not all the domains were studied in the same degree of detail; although the memory and executive domains were investigated in depth by up to six tests, only the Boston Naming Test was used for the language examination.

3.2. Diagnostic criteria for PD-MCI

As a response to the heterogeneity mentioned above, the Movement Disorder Society (MDS) commissioned a task force to develop formal diagnostic criteria for PD-MCI which were published in 2012 [84]. The criteria proposed by the MDS are intended to overcome most of the previously described limitations. The MDS task force proposes a uniform method to characterize and diagnose PD-MCI, providing a framework to advance the understanding of this pathology. The proposal of the task force sets out new objectives for the following years (**Table 2**).

I. Inclusion criteria

- Diagnosis of Parkinson's disease as based on the UK PD Brain Bank Criteria [124]
- Gradual decline, in the context of established PD, in cognitive ability reported by either the patient or informant, or observed by the clinician

- Cognitive deficits on either formal neuropsychological testing or a scale of global cognitive abilities
- Cognitive deficits are not sufficient to interfere significantly with functional independence, although subtle difficulties on complex functional tasks

II. Exclusion criteria

- Diagnosis of PD dementia based on MDS Task Force proposed criteria [123]
- Other primary explanations for cognitive impairment (e.g., delirium, stroke, major depression, metabolic abnormalities, adverse effects of medication, or head trauma)
- Other PD associated comorbid conditions (e.g., motor impairment or severe anxiety, depression, excessive daytime sleepiness, or psychosis) that, in the opinion of the clinician, significantly influence cognitive testing

Adapted with permission from Litvan et al. [84]. © 2012 Movement Disorder Society.

Table 2. MDS Criteria for the Diagnosis of PD-MCI.

The MDS criteria included a two-level operational schema that differs in the comprehensiveness of the neuropsychological testing. Level 1 criteria provide less diagnostic certainty than level 2: (A) Impairment on a scale of global cognitive abilities or impairment on a limited battery of neuropsychological tests. When a limited battery of tests is performed, impairment must be present in at least two tests for a diagnosis of PD-MCI (level 1); (B) Comprehensive neuropsychological testing that includes two tests in each of the five cognitive domains (attention and working memory, executive, language, memory, and visuospatial). Impairment should be present in at least two tests, either within a single cognitive domain or across different cognitive domains (level 2). In addition, impairment in neuropsychological tests may be demonstrated by performance approximately 1–2 standard deviations below age, education, gender, and culturally appropriate norms; or a significant decline demonstrated in serial cognitive testing; or a significant decline from estimated premorbid levels.

As proposed by the MDS task force, classification of PD-MCI subtypes is important for research purposes and for exploring whether impairments in different cognitive domains have a different neurobiological substrate and course. Comprehensive neuropsychological testing is required (level 2) for the PD-MCI sub-types classification. The use of two tests in each cognitive domain for the level 2 category examines all cognitive domains equally, can increase sensitivity and allow full subtyping of PD-MCI. The presence of two altered tests within a single cognitive domain, with the other domains unimpaired, represents a single domain subtype. Whether at least one test in two or more cognitive domains is impaired, then PD-MCI should be subtyped as multiple domain. The proposed MDS criteria recommend not using amnestic or nonamnestic terminology. Instead, specification of the affected domains is preferable so that potential differences among subtypes may be better analyzed in futures studies.

Up to now, only a few studies have provided data with the MDS PD-MCI criteria. Broeders et al. [85] examined a group of 123 newly diagnosed PD patients and found that PD-MCI was present in 35% of cases, when level 2 was applied (comprehensive assessment). In a more recent investigation, Stefanova et al. [86], applying level 2 of the MDS criteria, examined 111 early

PD patients and 105 healthy matched control subjects; PD-MCI was present in 24% of the patients. The differences in percentages compared to the study of Broeders et al. [85] can be explained by the clinical characteristics of PD patients; Stefanova et al. [86] included patients in stage 1 (Hoehn and Yahr] while the patient sample of the Broeders et al. [85] study were in stages 1 and 2. Pedersen et al. [87] examined a sample of 182 PD patients (Hoehn and Yahr stage 1–2), applying level 1 (brief assessment) of the MDS criteria and found that 20.3% of patients met MCI criteria. Other authors evaluated patients who had a mean PD duration of 5.2 and 14.1 years and found that PD-MCI was present in 33–42.6% of the patients respectively, when level 2 was used [88, 89]. Recently, Galtier et al. [90] showed that 60.5% of the patients were diagnosed with PD-MCI according to level 2 MDS criteria. The percentage of PD-MCI in this study was slightly higher than that obtained in previous studies. These differences could be explained by the tests used to assess the linguistic domain. The authors included an assessment of language comprehension, unlike the methodology used in previous investigations. Most of the studies that applied the MDS task force criteria used −1.5 SD cut-off [85, 87, 89, 90]. Goldman et al. [91], using a cut-off of 2 SD below norms, reported that 61.8% of patients (mean PD duration of 9.3 years) were classified as PD-MCI with level 2 of the MDS criteria. The subtype categorization showed the high predominance of the multiple-domain PD-MCI with percentages of between 84 and 96% [90, 92, 93].

4. Relationship between cognitive impairment in PD and clinical variables

There are many research studies which have studied the relationship between cognitive impairment and potential predictor variables. Cognitive performance has been related to the neurological impairment, duration of illness, age at onset of PD, depressive symptoms and educational level, among others. As we shall see, the results are diverse which could once again be interpreted as a reflection of the heterogeneity of cognitive impairment in PD.

Regarding neurological impairment, different investigations have opted for correlation analysis and found that the degree of neurological impairment was associated with poor performance in visuospatial functions [28, 94], processing speed [95], working memory [24], procedural learning [37] and executive functions [96, 97]. However, other authors have not confirmed these results finding no relationship between the neurological impairment and different cognitive functions, such as processing speed [98], visuospatial functions [99], or procedural learning [100, 101]. Neither has an association with declarative memory [53, 100, 102] or linguistic functions (comprehension sentences, verbs generation) [67, 103–105] been found.

Other investigations compared PD patients with different levels of neurological impairment according to the Hoehn and Yahr scale. Although these studies are less frequent, patients with mid-late PD (according to Hoehn and Yahr stage) often present more affectation in different cognitive domains. The investigation conducted by Huber et al. [8] was one of the first studies that examined cognitive performance by comparing patients with different stages of PD. Moderate-to-late stage patients performed poorly in visuospatial functions, memory, executive functions, and naming. The results of Huber et al. [8] are clear evidence that the deterioration in the PD is not homogeneous, but that it is linked to the severity of the disease. Other authors also found differences in cognitive functions related to neurological impairment. For example, late disease stage patients showed poor performance in immediate memory (verbal and visual) [106], and executive functions (alternating series) [20].

Quite a few investigations pay attention to the relationship between illness duration and cognitive impairment. Research studies using correlation analysis showed that disease duration was not associated to processing speed [95, 98], working memory [10, 102], procedural learning [37], visuospatial functions [107], executive functions [10, 96], or sentence comprehension [67, 108, 109]. The results are more heterogeneous for other cognitive functions such as memory; some authors showed that disease duration was related to poor performance in diverse memory tests [10], while others did not find similar results [53, 110].

Other authors have demonstrated that cognitive dysfunction occurs even at the time of PD diagnosis. Foltynie et al. [79] showed that 36% of newly diagnosed PD patients had signs of cognitive impairment based on their performance in a pattern recognition memory task and in the Tower of London task. Similarly, Muslimovic et al. [81] examined a sample of newly diagnosed PD patients and found poor performance in different cognitive tasks; the differences when compared to normative data could mainly be explained by measures of immediate memory and executive function.

The age at onset of the disease has been associated with an increased risk of cognitive impairment, in other words the older the age at onset, the greater risk of cognitive decline, as measured with the Mini-Mental State Examination [111]. The study of relationship between age at onset of the disease and different cognitive functions revealed that the older the patient was at onset, the more likely the patient was to perform poorly in declarative memory (verbal and visual), executive, visuospatial and language functions (naming) [10, 15, 112, 113].

Depression is among the most common neuropsychiatric disturbances in PD. Different studies have concluded that between 36 and 60% of patients show depressive symptoms [114–116]. Numerous investigations have focused on the association between cognitive impairment and depression in PD. Depression has been associated with poor performance in global cognition, as measured by instruments such as the Mini-Mental State Examination or the Dementia Rating Scale [116–118]. Some authors who have studied the relationship between depressive symptoms and specific cognitive functions showed that depression was related to poor performance in different measures of executive functions [11] and in the comprehension of complex sentences [62]. However, other authors did not find any connection between depression and different cognitive functions, including processing speed [95], visuospatial functions [99], declarative memory [48], procedural learning [101], or sentence comprehension [67].

Certain authors have compared PD patients with and without depression by means of a comprehensive neuropsychological assessment. The results showed that patients with depressive symptoms presented an altered performance in declarative memory and semantic fluency, without showing differences in verbal span, phonetic fluency, concept formation, or naming. However, when both groups of patients (with and without depression) were equated according to the Dementia Rating Scale no differences were found between the groups [119]. Ng et al. [120] recently looked into the influence of depression in cognitive functions using a longitudinal study. They examined eighty one PD patients who were classified into two groups; with and without depression, according to the score in the Geriatric Depression Scale (score ≥5 was required for depression diagnosis). The results showed that PD patients with depression had a slightly lower performance in global cognition, as measured by the Mini-Mental State Examination and the Montreal Cognitive Assessment test, although these differences did not reach statistical significance. On the other hand, no differences were found between patients with and without depression in a set of neuropsychological tests that included measures of attention, memory, executive, visuospatial, and language functions. An 18 month longitudinal study was conducted, and similar results to the baseline were found; both groups of patients did not differ in global cognition and cognitive measures. Therefore, although the depression in PD appears to have some effect on global cognition and some specific cognitive functions, the available results suggest that both depression and cognitive impairment evolve independently in this pathology.

As regards the study of clinical variables associated with PD-MCI, according to the new MDS task force criteria, the available data are still limited. The study of Pedersen et al. [87] found that patients with PD-MCI were older, had less education, longer disease duration and higher Hoehn and Yahr stage than patients without PD-MCI. Hobson and Meara [93] showed that PD-MCI was associated to increasing age and worsening motor function. Galtier et al. [90] reported that PD-MCI was associated with lower education and higher neurological impairment, as measured by the Hoehn and Yahr scale, although they did not find age of onset or duration to be important factors.

5. Dementia in PD

As we have seen in first section of the present chapter, the interest in dementia associated to PD patients dates back to the 1960s and over the last 30 years there have a large number of studies into the epidemiology of PDD. Aarsland et al. [121] conducted a review of 4336 patients in 27 studies and showed that the mean prevalence of PDD was 40%. The prevalence of dementia increased from 28% after 5 years of follow-up, to 48% at 15 years, and up to 83% after 20 years. Moreover, PDD has been associated with increased mortality; after 20 years of follow-up of newly diagnosed PD patients 100 of 136 (74%) have died [122].

The Movement Disorder Society (MDS) recruited a Task Force to define the clinical diagnostic criteria for PDD which were published in 2007 [123]. The defining feature of PDD is that dementia develops in the context of established PD. Hence, diagnosis of idiopathic PD (based on the UK PD Brain Bank Criteria) [124] before the development of dementia symptoms is the essential first step in the diagnosis. Diagnosis of dementia must be based on the

http://dx.doi.org/10.5772/62888

presence of deficits in at least two of the four core cognitive domains (attention, memory, executive, and visuospatial functions) as shown in clinical and cognitive examination, and be severe enough to affect normal functioning. Neuropsychiatric and behavioral symptoms are frequent, but are not invariable (**Table 3**). Clinical diagnostic criteria for probable and possible PDD are proposed by the MDS (**Table 4**).

I. Core features

1. Diagnosis of Parkinson's disease according to Queen Square Brain Bank criteria

2. A dementia syndrome with insidious onset and slow progression, developing within the context of established Parkinson's disease and diagnosed by history, clinical, and mental examination, defined as:

    - Impairment in more than one cognitive domain
    - Representing a decline from premorbid level
    - Deficits severe enough to impair daily life (social, occupational, or personal care), independent of the impairment ascribable to motor or autonomic symptoms

II. Associated clinical features

1. Cognitive features:

    - Attention: Impaired. Impairment in spontaneous and focused attention, poor performance in attentional tasks; performance may fluctuate during the day and from day to day
    - Executive functions: Impaired. Impairment in tasks requiring initiation, planning, concept formation, rule finding, set shifting or set maintenance; impaired mental speed (bradyphrenia).
    - Visuospatial functions: Impaired. Impairment in tasks requiring visual-spatial orientation, perception, or construction
    - Memory: Impaired. Impairment in free recall of recent events or in tasks requiring learning new material, memory usually improves with cueing, recognition is usually better than free recall
    - Language: Core functions largely preserved. Word finding difficulties and impaired comprehension of complex sentences may be present

2. Behavioral features:

    - Apathy: decreased spontaneity; loss of motivation, interest, and effortful behavior
    - Changes in personality and mood including depressive features and anxiety
    - Hallucinations: mostly visual, usually complex, formed visions of people, animals or objects
    - Delusions: usually paranoid, such as infidelity, or phantom boarder (unwelcome guests living in the home) delusions
    - Excessive daytime sleepiness

III. Features which do not exclude PD-D, but make the diagnosis uncertain

- Co-existence of any other abnormality which may by itself cause cognitive impairment, but judged not to be the cause of dementia, e.g. presence of relevant vascular disease in imaging
- Time interval between the development of motor and cognitive symptoms not known

IV. Features suggesting other conditions or diseases as cause of mental impairment, which, when present make it impossible to reliably diagnose PDD

- The cognitive and behavioral symptoms appearing solely in the context of other conditions such as:

  Acute confusion due to

  a. Systemic diseases or abnormalities

  b. Drug intoxication

  Major Depression according to DSM IV

- Features compatible with "Probable Vascular dementia" criteria according to NINDS-AIREN

Adapted with permission from Emre et al. [123]. © 2007 Movement Disorder Society.

Table 3. Features of PDD.

Probable PDD

1. Core features: Both must be present

2. Associated clinical features:

- Typical profile of cognitive deficits including impairment in at least two of the four core cognitive domains (impaired attention which may fluctuate, impaired executive functions, impairment in visuo-spatial functions, and impaired free recall memory which usually improves with cueing)
- The presence of at least one behavioral symptom (apathy, depressed or anxious mood, hallucinations, delusions, excessive daytime sleepiness) supports the diagnosis of Probable PDD, lack of behavioral symptoms, however, does not exclude the diagnosis

3. None of the group III features present

4. None of the group IV features present

Possible PDD

1. Core features: Both must be present

2. Associated clinical features:

- Atypical profile of cognitive impairment in one or more domains, such as prominent or receptive-type (fluent) aphasia, or pure storage-failure type amnesia (memory does not improve with cueing or in recognition tasks) with preserved attention
- Behavioral symptoms may or may not be present

OR

3.	One or more of the group III features present
4.	None of the group IV features present

Adapted with permission from Emre et al. [123]. © 2007 Movement Disorder Society.

Table 4. Criteria for the diagnosis of probable and possible PDD.

All epidemiological studies assessing the progression to dementia in PD have observed a high frequency of cognitive defects in patients without dementia; neuropsychological defects indicative of predominant posterior cortical dysfunction have been associated to dementia [125]. Along these lines, some investigations have examined whether cognitive performance in the first stages of the disease could predict the future development of dementia. The results obtained by different authors show that memory domain performance was a significant predictor to develop PDD [87, 90, 126, 127], although other cognitive domains such as attention [87], executive [128], visuospatial [82], and language [126] have also been identified as predictors of the development of dementia. Once again, these outcomes can be considered as evidence of the neuropathological heterogeneity associated with the evolution of PD. Over time, progression of cognitive impairment in PD is explained by the deterioration of the previously affected cognitive domains, but new symptoms and new cognitive defects seem to have a special impact on the conversion to PDD. In a longitudinal study, patients who developed PDD were characterized by the presence of defects in language functions; the comparison between patients with PDD, Alzheimer's disease, and dementia with Lewy bodies showed that the three groups had the same degree of difficulty in confrontation naming [129].

On the other hand, different clinical and demographic variables have been associated with the development of PDD and the most consistently reported are older age, lower education, greater severity of motor symptoms and REM sleep behavior disorder [126, 130–133]. Visual hallucinations have also been considered as a risk factor to develop dementia. In an 8-year prospective study, the presence of visual hallucinations at baseline proved a significant predictor of PDD [134]. A recent investigation with a sample of PD-MCI patients showed that 50% of patients with visual hallucinations developed PDD, in contrast to 25% of patients without hallucinations [135].

Recent studies have demonstrated that PD-MCI diagnosis is also associated with the development of dementia. The results described by different authors showed that patients who were diagnosed with PD-MCI have an increased risk of developing PDD in the years following diagnosis. In a 3 year longitudinal study with early PD patients, significantly more patients with PD-MCI than PD patients with normal cognition progressed to dementia; among patients with PD-MCI 27% developed PDD (annual progression rate of 9%), whereas only 0.7% of patients with normal cognition developed PDD [87]. Domellöf et al. [88] conducted a 5 year longitudinal study which included 115 PD patients with neuropsychological testing. Of the 115 patients, 31 (27%) developed PDD, which corresponds to an incidence rate of 62.6 per 1000 person-years. Forty-nine (42.6%) patients were classified as having MCI according to MDS criteria, of which 25 (51%) developed PDD within 5 years, corresponding to an incidence rate of 142 per 1000 person-years. Similarly, Galtier et al. [90] showed that 42.3% of PD-MCI patients had dementia in a six to eight follow up study, whereas in the group of PD patients with normal cognition only 23.5% developed dementia during the follow up study. In addition, a 16 year longitudinal study showed that 91% of PD-MCI patients had progressed to PDD [93]. Santangelo et al. [136] examined 76 patients who underwent neuropsychological testing at baseline (Hoehn and Yahr stage 1–2), and at 2 and 4 years; 32.9% of PD patients had developed PD-MCI at baseline (level 2). No patient went from PD-MCI to dementia after 2 years, while 5.5% developed dementia after 4 years. The percentage of conversion to PDD is lower than that reported in previous studies. The authors considered that a possible explanation for this discrepancy might be found in the characteristics of our patients, who were relatively young and had mild disease severity compared to other studies stated above.

6. Conclusions

In summary, the study of cognitive functions in PD has awakened much scientific and research interest during the last 60 years. PD patients may even show cognitive deficits in the early stages of the pathology, as has been confirmed in studies with newly diagnosed patients. Cognitive impairment in PD is associated with alterations in different cognitive domains including deficits in attention, executive, memory, visuospatial and language functions. However, the heterogeneity in the manifestations and progression of these deficits is a characteristic of the pathology. In addition, different clinical and demographic variables have been linked to the evolution of cognitive impairment, with some of the most relevant being neurological impairment, disease duration, older age and educational level. Diagnostic criteria for PD-MCI and PDD have recently been developed and provide a uniform method to characterize the evolution of cognitive impairment in PD and advance the understanding of this pathology. The results demonstrate that PD-MCI is common in PD patients affecting around 25% in the first stages and increasing to over 50% according to the progression of the disease. Moreover, PD-MCI is considered a risk factor in the development of PDD, with a high conversion rate to dementia in the years following the PD-MCI diagnosis.

Author details

Ivan Galtier*, Antonieta Nieto and Jose Barroso

*Address all correspondence to: igaltier@ull.edu.es

School of Psychology, University of La Laguna, Tenerife, Spain

http://dx.doi.org/10.5772/62888

References

[1] Parkinson J. An Essay on the Shaking Palsy. London: Sherwood, Neely and Jones; 1817. 88 p.

[2] Charcot JM. [Lectures on the diseases of the nervous system]. 2° Edition. Paris: Delahaye et Lecrosnier; 1875.

[3] Reitan RM, Boll TJ. Intellectual and cognitive functions in Parkinson's disease. J Consult Clin Psychol. 1971;37(3):364–9.

[4] Cummings JL, Benson DF. Subcortical dementia. Review of an emerging concept. Arch Neurol. 1984;41(8):874–9.

[5] Huber SJ, Shuttleworth EC, Paulson GW. Dementia in Parkinson's disease. Arch Neurol. 1986;43(10):987–90.

[6] Levin BE, Llabre MM, Weiner WJ. Cognitive impairments associated with early Parkinson's disease. Neurology. 1989;39(4):557–61.

[7] Matthews CG, Haaland KY. The effect of symptom duration on cognitive and motor performance in parkinsonism. Neurology. 1979;29(7):951–6.

[8] Huber SJ, Freidenberg DL, Shuttleworth EC, Paulson GW, Christy JA. Neuropsychological impairments associated with severity of Parkinson's disease. J Neuropsychiatry Clin Neurosci. 1989;1(2):154–8.

[9] Pillon B, Dubois B, Lhermitte F, Agid Y. Heterogeneity of cognitive impairment in progressive supranuclear palsy, Parkinson's disease, and Alzheimer's disease. Neurology. 1986;36(9):1179–85.

[10] Pillon B, Dubois B, Bonnet AM, Esteguy M, Guimaraes J, Vigouret JM, et al. Cognitive slowing in Parkinson's disease fails to respond to levodopa treatment: the 15-objects test. Neurology. 1989;39(6):762–8.

[11] Starkstein SE, Bolduc PL, Preziosi TJ, Robinson RG. Cognitive impairments in different stages of Parkinson's disease. J Neuropsychiatry Clin Neurosci. 1989;1(3):243–8.

[12] Lees AJ, Smith E. Cognitive deficits in the early stages of Parkinson's disease. Brain. 1983;106 (Pt 2):257–70.

[13] Akamatsu T, Fukuyama H, Kawamata T. The effects of visual, auditory, and mixed cues on choice reaction in Parkinson's disease. J Neurol Sci. 2008;269(1–2):118–25.

[14] Dubois B, Pillon B, Legault F, Agid Y, Lhermitte F. Slowing of cognitive processing in progressive supranuclear palsy. A comparison with Parkinson's disease. Arch Neurol. 1988;45(11):1194–9.

[15] Hietanen M, Teräväinen H. Cognitive performance in early Parkinson's disease. Acta Neurol Scand. 1986;73(2):151–9.

[16] Jahanshahi M, Brown RG, Marsden CD. Simple and choice reaction time and the use of advance information for motor preparation in Parkinson's disease. Brain. 1992;115 (Pt 2:539–64.

[17] Jordan N, Sagar HJ, Cooper JA. Cognitive components of reaction time in Parkinson's disease. J Neurol Neurosurg Psychiatry. 1992;55(8):658–64.

[18] Kutukcu Y, Marks WJ, Goodin DS, Aminoff MJ. Simple and choice reaction time in Parkinson's disease. Brain Res. 1999 9;815(2):367–72.

[19] Camicioli RM, Wieler M, de Frias CM, Martin WRW. Early, untreated Parkinson's disease patients show reaction time variability. Neurosci Lett. 2008;441(1):77–80.

[20] de Frias CM, Dixon RA, Fisher N, Camicioli R. Intraindividual variability in neurocognitive speed: a comparison of Parkinson's disease and normal older adults. Neuropsychologia. 2007;45(11):2499–507.

[21] Gauntlett-Gilbert J, Brown VJ. Reaction time deficits and Parkinson's disease. Neurosci Biobehav Rev. 1998;22(6):865–81.

[22] Dujardin K, Denève C, Ronval M, Krystkowiak P, Humez C, Destée A, et al. Is the paced auditory serial addition test (PASAT) a valid means of assessing executive function in Parkinson's disease? Cortex. 2007;43(5):601–6.

[23] Galtier I, Nieto A, Barroso J, Lorenzo N. [Visuospatial learning impairment in Parkinson Disease]. Psicothema. 2009;21:21–6.

[24] Kemps E, Szmalec A, Vandierendonck A, Crevits L. Visuo-spatial processing in Parkinson's disease: evidence for diminished visuo-spatial sketch pad and central executive resources. Parkinsonism Relat Disord. 2005;11(3):181–6.

[25] Siegert RJ, Weatherall M, Taylor KD, Abernethy DA. A meta-analysis of performance on simple span and more complex working memory tasks in Parkinson's disease. Neuropsychology. 2008;22(4):450–61.

[26] Beato R, Levy R, Pillon B, Vidal C, du Montcel ST, Deweer B, et al. Working memory in Parkinson's disease patients: clinical features and response to levodopa. Arq Neuropsiquiatr. 2008;66(2A):147–51.

[27] Uc EY, Rizzo M, Anderson SW, Qian S, Rodnitzky RL, Dawson JD. Visual dysfunction in Parkinson disease without dementia. Neurology. 2005;65(12):1907–13.

[28] Bruna O, Roig C, Junqué C, Vendrell P. [Relationship between visuospatial impairment and oculomotor parameters in Parkinson's disease]. Psicothema. 2000;12:187–91.

[29] Sanchez Rodriguez JL. [Neuropsychological deficit in Parkinson's disease. Its relation with clinical variables]. Rev Neurol. 2002;35(4):310–7.

[30] Witt K, Nuhsman A, Deuschl G. Dissociation of habit-learning in Parkinson's and cerebellar disease. J Cogn Neurosci. 2002;14(3):493–9.

[31] Lezak MD. Neuropsychological Assessment. 3rd edition. New York: Oxford University Press; 1995.

[32] Liozidou A, Potagas C, Papageorgiou SG, Zalonis I. The role of working memory and information processing speed on Wisconsin card sorting test performance in Parkinson disease without dementia. J Geriatr Psychiatry Neurol. 2012;25(4):215–21.

[33] Paolo AM, Axelrod BN, Tröster AI, Blackwell KT, Koller WC. Utility of a Wisconsin card sorting test short form in persons with Alzheimer's and Parkinson's disease. J Clin Exp Neuropsychol. 1996;18(6):892–7.

[34] Henry JD, Crawford JR. A meta-analytic review of verbal fluency performance following focal cortical lesions. Neuropsychology. 2004;18(2):284–95.

[35] Bouquet CA, Bonnaud V, Gil R. Investigation of supervisory attentional system functions in patients with Parkinson's disease using the Hayling task. J Clin Exp Neuropsychol. 2003;25(6):751–60.

[36] Mimura M, Oeda R, Kawamura M. Impaired decision-making in Parkinson's disease. Parkinsonism Relat Disord. 2006;12(3):169–75.

[37] Muslimovic D, Post B, Speelman JD, Schmand B. Motor procedural learning in Parkinson's disease. Brain. 2007;130(Pt 11):2887–97.

[38] Brand M, Labudda K, Kalbe E, Hilker R, Emmans D, Fuchs G, et al. Decision-making impairments in patients with Parkinson's disease. Behav Neurol. 2004;15(3–4):77–85.

[39] Schneider JS. Behavioral persistence deficit in Parkinson's disease patients. Eur J Neurol. 2007;14(3):300–4.

[40] Troyer AK, Moscovitch M, Winocur G, Leach L, Freedman M. Clustering and switching on verbal fluency tests in Alzheimer's and Parkinson's disease. J Int Neuropsychol Soc. 1998;4(2):137–43.

[41] Henry JD, Crawford JR. Verbal fluency deficits in Parkinson's disease: a meta-analysis. J Int Neuropsychol Soc. 2004;10(4):608–22.

[42] Signorini M, Volpato C. Action fluency in Parkinson's disease: a follow-up study. Mov Disord. 2006;21(4):467–72.

[43] Hsieh Y-H, Chen K-J, Wang C-C, Lai C-L. Cognitive and motor components of response speed in the stroop test in Parkinson's disease patients. Kaohsiung J Med Sci. 2008;24(4): 197–203.

[44] el-Awar M, Becker JT, Hammond KM, Nebes RD, Boller F. Learning deficit in Parkinson's disease. Comparison with Alzheimer's disease and normal aging. Arch Neurol. 1987;44(2):180–4.

[45] Revonsuo A, Portin R, Koivikko L, Rinne JO, Rinne UK. Slowing of information processing in Parkinson's disease. Brain Cogn. 1993;21(1):87–110.

[46] Stefanova ED, Kostic VS, Ziropadja LJ, Ocic GG, Markovic M. Declarative memory in early Parkinson's disease: serial position learning effects. J Clin Exp Neuropsychol. 2001;23(5):581–91.

[47] Galtier I, Nieto A, Lorenzo JN, Barroso J. Cognitive impairment in Parkinson's disease: more than a frontostriatal dysfunction. Span J Psychol. 2014;17:1–8.

[48] Higginson CI, Wheelock VL, Carroll KE, Sigvardt KA. Recognition memory in Parkinson's disease with and without dementia: evidence inconsistent with the retrieval deficit hypothesis. J Clin Exp Neuropsychol. 2005;27(4):516–28.

[49] Kelly SW, Jahanshahi M, Dirnberger G. Learning of ambiguous versus hybrid sequences by patients with Parkinson's disease. Neuropsychologia. 2004;42(10):1350–7.

[50] Vingerhoets G, Vermeule E, Santens P. Impaired intentional content learning but spared incidental retention of contextual information in non-demented patients with Parkinson's disease. Neuropsychologia. 2005;43(5):675–81.

[51] Whittington CJ, Podd J, Kan MM. Recognition memory impairment in Parkinson's disease: power and meta-analyses. Neuropsychology. 2000;14(2):233–46.

[52] Uekermann J, Daum I, Peters S, Wiebel B, Przuntek H, Müller T. Depressed mood and executive dysfunction in early Parkinson's disease. Acta Neurol Scand. 2003;107(5): 341–8.

[53] Pillon B, Ertle S, Deweer B, Sarazin M, Agid Y, Dubois B. Memory for spatial location is affected in Parkinson's disease. Neuropsychologia. 1996;34(1):77–85.

[54] Pillon B, Deweer B, Vidailhet M, Bonnet AM, Hahn-Barma V, Dubois B. Is impaired memory for spatial location in Parkinson's disease domain specific or dependent on "strategic" processes? Neuropsychologia. 1998;36(1):1–9.

[55] Critchley EM. Speech disorders of Parkinsonism: a review. J Neurol Neurosurg Psychiatry. 1981;44(9):751–8.

[56] Ho AK, Iansek R, Bradshaw JL. The effect of a concurrent task on Parkinsonian speech. J Clin Exp Neuropsychol. 2002;24(1):36–47.

[57] Lloyd AJ. Comprehension of prosody in Parkinson's disease. Cortex. 1999;35(3):389–402.

[58] Cummings JL, Darkins A, Mendez M, Hill MA, Benson DF. Alzheimer's disease and Parkinson's disease: comparison of speech and language alterations. Neurology. 1988;38(5):680–4.

[59] Illes J, Metter EJ, Hanson WR, Iritani S. Language production in Parkinson's disease: acoustic and linguistic considerations. Brain Lang. 1988;33(1):146–60.

[60] Murray LL. Spoken language production in Huntington's and Parkinson's diseases. J Speech Lang Hear Res. 2000;43(6):1350–66.

[61] Goldman WP, Baty JD, Buckles VD, Sahrmann S, Morris JC. Cognitive and motor functioning in Parkinson disease: subjects with and without questionable dementia. Arch Neurol. 1998;55(5):674–80.

[62] Skeel RL, Crosson B, Nadeau SE, Algina J, Bauer RM, Fennell EB. Basal ganglia dysfunction, working memory, and sentence comprehension in patients with Parkinson's disease. Neuropsychologia. 2001;39(9):962–71.

[63] Bertella L, Albani G, Greco E, Priano L, Mauro A, Marchi S, et al. Noun verb dissociation in Parkinson's disease. Brain Cogn. 2002;48(2–3):277–80.

[64] Cotelli M, Borroni B, Manenti R, Zanetti M, Arévalo A, Cappa SF, et al. Action and object naming in Parkinson's disease without dementia. Eur J Neurol. 2007;14(6):632–7.

[65] Rodríguez-Ferreiro J, Menéndez M, Ribacoba R, Cuetos F. Action naming is impaired in Parkinson disease patients. Neuropsychologia. 2009;47(14):3271–4.

[66] Grossman M. Sentence processing in Parkinson's disease. Brain Cogn. 1999;40(2):387–413.

[67] Grossman M, Carvell S, Stern MB, Gollomp S, Hurtig HI. Sentence comprehension in Parkinson's disease: the role of attention and memory. Brain Lang. 1992;42(4):347–84.

[68] Grossman M, Kalmanson J, Bernhardt N, Morris J, Stern MB, Hurtig HI. Cognitive resource limitations during sentence comprehension in Parkinson's disease. Brain Lang. 2000;73(1):1–16.

[69] Grossman M, Zurif E, Lee C, Prather P, Kalmanson J, Stern MB, et al. Information processing speed and sentence comprehension in Parkinson's disease. Neuropsychology. 2002;16(2):174–81.

[70] Lee C, Grossman M, Morris J, Stern MB, Hurtig HI. Attentional resource and processing speed limitations during sentence processing in Parkinson's disease. Brain Lang. 2003;85(3):347–56.

[71] Reisberg B, Ferris SH, de Leon MJ, Crook T. The Global Deterioration Scale for assessment of primary degenerative dementia. Am J Psychiatry. 1982;139(9):1136–9.

[72] Reisberg B, Ferris SH, de Leon MJ, Franssen ESE, Kluger A, Mir P, et al. Stage-specific behavioral, cognitive, and in vivo changes in community residing subjects with age-associated memory impairment and primary degenerative dementia of the Alzheimer type. Drug Dev Res. 1988;15(2–3):101–14.

[73] Petersen RC, Stevens JC, Ganguli M, Tangalos EG, Cummings JL, DeKosky ST. Practice parameter: early detection of dementia: mild cognitive impairment (an evidence-based review). Report of the Quality Standards Subcommittee of the American Academy of Neurology. Neurology. 2001;56(9):1133–42.

[74] Winblad B, Palmer K, Kivipelto M, Jelic V, Fratiglioni L, Wahlund L-O, et al. Mild cognitive impairment—beyond controversies, towards a consensus: report of the

International Working Group on Mild Cognitive Impairment. J Intern Med. 2004;256(3): 240–6.

[75] Janvin C, Aarsland D, Larsen JP, Hugdahl K. Neuropsychological profile of patients with Parkinson's disease without dementia. Dement Geriatr Cogn Disord. 2003;15(3): 126–31.

[76] Litvan I, Aarsland D, Adler CH, Goldman JG, Kulisevsky J, Mollenhauer B, et al. MDS Task Force on mild cognitive impairment in Parkinson's disease: critical review of PD-MCI. Mov Disord. 2011;26(10):1814–24.

[77] Caviness JN, Driver-Dunckley E, Connor DJ, Sabbagh MN, Hentz JG, Noble B, et al. Defining mild cognitive impairment in Parkinson's disease. Mov Disord. 2007;22(9): 1272–7.

[78] Sollinger AB, Goldstein FC, Lah JJ, Levey AI, Factor S a. Mild cognitive impairment in Parkinson's disease: subtypes and motor characteristics. Parkinsonism Relat Disord. Elsevier Ltd; 2010;16(3):177–80.

[79] Foltynie T, Brayne CEG, Robbins TW, Barker R a. The cognitive ability of an incident cohort of Parkinson's patients in the UK. The CamPaIGN study. Brain. 2004;127(Pt 3): 550–60.

[80] Janvin CC, Larsen JP, Salmon DP, Galasko D, Hugdahl K, Aarsland D. Cognitive profiles of individual patients with Parkinson's disease and dementia: comparison with dementia with Lewy bodies and Alzheimer's disease. Mov Disord. 2006;21(3):337–42.

[81] Muslimovic D, Post B, Speelman JD, Schmand B. Cognitive profile of patients with newly diagnosed Parkinson disease. Neurology. 2005;65(8):1239–45.

[82] Williams-Gray CH, Foltynie T, Brayne CEG, Robbins TW, Barker R a. Evolution of cognitive dysfunction in an incident Parkinson's disease cohort. Brain. 2007;130(Pt 7): 1787–98.

[83] Hoops S, Nazem S, Siderowf AD, Duda JE, Xie SX, Stern MB, et al. Validity of the MoCA and MMSE in the detection of MCI and dementia in Parkinson disease. Neurology. 2009;73(21):1738–45.

[84] Litvan I, Goldman JG, Tröster AI, Schmand BA, Weintraub D, Petersen RC, et al. Diagnostic criteria for mild cognitive impairment in Parkinson's disease: Movement Disorder Society Task Force guidelines. Mov Disord. 2012;27(3):349–56.

[85] Broeders M, de Bie RMA, Velseboer DC, Speelman JD, Muslimovic D, Schmand B. Evolution of mild cognitive impairment in Parkinson disease. Neurology. 2013;81(4): 346–52.

[86] Stefanova E, Žiropadja L, Stojković T, Stanković I, Tomić A, Ječmenica-Lukić M, et al. Mild Cognitive Impairment in Early Parkinson's Disease Using the Movement

Disorder Society Task Force Criteria: Cross-Sectional Study in Hoehn and Yahr Stage 1. Dement Geriatr Cogn Disord. 2015;40(3–4):199–209.

[87] Pedersen KF, Larsen JP, Tysnes O-B, Alves G. Prognosis of mild cognitive impairment in early parkinson disease: the Norwegian ParkWest Study. JAMA Neurol. 2013;70(5):580–6.

[88] Domellöf ME, Ekman U, Forsgren L, Elgh E. Cognitive function in the early phase of Parkinson's disease, a five-year follow-up. Acta Neurol Scand. 2015;132(2):79–88.

[89] Marras C, Armstrong MJ, Meaney C a., Fox S, Rothberg B, Reginold W, et al. Measuring mild cognitive impairment in patients with Parkinson's disease. Mov Disord. 2013;28(5):626–33.

[90] Galtier I, Nieto A, Lorenzo JN, Barroso J. Mild cognitive impairment in Parkinson's disease: diagnosis and progression to dementia. J Clin Exp Neuropsychol. 2016;38(1): 40–50.

[91] Goldman JG, Holden S, Bernard B, Ouyang B, Goetz CG, Stebbins GT. Defining optimal cutoff scores for cognitive impairment using movement disorder society task force criteria for mild cognitive impairment in Parkinson's disease. Mov Disord. 2013;28(14): 1972–9.

[92] Goldman JG, Holden S, Ouyang B, Bernard B, Goetz CG, Stebbins GT. Diagnosing PD-MCI by MDS Task Force criteria: how many and which neuropsychological tests? Mov Disord. 2015;30(3):402–6.

[93] Hobson P, Meara J. Mild cognitive impairment in Parkinson's disease and its progression onto dementia: a 16-year outcome evaluation of the Denbighshire cohort. Int J Geriatr Psychiatry. 2015;30(10):1048–55.

[94] Alegret M, Junqué C, Pueyo R, Valldeoriola F, Vendrell P, Tolosa E, et al. MRI atrophy parameters related to cognitive and motor impairment in Parkinson's disease. Neurol (Barcelona, Spain). 2001;16(2):63–9.

[95] Deroost N, Kerckhofs E, Coene M, Wijnants G, Soetens E. Learning sequence movements in a homogenous sample of patients with Parkinson's disease. Neuropsychologia. 2006;44(10):1653–62.

[96] Alevriadou A, Katsarou Z, Bostantjopoulou S, Kiosseoglou G, Mentenopoulos G. Wisconsin card sorting test variables in relation to motor symptoms in Parkinson's disease. Percept Mot Skills. 1999;89(3 Pt 1):824–30.

[97] Pereira JB, Junqué C, Martí MJ, Ramirez-Ruiz B, Bartrés-Faz D, Tolosa E. Structural brain correlates of verbal fluency in Parkinson's disease. Neuroreport. 2009;20(8):741–4.

[98] Morris RG, Downes JJ, Sahakian BJ, Evenden JL, Heald A, Robbins TW. Planning and spatial working memory in Parkinson's disease. J Neurol Neurosurg Psychiatry. 1988;51(6):757–66.

[99] Crucian GP, Barrett AM, Schwartz RL, Bowers D, Triggs WJ, Friedman W, et al. Cognitive and vestibulo-proprioceptive components of spatial ability in Parkinson's disease. Neuropsychologia. 2000;38(6):757–67.

[100] Vakil E, Herishanu-Naaman S. Declarative and procedural learning in Parkinson's disease patients having tremor or bradykinesia as the predominant symptom. Cortex. 1998;34(4):611–20.

[101] Sommer M, Grafman J, Clark K, Hallett M. Learning in Parkinson's disease: eyeblink conditioning, declarative learning, and procedural learning. J Neurol Neurosurg Psychiatry. 1999;67(1):27–34.

[102] Dalrymple-Alford JC, Kalders AS, Jones RD, Watson RW. A central executive deficit in patients with Parkinson's disease. J Neurol Neurosurg Psychiatry. 1994;57(3):360–7.

[103] Colman KSF, Koerts J, van Beilen M, Leenders KL, Post WJ, Bastiaanse R. The impact of executive functions on verb production in patients with Parkinson's disease. Cortex. 2009;45(8):930–42.

[104] Crescentini C, Mondolo F, Biasutti E, Shallice T. Supervisory and routine processes in noun and verb generation in nondemented patients with Parkinson's disease. Neuropsychologia. 2008;46(2):434–47.

[105] Péran P, Rascol O, Démonet J-F, Celsis P, Nespoulous J-L, Dubois B, et al. Deficit of verb generation in nondemented patients with Parkinson's disease. Mov Disord. 2003;18(2):150–6.

[106] Whittington CJ, Podd J, Stewart-Williams S. Memory deficits in Parkinson's disease. J Clin Exp Neuropsychol. 2006;28(5):738–54.

[107] Girotti F, Soliveri P, Carella F, Geminiani G, Aiello G, Caraceni T. Role of motor performance in cognitive processes of Parkinsonian patients. Neurology. 1988;38(4): 537–40.

[108] Natsopoulos D, Grouios G, Bostantzopoulou S, Mentenopoulos G, Katsarou Z, Logothetis J. Algorithmic and heuristic strategies in comprehension of complement clauses by patients with Parkinson's disease. Neuropsychologia. 1993;31(9):951–64.

[109] Natsopoulos D, Katsarou Z, Alevriadou A, Grouios G, Bostantzopoulou S, Mentenopoulos G. Deductive and inductive reasoning in Parkinson's disease patients and normal controls: review and experimental evidence. Cortex. 1997;33(3):463–81.

[110] Flowers KA, Pearce I, Pearce JM. Recognition memory in Parkinson's disease. J Neurol Neurosurg Psychiatry. 1984;47(11):1174–81.

[111] Aarsland D, Andersen K, Larsen JP, Perry R, Wentzel-Larsen T, Lolk A, et al. The rate of cognitive decline in Parkinson disease. Arch Neurol. 2004;61(12):1906–11.

[112] Dubois B, Pillon B, Sternic N, Lhermitte F, Agid Y. Age-induced cognitive disturbances in Parkinson's disease. Neurology. 1990;40(1):38–41.

[113] Locascio JJ, Corkin S, Growdon JH. Relation between clinical characteristics of Parkinson's disease and cognitive decline. J Clin Exp Neuropsychol. 2003;25(1):94–109.

[114] Cummings JL. Depression and Parkinson's disease: a review. Am J Psychiatry. 1992;149(4):443–54.

[115] Shulman LM, Taback RL, Bean J, Weiner WJ. Comorbidity of the nonmotor symptoms of Parkinson's disease. Mov Disord. 2001;16(3):507–10.

[116] Rojo A, Aguilar M, Garolera MT, Cubo E, Navas I, Quintana S. Depression in Parkinson's disease: clinical correlates and outcome. Parkinsonism Relat Disord. 2003;10(1):23–8.

[117] Starkstein SE, Bolduc PL, Mayberg HS, Preziosi TJ, Robinson RG. Cognitive impairments and depression in Parkinson's disease: a follow up study. J Neurol Neurosurg Psychiatry. 1990;53(7):597–602.

[118] Cubo E, Bernard B, Leurgans S, Raman R. Cognitive and motor function in patients with Parkinson's disease with and without depression. Clin Neuropharmacol. 2000;23(6):331–4.

[119] Tröster AI, Stalp LD, Paolo AM, Fields JA, Koller WC. Neuropsychological impairment in Parkinson's disease with and without depression. Arch Neurol. 1995;52(12): 1164–9.

[120] Ng A, Chander RJ, Tan LCS, Kandiah N. Influence of depression in mild Parkinson's disease on longitudinal motor and cognitive function. Parkinsonism Relat Disord. 2015;21(9):1056–60.

[121] Aarsland D, Zaccai J, Brayne C. A systematic review of prevalence studies of dementia in Parkinson's disease. Mov Disord. 2005;20(10):1255–63.

[122] Hely MA, Reid WGJ, Adena MA, Halliday GM, Morris JGL. The Sydney multicenter study of Parkinson's disease: the inevitability of dementia at 20 years. Mov Disord. 2008;23(6):837–44.

[123] Emre M, Aarsland D, Brown R, Burn DJ, Duyckaerts C, Mizuno Y, et al. Clinical diagnostic criteria for dementia associated with Parkinson's disease. Mov Disord. 2007;22(12):1689–707; quiz 1837.

[124] Hughes AJ, Daniel SE, Kilford L, Lees AJ. Accuracy of clinical diagnosis of idiopathic Parkinson's disease: a clinico-pathological study of 100 cases. J Neurol Neurosurg Psychiatry. 1992;55(3):181–4.

[125] Williams-Gray CH, Evans JR, Goris A, Foltynie T, Ban M, Robbins TW, et al. The distinct cognitive syndromes of Parkinson's disease: 5 year follow-up of the CamPaIGN cohort. Brain. 2009;132(Pt 11):2958–69.

[126] Hobson P, Meara J. Risk and incidence of dementia in a cohort of older subjects with Parkinson's disease in the United Kingdom. Mov Disord. 2004;19(9):1043–9.

[127] Levy G, Jacobs DM, Tang M-X, Côté LJ, Louis ED, Alfaro B, et al. Memory and executive function impairment predict dementia in Parkinson's disease. Mov Disord. 2002;17(6): 1221–6.

[128] Woods SP, Tröster AI. Prodromal frontal/executive dysfunction predicts incident dementia in Parkinson's disease. J Int Neuropsychol Soc. 2003;9(1):17–24.

[129] Noe E, Marder K, Bell KL, Jacobs DM, Manly JJ, Stern Y. Comparison of dementia with Lewy bodies to Alzheimer's disease and Parkinson's disease with dementia. Mov Disord. 2004;19(1):60–7.

[130] Gjerstad MD, Aarsland D, Larsen JP. Development of daytime somnolence over time in Parkinson's disease. Neurology. 2002;58(10):1544–6.

[131] Hughes TA, Ross HF, Musa S, Bhattacherjee S, Nathan RN, Mindham RH, et al. A 10-year study of the incidence of and factors predicting dementia in Parkinson's disease. Neurology. 2000;54(8):1596–602.

[132] Levy G, Schupf N, Tang M-X, Cote LJ, Louis ED, Mejia H, et al. Combined effect of age and severity on the risk of dementia in Parkinson's disease. Ann Neurol. 2002;51(6): 722–9.

[133] Mahieux F, Fénelon G, Flahault A, Manifacier MJ, Michelet D, Boller F. Neuropsychological prediction of dementia in Parkinson's disease. J Neurol Neurosurg Psychiatry. 1998;64(2):178–83.

[134] Aarsland D, Andersen K, Larsen JP, Lolk A, Kragh-Sørensen P. Prevalence and characteristics of dementia in Parkinson disease: an 8-year prospective study. Arch Neurol. 2003;60(3):387–92.

[135] Gasca-Salas C, Clavero P, García-García D, Obeso JA, Rodríguez-Oroz MC. Significance of visual hallucinations and cerebral hypometabolism in the risk of dementia in Parkinson's disease patients with mild cognitive impairment. Hum Brain Mapp. 2016;37(3):968–77.

[136] Santangelo G, Vitale C, Picillo M, Moccia M, Cuoco S, Longo K, et al. Mild cognitive impairment in newly diagnosed Parkinson's disease: a longitudinal prospective study. Parkinsonism Relat Disord. 2015;21(10):1219–26.

Chapter 9

Brain Network Metabolic Changes in Patients with Parkinsonian Tremors

Hideo Mure, David Eidelberg and Satoshi Goto

Additional information is available at the end of the chapter

http://dx.doi.org/10.5772/63159

Abstract

Functional neuroimaging and modern multivariate analysis techniques have greatly contributed to research into the pathophysiology, diagnosis, and new treatments of neurodegenerative diseases, such as Parkinson's disease (PD). The pathogenesis of PD symptoms, especially akinesia and rigidity, is associated with abnormalities of cortico-striato-pallido-thalamocortical circuits. Although a resting tremor is one of the cardinal features of PD, the pathophysiology underlying this symptom is unclear and is thought to differ from those of akinesia and rigidity. The application of network analyses to metabolic positron emission tomography scans of patients with PD has provided valuable information concerning functional neural connectivity and identified the patterns of covariance that are specific to the motor manifestations and many nonmotor features of the disease, such as cognitive dysfunction. Functional imaging methods have revealed PD-specific brain activation patterns, including a parkinsonian tremor-related network. Network-based algorithms might aid in the clinical diagnosis of patients with PD from early symptoms and provide objective evidence of treatment responses.

Keywords: parkinson's disease, tremor, metabolic brain networks, positron emission tomography, deep brain stimulation

1. Introduction

A resting tremor, which results from a striatal dopamine (DA) deficiency, is one of the most common motor symptoms of Parkinson's disease (PD). A tremor-dominant type of PD is exhibited by 36 to 49% of patients with PD [1]. Clinical and pathophysiological studies have revealed that the PD tremor has distinct characteristics compared with other major parkinsonian signs, such as akinesia (bradykinesia) and rigidity [2, 3]. Studies that used the Unified Parkinson's Disease Rating Scale (UPDRS) have shown that the severity of patients' akinesia and rigidity symptoms correlates with the severity of striatal DA loss and the clinical progression of the disease, while the severity of their tremor did not [4–7]. Although levodopa therapy is still the gold standard in the treatment of PD, it is more effective on akinesia and rigidity symptoms than it is on tremor. Furthermore, patients with the tremor-dominant type of PD have a better prognosis compared to those with the akinesia-rigid type [8]. The thalamic ventral intermediate (Vim) nucleus is considered the optimal target for stereotactic intervention treatments of PD tremor. Indeed, ablation or deep brain stimulation (DBS) of the Vim nucleus effectively reduces PD tremor while it does not improve akinesia or rigidity.

To date, metabolic changes in the brain networks of patients with PD have been analyzed with a variety of neuroimaging techniques, including positron emission tomography (PET), single-photon emission computed tomography (SPECT), and functional magnetic resonance imaging (fMRI). Eidelberg and colleagues have applied multivariate analyses to [^{18}F]fluorodeoxyglucose (FDG)-PET scans in their studies of the brain networks of patients with PD, and they found a PD-related pattern (PDRP) of spatial covariance. They showed that patients with PD exhibit increased metabolism in the thalamus, globus pallidus, pons, and primary motor cortex and decreased metabolism in the lateral premotor cortex, supplementary motor area (SMA), and parietal association area. Interestingly, the scores for the PDRP expression of the individual patients with PD correlated with their UPDRS motor subscores for akinesia and rigidity, but not with their subscores for tremor. These findings suggested that PD tremors might be associated with different patterns of activation in these regions compared to those observed in the PDRP. Mure et al. (2011) identified a discrete PD-related tremor pattern (PDTP) in the FDG-PET scans of a cohort of patients with tremor-dominant PD who had undergone DBS in the thalamic Vim nucleus. They analyzed the scans that were obtained when the patients were on- and off-stimulation with an Ordinal Trends/Canonical Variates Analysis, which is a within-subject, network-mapping, and algorithm-guided principal component analysis (PCA) method. They found that the PDTP topography was characterized by increased metabolism in the cerebellar dentate nucleus and primary cortex and, to a lesser degree, in the putamen. In contrast to the PDRP, the scores for the PDTP expression correlated with the tremor amplitudes and UPDRS motor scores for tremor, but not with the UPDRS motor scores for akinesia and rigidity. In addition, the PDTP was modulated more by Vim-DBS than by subthalamic DBS. Thus, these findings suggested that PD tremors might be mediated by a distinct metabolic network that primarily involves cerebello-thalamo-cortical pathways.

In this chapter, we introduce the recent advancements that have been made in neuroimaging research for elucidating the pathogenesis of PD tremor and other PD symptoms. In addition, we emphasize the importance of quantitative analyses of the PDTP and PDRP in the development of objective methods for precisely diagnosing PD and evaluating the effects of treatments on PD tremor.

2. Functional neuroimaging techniques: a brief overview

Functional neuroimaging is used in studies with the goal of elucidating the pathophysiology of neurological disorders. Representative functional neuroimaging techniques are fMRI, SPECT, and PET. The fMRI technique, which is employed more because injections of radiotracers are not required, measures changes in the relative amounts of deoxyhemoglobin in different regions of the brain. The interactions of deoxyhemoglobin with the water molecules surrounding blood vessels result in proton signals that produce blood-oxygenation-level-dependent (BOLD) contrast in the scans. Increases in regional blood flow result in relative decreases in deoxyhemoglobin and an increase in the BOLD signals. When neurons are active, the supply of oxygenated blood to the active region increases [9]. Thus, increases in BOLD signals are associated with local neuronal activity [9]. However, in contrast to imaging with radiotracers, fMRI has a poor signal-to-noise ratio, and its signals are difficult to quantify.

Radiotracer imaging techniques, such as PET and SPECT, are used to investigate the patterns of cerebral glucose metabolism, cerebral blood flow, and specific neurochemical systems. In general, even though SPECT imaging is less expensive and more widely available compared with PET imaging, PET has better spatial resolution and sensitivity. The most widely used PET radiotracer is FDG. Because FDG uptake reflects cerebral glucose metabolism, it is thought to measure regional synaptic activity [10]. [^{15}O]-labeled water ($H_2{}^{15}O$) PET can be used to quantify regional cerebral blood flow (rCBF). As described above, increases in rCBF are thought to reflect neuronal activity increases [9]. DAergic function can be evaluated by measuring the storage capability of presynaptic DA with [^{18}F]-fluorodopa or presynaptic DA transporter binding with [^{123}I]-iodine-123-beta-carbomethoxy-3 beta-(4-iodophenyltropane) (CIT) and [^{18}F]-fluoropropyl CIT. Postsynaptic DA receptors can also be assessed with [^{11}C]-raclopride [11]. Given the prominent role of nigrostriatal pathology in PD, radioligand imaging of the DA system has been widely used in investigations of PD. However, many other neurochemical systems, such as the serotonergic, adrenergic, and cholinergic systems, can be examined with PET and SPECT imaging [12]. Because rCBF and cerebral metabolisms are affected in many neurodegenerative disorders, PET and SPECT imaging techniques have greatly contributed to the understanding of the abnormal brain circuitry underlying the pathophysiology of PD.

3. Metabolic network mapping

Network analyses of functional brain imaging data are an innovative approach for examining circuit abnormalities in neurodegenerative diseases. PD is related to the degeneration of nigral DAergic neurons, which also alters activity in the thalamus, pallidum, and cortex. These metabolic changes can be evaluated at the regional voxel level with standard univariate approaches, such as statistical parametric mapping [13]. Disease-related abnormalities in brain functional organization can also be assessed at the network level with multivariate analytical procedures. The Scaled Subprofile Model (SSM) is an innovative multivariate approach that is used to identify disease-specific brain networks [14]. SSM is a spatial covariance method that is based on a PCA and that is used to assess the subject-by-region effects in functional brain images [15, 16]. The details of this method have been reviewed elsewhere [15–17]. Briefly, the SSM is applied to multivoxel metabolic imaging data in a combined sample of scans from healthy subjects and patients. Once a pattern is identified that distinguishes one group from the other, its expression can be prospectively quantified on an individual basis [18, 19], and the resulting subject scores can be correlated with clinical and physiological measures of interest. The SSM/PCA and related multivariate techniques are well suited to the study of circuit disorders, which are neurological diseases with stereotyped disturbances in brain network organization. Resting state measures of regional glucose utilization provide an index of local synaptic activity as well as of the biochemical maintenance processes that dominate this condition. The effects of pathology on these functions have a greater influence on regional cerebral metabolism and blood flow than physiological and/or hemodynamic factors do. It was recognized early in imaging research that neurodegenerative processes are associated with disease-specific alterations in functional connectivity across the whole brain. Therefore, network approaches have increasingly been used to analyze the metabolic imaging data from subjects with brain disorders, and these data have had a growing impact on imaging neuroscience.

4. Metabolic brain networks in PD

4.1. The PDRP

Presynaptic nigrostriatal DA loss is associated with abnormalities of the cortico-striato-pallido-thalamocortical (CSPTC) loops. Applications of the SSM/PCA method to resting-state FDG-PET scans of patients with PD have consistently revealed an abnormal disease-related spatial covariance pattern in the CSPTC loops and related pathways [15, 20, 21]. This PDRP is characterized by increased pallido-thalamic and pontine metabolism that is associated with relative reductions in the premotor cortex, SMA, and parietal association cortices (**Figure 1a**). The presence of the PDRP has been verified by its reproducibility in another independent PD cohort [22], and it has been associated with standardized motor ratings in multiple patient cohorts (**Figure 1b**) [23–25]. In general, PDRP expression has been found to correlate with clinical ratings of akinesia and rigidity, but not with tremor ratings. Interestingly, longitudinal increases in the pattern of expression correlate with progression in the motor disability ratings and concurrent PET measurements of presynaptic nigrostriatal DA function [26, 27]. In addition, the clinical outcomes of individual patients are associated with the degree of PDRP expression that is observed during subthalamic nucleus (STN)-targeted surgical interventions, including ablation therapy and DBS. Moreover, in patients with untreated PD, the PDRP expression scores that are determined with measures of cerebral perfusion in radiotracer imaging, such as $H_2^{15}O$-PET and 99mTc-ethyl cysteinate dimer SPECT, closely correlate with the corresponding network values that are computed from scans of cerebral glucose metabolism (i.e., FDG-PET) from the same cohort [22, 28]. Thus, PDRP expression can be measured in rCBF scans that are obtained by PET, SPECT, or perfusion-weighted MRI methods, such as the arterial spin labeling technique [29, 30].

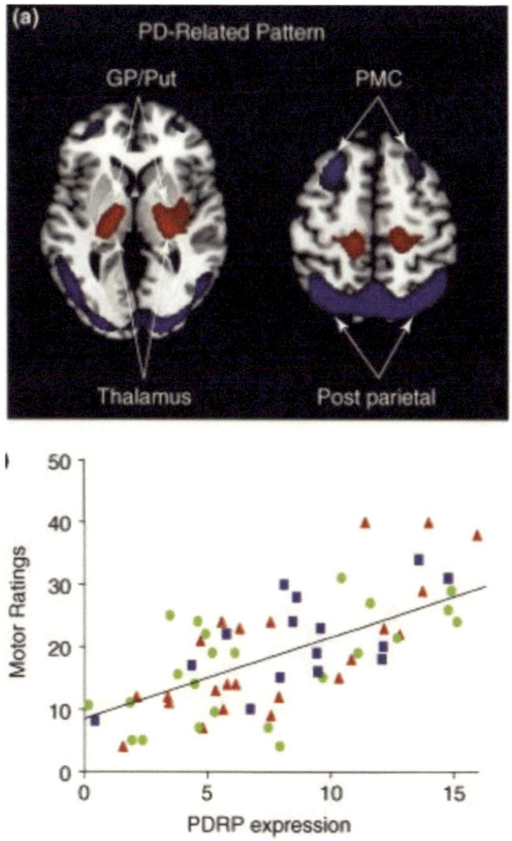

Figure 1. Neuroimaging analysis on Parkinson's disease-related pattern. (a) Parkinson's disease (PD)-related pattern (PDRP). This spatial covariance pattern of motor-related metabolism was identified by a multivariate analysis of [^{18}F]fluorodeoxyglucose (FDG)-positron emission tomography (PET) scans from 33 patients with PD and 33 age-matched normal control subjects. This pattern is characterized by hypermetabolism (red) in the thalamus, globus pallidus (GP)/putamen (Put), pons, and primary motor cortex and relative metabolic reductions (blue) in the lateral premotor (PMC) and posterior parietal cortex. (b) The scores of the PDRP expression in the subjects correlated with the motor subscale scores on the Unified Parkinson's Disease Rating Scale (UPDRS) from a combination of patients with PD from three independent cohorts ($n = 65$; $r = 0.68$; $p < 0.001$) [6, 23, 25]. (From Eidelberg D. Metabolic brain networks in neurodegenerative disorders: a functional imaging approach. *Trends Neurosci.* 2009;32:548-557, with permission from Elsevier).

4.2. The PD-related cognitive pattern (PDCP)

Although PD is clinically defined by its motor features, nonmotor symptoms that involve cognitive dysfunction can appear, even in early clinical stages [31]. Mild cognitive impairment (MCI) in early PD typically involves visuomotor processing, working memory, and/or aspects of executive performance [32, 33]. A FDG-PET study revealed decreased glucose metabolism in the frontal and occipital cortices of patients with PD with and without apparent cognitive impairments [34]. After applying a SSM/PCA analysis to FDG-PET data from a cohort of PD patients without dementia, Huang et al. identified a significant pattern of covariance that was related to cognitive performance [35]. This pattern, which was termed the PDCP, is characterized by metabolic decreases in the rostral SMA (pre-SMA), precuneus, and posterior parietal and prefrontal regions and increases in the dentate nucleus and cerebellar cortex (**Figure 2a**). The expression of PDCP in nondemented patients with PD correlates with the patients' ratings on neuropsychological tests of memory and executive functioning (**Figure 2b**). In addition, PDCP expression shows stepwise increases in accordance with worsening cognitive impairments (**Figure 2c**). In contrast to PDRP, the expression of PDCP is not modulated by antiparkinsonian motor symptom treatments, such as levodopa and DBS. Importantly, although both the PDRP and the PDCP increase in accordance with symptom duration, the rate of the increase in PDCP expression was slower than that of PDRP in the same subjects. These findings suggest that different neural systems underlie these two disease-related metabolic networks.

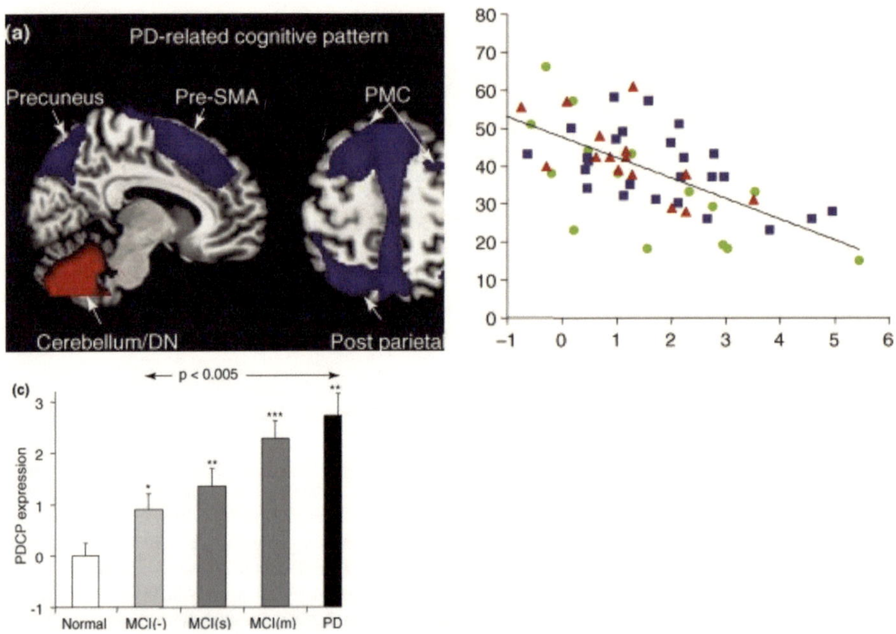

Figure 2. Neuroimaging analysis on Parkinson's disease-related cognitive pattern. (a) The PD-related cognitive pattern (PDCP). This spatial covariance pattern of cognition-related metabolism was identified by a network analysis of FDG-PET scans from 15 patients with nondemented PD [35]. This pattern is characterized by hypometabolism (blue) of the dorsolateral prefrontal cortex (PMC), rostral supplementary motor area (preSMA), precuneus, and posterior parietal regions and relative metabolic increases (red) in the dentate nucleus (DN) and cerebellar cortex. (b) The expression of PDCP correlates with the performances on neuropsychological tests of memory and executive functioning ($r = -0.67$, $p < 0.001$) of 56 patients with nondemented PD from two prospective validation groups and the original validation group [35]. (c) Bar graph of PDCP expression [mean ± standard error of the mean (SE)] in patients with PD with dementia (PDD), multiple-domain mild cognitive impairment [MCI(m)], single-domain mild cognitive impairment [MCI(s)], patients with PD without mild cognitive impairment [MCI(−)], and normal subjects. PDCP expression differed significantly across the patient and control groups and among the PD groups. The asterisks indicate significant increases in PDCP expression compared to normal controls. (From Eidelberg D. Metabolic brain networks in neurode-

generative disorders: a functional imaging approach. *Trends Neurosci.* 2009;32:548-557, Copyright 2009, with permission from Elsevier).

5. Parkisonian tremor and metabolic changes

5.1. Parkinsonian tremor

A resting tremor of 3–6 Hz is one of the cardinal features of PD that presents in 75 to 100% of patients during the course of the illness [36, 37]. The parkinsonian tremor is typically asymmetrical, at least initially, and it affects the upper limbs before involving the ipsilateral leg after about 2 years. Tremor of the lips, jaw, or tongue may also occur. Head or voice tremor is rare, which contrasts with observations of essential tremors. A postural tremor is also present in most cases, and it exhibits a wide range of severity [38]. However, kinetic tremor is uncommon [39]. An isolated lower-leg resting tremor is an uncommon symptom of neurological disease and an unusual presentation of PD, and such tremors are typically suspected to be caused by multiple system atrophy, psychogenic tremor, or drug-induced parkinsonism [40].

The pathophysiology of parkinsonian tremors is thought to be distinct from that of akinesia and rigidity [2, 3]. The clinical progression and mental status declines of patients with akinetic-rigidity-dominant PD are more rapid compared to patients with tremor-dominant PD [41]. Moreover, the loss of DAergic projections to the striatum correlates with the clinical ratings of bradykinesia and rigidity, but not with those of tremor [5, 42]. Indeed, DAergic therapy is less effective on parkinsonian tremor than it is on akinesia and rigidity.

The Vim nucleus of the thalamus has commonly been recognized as the optimal surgical target for the treatment of tremors. Neurons in this region receive projections from the deep cerebellar nuclei and discharge in synchrony with parkinsonian tremors [43]. Given that PD tremors can be modulated by the lesioning of other brain regions, such as the pons and cerebellum, the Vim nucleus is considered one of a number of interconnected nodes in a spatially distributed tremor circuit. Nevertheless, the precise anatomical and functional network underlying tremors is still unclear, particularly with respect to the relative contributions of the basal ganglia and cerebellum to this pathway [3, 44–47].

5.2. The PDTP

In order to identify the PDTP, FDG-PET scans were acquired in patients with tremor-predominant PD who underwent Vim-DBS. The PDTP was identified with an ordinal trends/canonical variates analysis, which is a within-subject network-mapping algorithm that is based on PCA methods [48], by comparing scans that were conducted during Vim-DBS OFF (i.e., tremor present) and Vim-DBS ON (i.e., tremor suppressed) [7]. This pattern is characterized by increased activity in the cerebellum and dorsal pons, primary motor cortex, and caudate and putamen (**Figure 3a**). Unlike PDRP, prospectively computed PDTP correlates with accelerometer measurements of the tremors and UPDRS tremor subscale scores, but not with UPDRS bradykinesia-rigidity subscale ratings (**Figure 3b** and **3c**). Interestingly, Vim-DBS was associated with changes in PDTP expression, but not PDRP expression. Although STN DBS decreased the activity in both networks, PDTP expression was reduced more by Vim than by STN stimulation (**Figure 4**). Moreover, while both the PDRP and the PDTP progressed over time, the rate of the PDTP increase was much slower than that of the PDRP. These findings suggest major differences between the tremor- and bradykinesia/rigidity-related brain networks in terms of their clinical correlates, treatment effects, and natural histories. The bradykinetic manifestations of PD have been associated with discrete functional abnormalities of the CSPTC pathways [49]. In contrast, tremor generation has been linked to abnormal activity in cerebello-thalamo-cortical pathways [44, 46, 47], and the role of the basal ganglia in the etiology of this symptom is still controversial [46, 50]. Indeed, prior $H_2{}^{15}O$ PET imaging studies have shown that both the lesioning and the stimulation of the thalamic Vim nucleus results in localized reductions in neural activity in the primary motor cortex and anterior cerebellum [51, 52]. Moreover, a magnetoencephalography study revealed a tremor-coherent oscillatory network involving the primary motor cortex, thalamus, and cerebellum [47]. These findings give support to the suggestions that PDTP topography and the cerebello-thalamo-cortical circuit are associated with parkinsonian tremors. Interestingly, the PDTP topography includes a significant contribution from the striatum, although the contribution is less than those of the other nodes of this network. In the primate, the striatum receives cerebellar output through the ventrolateral and intralaminar thalamic nuclei [53]. In aggregate, the regional nodes of the PD tremor network may be defined by the abnormal synchronization of firing, which results in localized increases in synaptic activity and concomitant increases in glucose metabolism. While the tremor-related metabolic changes that are observed are most prominent in the primary motor cortex and thalamus, these PDTP regions interconnect through the thalamic Vim nucleus and putamen [7].

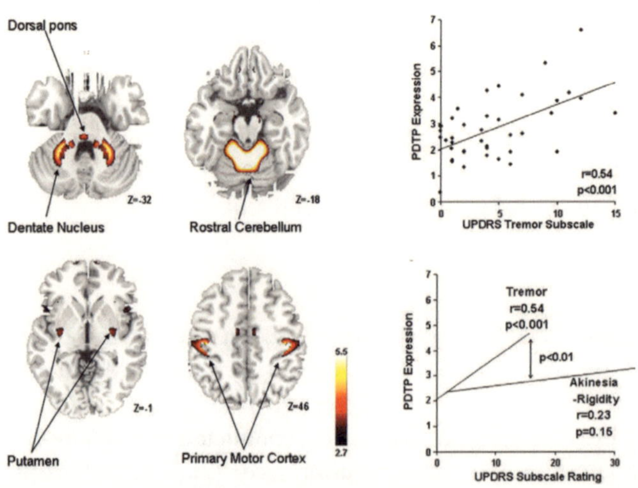

Figure 3. Neuroimaging analysis on Parkinson's disease tremor-related pattern. (a) PD tremor-related pattern (PDTP). This spatial covariance pattern was identified by an ordinal trends/canonical variate analysis of the FDG-PET data from nine patients with tremor-dominant PD who were scanned when they were on and off ventral intermediate nucleus (Vim) stimulation. The pattern is characterized by hypermetabolism in the primary motor cortex, anterior cer-

http://dx.doi.org/10.5772/63159

ebellum/dorsal pons, and putamen. (b) PDTP expression correlated with the UPDRS subscale ratings for tremor in 40 patients with PD ($r = 0.54$, $p < 0.001$). (c) The correlation of the PDTP scores with tremor was significantly greater in magnitude than that with the subscale ratings for akinesia-rigidity ($p < 0.01$; multiple regression analysis). (From Mure H. et. al., Parkinson's disease tremor-related metabolic network: characterization, progression, and treatment effects. *Neuroimage*. 2011;54:1244-1253 Copyright 2011, with permission from Elsevier).

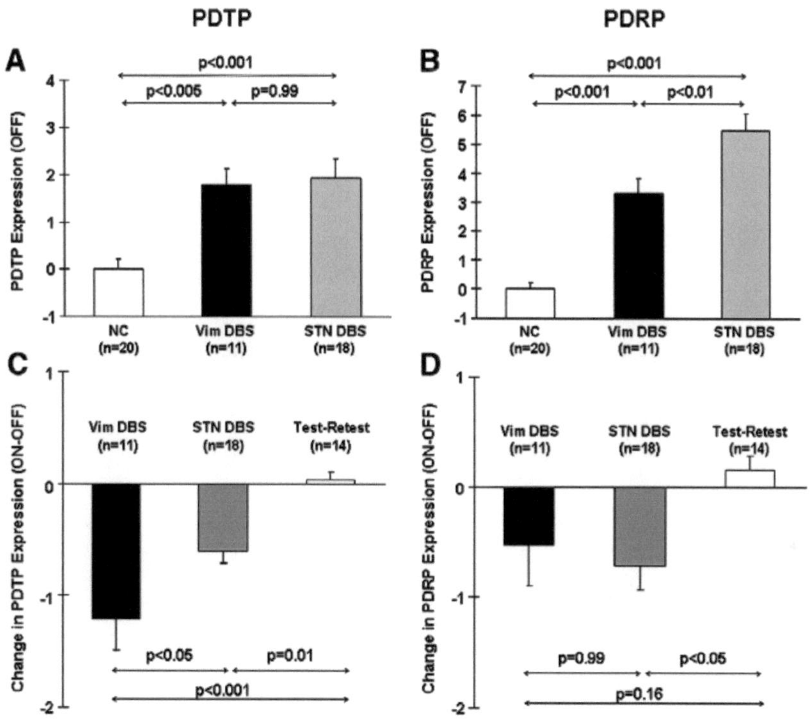

Figure 4. Changed activity of the metabolic network as a result of deep brain stimulation (DBS) for parkinsonian tremor. (a) Bar graphs showing the mean baseline PDTP expression (±SE) in patients who were treated with Vim-DBS (black), patients who were treated with subthalamic nucleus (STN) DBS (gray), and healthy control subjects (white). PDTP expression differed significantly across the three groups ($p < 0.001$; one-way ANOVA), with comparable increases in the baseline expression in both the Vim-DBS ($p < 0.005$) and STN DBS ($p < 0.001$) groups relative to the controls. (b) The baseline PDRP expression also differed across the three groups ($p < 0.001$), with higher expression in both treatment groups relative to the controls ($p < 0.001$). Nonetheless, PDRP expression was higher in the STN DBS group than in the Vim-DBS group ($p < 0.01$). (c) Treatment-mediated changes (ON-OFF) in PDTP expression (±SE) in the Vim-DBS patients (black), STN DBS patients (gray), and test-retest PD control subjects (white). The changes in PDTP expression differed across the three groups ($p < 0.001$; one-way ANOVA), with stimulation-mediated declines in network activity in both DBS groups (Vim: $p < 0.001$; STN: $p = 0.01$, relative to the test-retest control group). The PDTP changes were greater as a result of Vim stimulation compared with STN stimulation ($p < 0.05$). (d) There was also a significant group difference in the treatment-mediated PDRP changes ($p = 0.02$). The treatment-mediated reductions in PDRP expression were significant ($p < 0.05$) after STN stimulation, but not after Vim stimulation ($p = 0.16$). (From Mure H. et. al., Parkinson's disease tremor-related metabolic network: characterization, progression, and treatment effects. *Neuroimage*. 2011;54:1244-1253 Copyright 2011, with permission from Elsevier).

6. Concluding remarks

Neuroimaging study with the new multivariate network analysis is now used to elucidate the disease-related network abnormalities that involve the functional changes of certain brain regions in multiple neurodegenerative diseases. Particularly in PD, it has contributed to our understanding of the pathophysiology of the nigrostriatal dopaminergic system and of the non-dopaminergic system. Quantification of PD-related metabolic pattern could improve the accuracy and precision in diagnosing PD. Moreover, it also could provide an objective means of assessment of the PD therapies such as DBS.

Acknowledgements

This work was supported in part by grants from the Ministry of Education, Culture, Sports, Science, and Technology of Japan (grants-in-aid for Scientific Research no. 24390223, 26461272, and 26430054).

Author details

Hideo Mure[1], David Eidelberg[2] and Satoshi Goto[3*]

*Address all correspondence to: sgoto@tokushima-u.ac.jp

1 Department of Neurosurgery, Institute of Biomedical Sciences, Graduate School of Medical Science, Tokushima University, Japan

2 Center for Neurosciences, Feinstein Institute for Medical Research, North Shore-LIJ Health System, USA

3 Department of Neurodegenerative Disorders Research, Institute of Biomedical Sciences, Graduate School of Medical Science, Tokushima University, Japan

References

[1] Stebbins GT, Goetz CG, Burn DJ, Jankovic J, Khoo TK, Tilley BC. How to identify tremor dominant and postural instability/gait difficulty groups with the movement disorder society unified Parkinson's disease rating scale: comparison with the unified Parkinson's disease rating scale. *Mov Disord*. 2013;28:668–670.

[2] Fishman PS. Paradoxical aspects of parkinsonian tremor. *Mov Disord*. 2008;23:168–173.

[3] Zaidel A, Arkadir D, Israel Z, Bergman H. Akineto-rigid vs. tremor syndromes in parkinsonism. *Curr Opin Neurol*. 2009;22:387–393.

[4] Antonini A, Moeller JR, Nakamura T, Spetsieris P, Dhawan V, Eidelberg D. The metabolic anatomy of tremor in Parkinson's disease. *Neurology*. 1998;51:803–810.

[5] Benamer HT, Oertel WH, Patterson J, Hadley DM, Pogarell O, Hoffken H, Gerstner A, Grosset DG. Prospective study of presynaptic dopaminergic imaging in patients with mild parkinsonism and tremor disorders: part 1. Baseline and 3-month observations. *Mov Disord*. 2003;18:977–984.

[6] Eidelberg D, Moeller JR, Ishikawa T, Dhawan V, Spetsieris P, Chaly T, Robeson W, Dahl JR, Margouleff D. Assessment of disease severity in parkinsonism with fluorine-18-fluorodeoxyglucose and pet. *J Nucl Med*. 1995;36:378–383.

[7] Mure H, Hirano S, Tang CC, Isaias IU, Antonini A, Ma Y, Dhawan V, Eidelberg D. Parkinson's disease tremor-related metabolic network: characterization, progression, and treatment effects. *Neuroimage*. 2011;54:1244–1253.

[8] Jankovic J, McDermott M, Carter J, Gauthier S, Goetz C, Golbe L, Huber S, Koller W, Olanow C, Shoulson I, et al. Variable expression of parkinson's disease: a base-line analysis of the datatop cohort. The Parkinson study group. *Neurology*. 1990;40:1529–1534.

[9] Raichle ME, Mintun MA. Brain work and brain imaging. *Annu Rev Neurosci*. 2006;29:449–476.

[10] Eidelberg D, Moeller JR, Kazumata K, Antonini A, Sterio D, Dhawan V, Spetsieris P, Alterman R, Kelly PJ, Dogali M, Fazzini E, Beric A. Metabolic correlates of pallidal neuronal activity in parkinson's disease. *Brain*. 1997;120 (Pt 8):1315–1324.

[11] Niccolini F, Su P, Politis M. Dopamine receptor mapping with pet imaging in Parkinson's disease. *J Neurol*. 2014;261:2251–2263.

[12] Brooks DJ. Positron emission tomography and single-photon emission computed tomography in central nervous system drug development. *NeuroRx*. 2005;2:226–236.

[13] Moeller JR, Habeck CG. Reciprocal benefits of mass-univariate and multivariate modeling in brain mapping: applications to event-related functional mri, h(2) (15)o-, and fdg-pet. *Int J Biomed Imaging*. 2006;2006:79862.

[14] Moeller JR, Strother SC. A regional covariance approach to the analysis of functional patterns in positron emission tomographic data. *J Cereb Blood Flow Metab*. 1991;11:A121–135.

[15] Eidelberg D. Metabolic brain networks in neurodegenerative disorders: a functional imaging approach. *Trends Neurosci*. 2009;32:548–557.

[16] Spetsieris PG, Eidelberg D. Scaled subprofile modeling of resting state imaging data in Parkinson's disease: methodological issues. *Neuroimage*. 2011;54:2899–2914.

[17] Habeck C, Stern Y. Multivariate data analysis for neuroimaging data: overview and application to Alzheimer's disease. *Cell Biochem Biophys*. 2010;58:53–67.

[18] Ma Y, Eidelberg D. Functional imaging of cerebral blood flow and glucose metabolism in Parkinson's disease and Huntington's disease. *Mol Imaging Biol*. 2007;9:223–233.

[19] Spetsieris PG, Ma Y, Eckert T, Dhawan V, Eidelberg D. New strategies for automated differential diagnosis of degenerative brain disorders. *Conf Proc IEEE Eng Med Biol Soc*. 2007;2007:3421–3425.

[20] Eidelberg D, Moeller JR, Dhawan V, Spetsieris P, Takikawa S, Ishikawa T, Chaly T, Robeson W, Margouleff D, Przedborski S, et al. The metabolic topography of parkinsonism. *J Cereb Blood Flow Metab*. 1994;14:783–801.

[21] Moeller JR, Nakamura T, Mentis MJ, Dhawan V, Spetsieres P, Antonini A, Missimer J, Leenders KL, Eidelberg D. Reproducibility of regional metabolic covariance patterns: comparison of four populations. *J Nucl Med*. 1999;40:1264–1269.

[22] Ma Y, Tang C, Spetsieris PG, Dhawan V, Eidelberg D. Abnormal metabolic network activity in Parkinson's disease: test-retest reproducibility. *J Cereb Blood Flow Metab*. 2007;27:597–605.

[23] Asanuma K, Tang C, Ma Y, Dhawan V, Mattis P, Edwards C, Kaplitt MG, Feigin A, Eidelberg D. Network modulation in the treatment of Parkinson's disease. *Brain*. 2006;129:2667–2678.

[24] Feigin A, Antonini A, Fukuda M, De Notaris R, Benti R, Pezzoli G, Mentis MJ, Moeller JR, Eidelberg D. Tc-99m ethylene cysteinate dimer spect in the differential diagnosis of parkinsonism. *Mov Disord*. 2002;17:1265–1270.

[25] Lozza C, Baron JC, Eidelberg D, Mentis MJ, Carbon M, Marie RM. Executive processes in Parkinson's disease: Fdg-pet and network analysis. *Hum Brain Mapp*. 2004;22:236–245.

[26] Tang CC, Poston KL, Dhawan V, Eidelberg D. Abnormalities in metabolic network activity precede the onset of motor symptoms in Parkinson's disease. *J Neurosci*. 2010;30:1049–1056.

[27] Huang C, Tang C, Feigin A, Lesser M, Ma Y, Pourfar M, Dhawan V, Eidelberg D. Changes in network activity with the progression of Parkinson's disease. *Brain*. 2007;130:1834–1846.

[28] Hirano S, Asanuma K, Ma Y, Tang C, Feigin A, Dhawan V, Carbon M, Eidelberg D. Dissociation of metabolic and neurovascular responses to levodopa in the treatment of Parkinson's disease. *J Neurosci*. 2008;28:4201–4209.

[29] Ma Y, Huang C, Dyke JP, Pan H, Alsop D, Feigin A, Eidelberg D. Parkinson's disease spatial covariance pattern: noninvasive quantification with perfusion mri. *J Cereb Blood Flow Metab*. 2010;30:505–509.

[30] Melzer TR, Watts R, MacAskill MR, Pearson JF, Rueger S, Pitcher TL, Livingston L, Graham C, Keenan R, Shankaranarayanan A, Alsop DC, Dalrymple-Alford JC, Anderson TJ. Arterial spin labelling reveals an abnormal cerebral perfusion pattern in Parkinson's disease. *Brain*. 2011;134:845–855.

[31] Caviness JN, Driver-Dunckley E, Connor DJ, Sabbagh MN, Hentz JG, Noble B, Evidente VG, Shill HA, Adler CH. Defining mild cognitive impairment in Parkinson's disease. *Mov Disord*. 2007;22:1272–1277.

[32] Aarsland D, Bronnick K, Williams-Gray C, Weintraub D, Marder K, Kulisevsky J, Burn D, Barone P, Pagonabarraga J, Allcock L, Santangelo G, Foltynie T, Janvin C, Larsen JP, Barker RA, Emre M. Mild cognitive impairment in Parkinson disease: a multicenter pooled analysis. *Neurology*. 2010;75:1062–1069.

[33] Mure H, Tang CC, Argyelan M, Ghilardi MF, Kaplitt MG, Dhawan V, Eidelberg D. Improved sequence learning with subthalamic nucleus deep brain stimulation: evidence for treatment-specific network modulation. *J Neurosci*. 2012;32:2804–2813.

[34] Hosokai Y, Nishio Y, Hirayama K, Takeda A, Ishioka T, Sawada Y, Suzuki K, Itoyama Y, Takahashi S, Fukuda H, Mori E. Distinct patterns of regional cerebral glucose metabolism in Parkinson's disease with and without mild cognitive impairment. *Mov Disord*. 2009;24:854–862.

[35] Huang C, Mattis P, Tang C, Perrine K, Carbon M, Eidelberg D. Metabolic brain networks associated with cognitive function in Parkinson's disease. *Neuroimage*. 2007;34:714–723.

[36] Rajput AH, Rozdilsky B, Ang L. Occurrence of resting tremor in Parkinson's disease. *Neurology*. 1991;41:1298–1299.

[37] Hughes AJ, Daniel SE, Blankson S, Lees AJ. A clinicopathologic study of 100 cases of Parkinson's disease. *Arch Neurol*. 1993;50:140–148.

[38] Habibur R. Diagnosis and management of tremor. *Arch Intern Med*. 2000;160:2438–2444.

[39] Kraus PH, Lemke MR, Reichmann H. Kinetic tremor in Parkinson's disease—an underrated symptom. *J Neural Transm (Vienna)*. 2006;113:845–853.

[40] Hellmann MA, Melamed E, Steinmetz AP, Djaldetti R. Unilateral lower limb rest tremor is not necessarily a presenting symptom of Parkinson's disease. *Mov Disord*. 2010;25:924–927.

[41] Hoon DS, Fujimoto A, Shu S, Taback B. Assessment of genetic heterogeneity in tumors using laser capture microdissection. *Methods Enzymol*. 2002;356:302–309.

[42] Eidelberg D, Moeller JR, Ishikawa T, Dhawan V, Spetsieris P, Chaly T, Belakhlef A, Mandel F, Przedborski S, Fahn S. Early differential diagnosis of Parkinson's disease with 18f-fluorodeoxyglucose and positron emission tomography. *Neurology*. 1995;45:1995–2004.

[43] Lenz FA, Kwan HC, Martin RL, Tasker RR, Dostrovsky JO, Lenz YE. Single unit analysis of the human ventral thalamic nuclear group. Tremor-related activity in functionally identified cells. *Brain*. 1994;117(Pt 3):531–543.

[44] Volkmann J, Joliot M, Mogilner A, Ioannides AA, Lado F, Fazzini E, Ribary U, Llinas R. Central motor loop oscillations in parkinsonian resting tremor revealed by magnetoencephalography. *Neurology*. 1996;46:1359–1370.

[45] Deuschl G, Raethjen J, Lindemann M, Krack P. The pathophysiology of tremor. *Muscle Nerve*. 2001;24:716–735.

[46] Timmermann L, Florin E, Reck C. Pathological cerebral oscillatory activity in Parkinson's disease: a critical review on methods, data and hypotheses. *Expert Rev Med Devices*. 2007;4:651–661.

[47] Timmermann L, Gross J, Dirks M, Volkmann J, Freund HJ, Schnitzler A. The cerebral oscillatory network of parkinsonian resting tremor. *Brain*. 2003;126:199–212.

[48] Habeck C, Krakauer JW, Ghez C, Sackeim HA, Eidelberg D, Stern Y, Moeller JR. A new approach to spatial covariance modeling of functional brain imaging data: ordinal trend analysis. *Neural Comput*. 2005;17:1602–1645.

[49] DeLong MR, Wichmann T. Circuits and circuit disorders of the basal ganglia. *Arch Neurol*. 2007;64:20–24.

[50] Deuschl G, Raethjen J, Baron R, Lindemann M, Wilms H, Krack P. The pathophysiology of parkinsonian tremor: a review. *J Neurol*. 2000;247(Suppl. 5):V33–V48.

[51] Deiber MP, Pollak P, Passingham R, Landais P, Gervason C, Cinotti L, Friston K, Frackowiak R, Mauguiere F, Benabid AL. Thalamic stimulation and suppression of parkinsonian tremor. Evidence of a cerebellar deactivation using positron emission tomography. *Brain*. 1993;116(Pt 1):267–279.

[52] Fukuda M, Barnes A, Simon ES, Holmes A, Dhawan V, Giladi N, Fodstad H, Ma Y, Eidelberg D. Thalamic stimulation for parkinsonian tremor: correlation between regional cerebral blood flow and physiological tremor characteristics. *Neuroimage*. 2004;21:608–615.

[53] Hoshi E, Tremblay L, Feger J, Carras PL, Strick PL. The cerebellum communicates with the basal ganglia. *Nat Neurosci*. 2005;8:1491–1493.

Chapter 10

Animal Models of Parkinson's Disease

Javier Blesa, Ines Trigo-Damas,
Ana Quiroga-Varela and
Natalia Lopez-Gonzalez del Rey

Additional information is available at the end of the chapter

http://dx.doi.org/10.5772/63328

Abstract

Parkinson's disease (PD) is a neurodegenerative disorder characterized by the degeneration of dopaminergic neurons in the substantia nigra pars compacta, the consequent dopamine deficit in the striatum and the accumulation of aggregated α-synuclein (α-syn) in specific brain regions. The underlying pathophysiology of PD remains poorly understood. Animal models are the best tools to study the pathogenesis of PD. Most studies in PD animal models have focused on the motor features associated with dopamine depletion but still the molecular basis of PD and the molecular pathways of cell death remain unknown. While cellular models have helped to identify specific events, in vivo animal models have simulated most, although not all, of the hallmarks of PD and are useful for testing new neuroprotective approaches. In this chapter, we provide a summary of the most used PD animal models, including their advantages and limitations. Classically, in vivo PD animal models can be divided into those using environmental or synthetic neurotoxins (toxin-based models) or those utilizing the in vivo expression of PD-related mutations (genetic models). These models include 6-hydroxydopamine (6-OHDA), 1-methyl-1,2,3,6-tetrahydropyridine (MPTP), rotenone, and paraquat, as well as genetic models such as those related to α-syn, PINK1, Parkin, DJ-1, and LRRK2.

Keywords: MPTP, 6-OHDA, Rotenone, Paraquat, α-syn, LRRK2, Parkin, DJ1

1. Introduction

Parkinson's disease (PD) is a common neurodegenerative disorder characterized by the classical motor symptoms: resting tremor, bradykinesia, akinesia, rigidity, and postural instability. PD is characterized by the loss of ~50–70% of the dopaminergic neurons in the substantia nigra pars compacta (SNpc) and the consequent loss of dopamine (DA) in the striatum, and the presence of intracytoplasmic inclusions called Lewy bodies (LB) that are composed mainly of α-synuclein (α-syn) and ubiquitin [1]. Although the complete PD pathogenesis is not well understood, thanks to the use of animal models, we have gained a better understanding of its etiology, pathology, and molecular mechanisms. Importantly, none of the current available models is able to fully recapitulate PD symptoms and pathology [2].

The use of animal models in PD (both in vitro and in vivo) has greatly augmented thanks to new strategies for producing sophisticated models, such as the temporal- and/or cell-specific expression of mutated genes in vertebrates [3], human pluripotent cells coaxed into a specific type of neurons [4], and a host of different invertebrate organisms such as Drosophila [5], Medaka fish [6], or *Caenorhabditis elegans* [7]. Current PD experimental models can still be categorized into two main groups: toxic and genetic (or both of them combined). Over the years, a collection of strategies have been used to produce other animal models to model PD. Some of them included those based neither on neurotoxins nor on genetic mutations that are directly linked to familial PD. Some of these models lack transcription factors that are required for the survival of dopaminergic neurons, such as sonic hedgehog [8], nuclear receptor related protein-1 (Nurr1) [9], pituitary homeobox 3 (Pitx3) [10], or engrailed 1 [11]. Even so, the reproducibility and reliability of most of these new models are still under debate.

Therefore, the neurotoxins covered in this chapter focus on models produced by 6-hydroxydopamine (6-OHDA) and 1-methyl-1,2,3,6-tetrahydropyridine (MPTP) administration, and paraquat and rotenone which are more recent additions to the stable of toxic agents used to model PD. The recent identification of different genetic mutations related to PD (mainly SNCA (α-syn, PARK1, and 4), PRKN (parkin RBR E3 ubiquitin protein ligase, PARK2), PINK1 (PTEN-induced putative kinase 1, PARK6), DJ-1 (PARK7), and LRRK2 (leucine-rich repeat kinase 2, PARK8) has led to the development of a range of genetic models [12]. Although the expression of all these proteins in invertebrate models offers experimental advantages and can potentially address some important questions regarding the cellular processes underlying PD, in this chapter, we focus on the different expression of these proteins in mammalian models. Also, although the aforementioned genes are mutated in PD and are not overexpressed or knocked out (KO), these animal models are relevant in the way that may reveal specific molecular events that lead to the death of dopaminergic neurons.

In this chapter, we describe the classical and the most useful animal models to model PD. Readers with minimal knowledge of PD will eventually find out the different possibilities offered by each of these models, and their strengths and limitations.

2. Neurotoxic models

2.1. 6-OHDA (2,4,5-trihydroxyphenethylamine)

The classic and more often used neurotoxic in animal models of PD is 6-OHDA [13, 14]. Most animals are sensitive to 6-OHDA intoxication, including monkeys, cats, dogs, and rats. The rats were the more frequently used [15, 16]. Its effect was first described in the 1950s during the study of central nervous system; 6-OHDA caused a noradrenaline depletion for several months and a selective loss of noradrenergic terminals [17, 18] and was firstly isolated by Ungersted to lesion the nigrostriatal pathway in the rat decades ago [19].

Although 6-OHDA is structurally similar to DA (and noradrenaline), the presence of an additional hydroxyl group makes it toxic to dopaminergic neurons. Also, this compound does not cross the blood-brain barrier, and it makes necessary the direct injection in the brain, normally in subtantia nigra pars compacta, medium forebrain bundle, or striatum [17, 20, 21]. Lesion size depends on the amount of 6-OHDA, site of injection, and species. Typically, 6-OHDA is administered in a unilateral manner and its results are very attractive since the intact side can be used as control. Furthermore, even if there is success rate in ventricular administration [22], the bilateral administration normally leads to severe adipsia, aphagia, and also death [23, 24]. When administered intrastriatally, the 6-OHDA provokes a progressive and retrograde neuronal loss in SNpc and ventral tegmental area (VTA). Actually, in animals with full lesions (>90%) it is also observed the typical pattern seen in PD patients, with a greater loss in SNpc compared to VTA [21, 25]. Although 6-OHDA interacts with α-syn, it does not induce the formation of LB inclusions [17, 26]. The motor evaluation in these animal models is usually performed after the administration of drugs such as apomorphine which induces rotational behavior, but novel tests lacking the use of any drug have also been developed in rodents [27]. One use of this model is to ascertain whether the nigrostriatal degeneration is retrograde, i.e., tyrosine hydroxylase (TH) terminals die before the TH-neurons in SNpc as it happens in patients [21, 28] (**Figure 1**).

This model is a good model on the base that it can replicate parkinsonian features as DA depletion, nigral DA cell loss, and behavior deficits. Nevertheless, it does not affect other regions in the brain as olfactory bulbs, lower brainstem areas, or locus coeruleus.

2.2. MPTP (1-methyl-4-phenyl-1,2,5,6-tetrahydropyridine)

Even if the discovery of MPTP in 1982 due to an error in drug synthesis process could cause some mayhem in certain circles, for PD researchers it was an invaluable gift. Its toxicity was discovered after some young addicts developed idiopathic PD when they injected the compound intravenously. MPTP can be considered a gold standard for toxin-based animal models since it mimics some of the hallmarks of PD such as damage to the nigrostriatal DA pathway with a profound loss of DA in the striatum and SNpc, oxidative stress, reactive oxygen species, energy failure, and inflammation [29, 30]. However, MPTP does not induce the formation of LB, definitive characteristic of PD [31, 32]. Some studies have attempted to demonstrate the production of LB-like inclusions after MPTP administration, but those findings are not easy to replicate and make necessary to play with different dosing and timing schedules [33, 34].

MPTP is not a dopaminergic toxin, but its high lipophilia makes it to cross the blood-brain barrier after systemic administration. Once astrocytes enter the brain, they are metabolized to MPP+ by monoamine oxidase-B (MAO-B). MPP+ enters the dopaminergic neurons through the DA transporter (DAT), and once in the cytoplasm it binds to VMAT2 or it is stored in the vesicles in the mitochondria, where it inhibits the complex I of the mitochondrial electron transport chain leading to neuronal death by oxidative stress [35–37]. Thus, in mice lacking DAT, MPTP is not toxic [38]. Since the storage vesicles have a limited capacity, MPP+ most likely pushes DA out into the intercellular space where it can be metabolized to a number of compounds some of which are toxic, such as DOPAL [39] and where it can be subjected to superoxide radical (5-cysteinyl-DA) and hydroxyl radical attack (6-OHDA) (**Figure 1**). Principally, MPTP is used in primates and mice, and it is still unknown why it is not toxic in rats [40, 41]. And in primates, the resemblance with human PD features goes beyond the loss of dopaminergic neurons in the SNpc. In these animals, it also causes a greater loss of DA in SNpc than in VTA or retrorubral field [42, 43]. The classic way of administration is intravenous and systematic [44]. Some researchers also use an alternative route and they inject unilaterally in the internal carotid. This technique presents the same benefits as described before but it's more difficult to perform [45]. In primates, traditionally, the animals have been treated with high doses of MPTP, and acute models were obtained. However, in the recent years, researchers have introduced new administration protocols in order to obtain more progressive models, which would mimic more exactly the pathology in PD patients. These progressive models would give a chance to study the compensatory mechanism which takes place before the onset of the symptoms [43, 46, 47]. Additionally, in primates treated with low doses of MPTP, a greater degeneration of dopaminergic nerve terminals has been observed in the putamen than in the caudate nucleus [43, 48]. Interestingly, in primates, there is a high variability in the animal's susceptibility to MPTP and normally older animals are the most susceptible ones [49]. Also, primates treated with MPTP usually respond well to anti-parkinsonian treatments such as L-DOPA or apomorphine, and they also develop dyskinesias after long-term treatment.

The MPTP model in primates can be used in order to study other features of the PD as the nonmotor symptoms, which have recently become a target for researchers since mice do not develop a level of impairment similar to the humans [50, 51]. In the electrophysiological field, this model has also contributed to many advances including deep brain stimulation, currently the major surgical method to alleviate PD symptoms in patients [52, 53]. In the present, MPTP is more often used in mice than monkeys, mainly because of economic and practical reasons. Mice allow researchers to understand better the molecular mechanisms involved in cell death, to explore the neuronal death process or other pathological effects of PD. One remarkable aspect of the research in mice is the possibility of working with genetically modified animals [54, 55]. In sum, MPTP can be considered as the standard bearer for toxin-based PD animal models.

2.3. Rotenone

Rotenone is the most intoxicating member of the rotenoid family and is typically found in tropical plants. It is both an herbicide and insecticide having a half-life of 3–5 days depending on light conditions and degrades quickly in soil and water [56]. The toxicity of rotenone comes from its high lipophilia, and it can easily cross the blood-brain barrier (**Figure 1**). It is mainly used in rats since, so far, the studies attempting to lesion in mice or monkeys have not been successful [57, 58]. Recently, some studies have tested the toxicity of rotenone when administrated intragastric [59] or directly in the brain [60]. The administration of rotenone can be done via different routes. The most commonly used regime has typically been the systemic administration using osmotic pumps in rats, especially in Lewis rats which present a higher susceptibility to the toxic than other strains [61]. Oral administration is considered the least effective one [61, 62]. Intraperitoneal injections might induce behavioral and neurochemical deficits, and it also presents a high mortality [60]. In the case of intravenous administration, rotenone may lead to loss of nigrostriatal DA neurons and it is able to induce α-syn aggregation and LB formation, apart from other features such as oxidative stress or gastrointestinal problems [63]. It is the last aspect that makes this model so attractive, since it seems to replicate almost all of the hallmarks of PD [64]. Similar to what happens in PD, rotenone intoxication is associated with 35% reduction in serotonin, 26% in noradrenergic, and 29% in cholinergic neurons [65].

On the contrary, there is some controversy about the use of rotenone as a model of PD since in spite of the DA oxidation there is not much evidence of depletion of DA in the nigrostriatal system [66], and there are no well-documented cases of PD patients from rotenone intoxication. This makes the model not very advantageous compared to other toxic-based ones, such as 6-OHDA and MPTP.

2.4. Paraquat (N,N-dimethyl-4-4-4-bypiridinium)

Paraquat (PQ) is an herbicide that exhibits similar structure to MPP+, and this is the reason why it was suggested that it could have a parkinsonian toxic effect. However, so far, only 95 cases of PD patients linked to PQ have been reported [67] even if being widely used in agriculture. Typically, PQ exerts its deleterious effect through oxidative stress mediated by redox cycling and generating reactive oxygen species, more exactly, superoxide radical, hydrogen peroxide, and the hydroxyl radical, which in turn would lead to the damage of lipids, proteins, RNA, and DNA [68, 69]. The evidence of PQ toxicity in the nigrostriatal DA system is somehow ambiguous. Some studies carried out in mice have been able to demonstrate that systemic administration can reduce motor activity, and there is a dose-dependent loss of TH-positive striatal fibers and SNc neurons [70, 71]. In contrast, other researchers claimed that there are no PQ-induced changes after administration [72]. Interestingly, in a recent study, Rappold et al. [73] could evidence that when administered in high doses, PQ can employ the organic cationic transporter-3 (OCT-3) and the DAT becomes toxic to neurons in SNpc. They also suggest that PQ damages are caused by radicalized PQ and facilitated by glial cells, as it does MPP+. One of the most striking aspects of PQ with respect to PD is its ability to induce LB-like structures in dopaminergic neurons of the SNpc [74] mimicking the PD-like pathology. Nevertheless, how oxidative stress and cell death are linked because of PQ remains unknown, limiting the research to the study of the process of LB formation in dopaminergic neurons (**Figure 1**).

Additionally, PQ is not the only pesticide or agricultural chemical known to provoke damage in the dopaminergic system. Maneb (manganese ethylenebisdithiocarbamate) or ziram are other examples of compounds that when exposed to them have a greater risk of developing

PD [75, 76]. In any case, results from studies using pesticides give credence to the theory that environmental pesticides can cause PD [77, 78]. However, further studies are required to determine the precise involvement of these compounds in the etiology of PD.

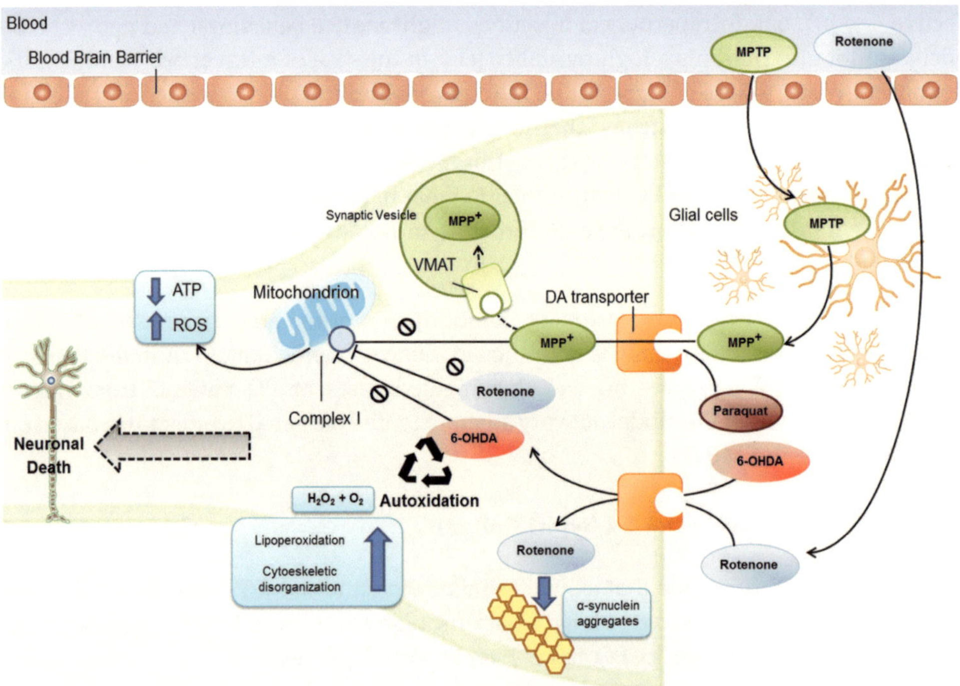

Figure 1. Pathogenesis of toxin-induced models. MPTP crosses the blood-brain barrier and is metabolized to 1-methyl-4-phenylpyridinium (MPP^+) by the enzyme monoamine oxidase B (MAO-B) in glial cells and then to the active toxic compound. MPP^+ is then taken up by dopamine transporter where it impairs mitochondrial respiration by inhibiting complex I of the electron transport chain, causing oxidative stress and activation of programmed cell death molecular pathways. Both paraquat and 6-hydroxydopamine (6-OHDA) easily cross cell membrane through the dopamine transporter and may also exert their toxicities, in part, by targeting mitochondria with the subsequent production of ROS and quinones causing the degeneration of the nigrostriatal dopaminergic neurons. Rotenone is extremely hydrophobic and penetrates easily the cellular membrane inducing the formation of α-synuclein aggregates and mitochondrial impairment with the subsequent production of ROS and quinones.

3. Genetic models

Although PD is mainly a sporadic disorder, about 10% of all PD cases are caused by genetic mutations [79]. Animal models of these mutations are important as they represent potential therapeutic targets. Having said that, the pathological and behavioral phenotypes of these genetic models are often quite different from the human condition [80]. For example, almost all of these genetic models failed to find significant loss of dopaminergic neurons, the main pathological hallmark of PD [81–84]. Below, we describe different genetic models that reproduce the most known mutations observed in familial PD (**Figure 2**).

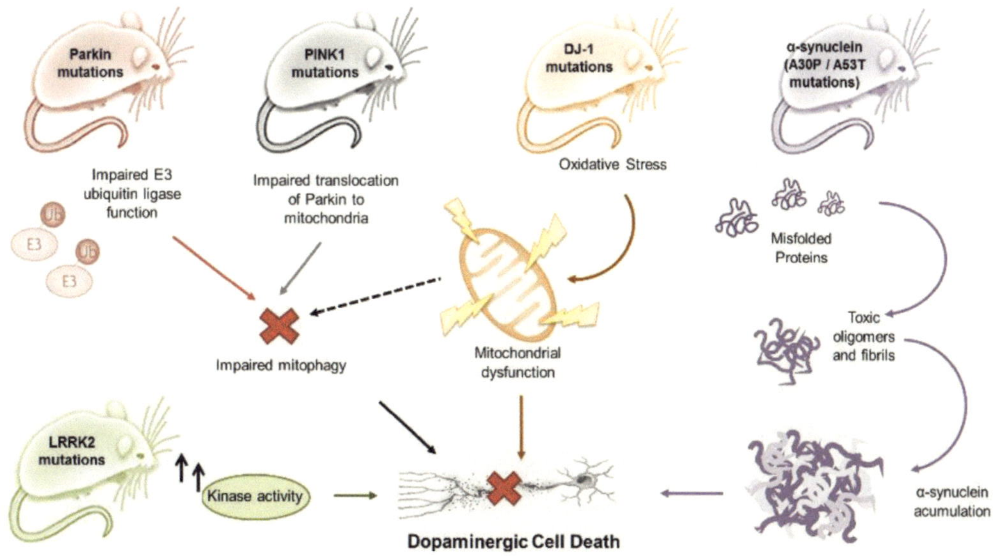

Figure 2. Genetic animal models in Parkinson disease (PD). Many genetic mouse models have been developed in order to understand PD pathogenesis and identify potential therapeutic targets. Genetic models are adjusted based on genetic mutations identified in the human disease. These genes are part of signaling pathways important for neuronal dopaminergic function. These models contribute to know mechanisms on disease onset or progression of PD or to understand the case and effect of these genetic mutations.

3.1. α-syn

SNCA (α-syn) was the first gene linked to a dominant-type, familial PD, called Park1 [85]. The duplication or triplication of α-syn is sufficient to cause PD, suggesting that the level of α-syn expression is a critical determinant of PD progression [86]. Three missense mutations of α-syn, encoding the substitutions A30P, A53T, and E46K, have been identified in familial PD so far [87, 88]. The pathological accumulation of misfolded α-syn plays an essential role in the pathogenesis of PD since α-syn is the main component of LB. While LBs are found principally in nigral neurons of PD patients, they are also found in other brain regions such as locus coeruleus, nucleus basalis of Meynert, hypothalamus, cerebral cortex, and cranial nerve motor nuclei [89]. Numerous animal models have been developed trying to replicate α-syn neurodegeneration and propagation. These include transgenic mice (KO and overexpression), grafting models, intracerebral protein injections, or virally induced expression of α-syn. The main handicap of these models is that no significant nigrostriatal degeneration has been found in most of them, although some of these mice showed decreased striatal levels of TH or DA and behavioral impairments [80].

In general, the models of α-syn overexpression in mice produced some behavioral alterations in both the A30P and A53T mice [90–92]. Also, depending on the promoter, some models showed loss of terminals and DA in the striatum [93–98] although almost of them failed to reproduce the dopaminergic cell loss characteristic of PD [2, 94, 99–101]. Only the TH promoter led to dopaminergic cell loss in a few studies [102, 103]. Janezic et al. [104] generated bacterial artificial chromosome (BAC) transgenic mice (SNCA-OVX) that express WT human α-syn and display an age-dependent loss of SNc DA neurons preceded by early deficits in DA release from terminals in the dorsal striatum, protein aggregation, and reduced firing of SNc DA neurons [104]. Regarding viral vectors injections, largely lentiviruses and adeno-associated viruses (AAVs), have been used to drive exogenous α-syn in mice, rats, and primates [105–109]. In this case, viral vector-mediated α-syn models display α-syn pathology and clear dopaminergic neurodegeneration. The injection of human mutant α-syn by AAVs into the SNpc of rats induces a progressive, age-dependent loss of DA neurons, motor impairment, α-syn cytoplasmic inclusions, and degenerative changes in striatal axons both in rats [110, 111] and mice [109, 112]. In the last years, the suggested prion-like behavior of α-syn has been examined in animal models of PD. These models not only explore the pathology and spreading of α-syn but the cell-to-cell transfer. Importantly, to date, numerous studies have demonstrated that α-syn may be transmissible from cell to cell in animal models in different ways using different approaches [33, 113–120].

Thus, despite the limitations of these α-syn models, some of them could be useful to elucidate the role of a-α-syn in PD and the suggested prion-like mechanism of propagation of this protein [121].

3.2. LRKK2

Mutations in LRRK2 are known to cause a late-onset autosomal dominant form of PD [122]. The most frequent mutations are the G2019S and the R1441C [123]. Many different LRRK2 rodent models have been developed with different approaches but as it happens with α-syn, although they show α-syn or ubiquitin accumulation, progressive motor impairments, and slight reduction of striatal DA, they do not display functional disruption of the nigrostriatal dopaminergic neurons [82, 124–128]. Similarly, overexpression of G2019S or R1441C LRRK2 leads to none or slight loss of dopaminergic neurons in the SNpc and no alteration in striatal DA levels or locomotor activity in both mice and rats [129–131].

BAC transgenic mice expressing mutated LRKK2 have also been developed showing no nigrostriatal degeneration [132–134]. On the contrary, a rat LRRK2 model with neuron-specific, adenoviral mediated expression of LRRK2 G2019S in the nigrostriatal system has been produced, which develops a progressive degeneration of nigral dopaminergic neurons [135]. Additionally, using viral vector-based models, Lee and colleagues [28] reported that the expression of G2019S LRRK2 resulted in a 50% neuronal loss in the ipsilateral SNc associated with reduced striatal dopaminergic fibers [136]. In summary, we can conclude that the transgenic LRRK2 animal models are not a useful model for studying the pathology of PD.

3.3. Pink1 and Parkin

Homozygous mutations in the Parkin and PINK1 genes were discovered in families with autosomal recessive PD [137]. In fact, parkin mutations are the most common cause of autosomal recessive PD. Likewise, mutations in PINK1 are the second most common. Despite this early onset, patients with these mutations have an indistinguishable phenotype from that of sporadic patients. Many PINK1 and parkin KO mice have been generated, and the phenotypes of these mice are very similar. PINK1 and Parkin KO mice have an age-dependent, moderate reduction in striatal DA levels accompanied by low locomotor activity, but do not exhibit major abnormalities in the DA neurons or striatal DA levels, and they do not show LB formation either [81, 138–145]. A new approach consisting in overexpression of T240R-parkin and of human WT parkin in rats leads to progressive and dose-dependent DA cell death [146]. Noteworthy, the Parkin-Q311X-DAT-BAC mice exhibit multiple late onsets and progressive hypokinetic motor deficits, age-dependent DA neuron degeneration in the SNc, and a significant reduction in striatal DA and dopaminergic terminals in the striatum [147]. Overall, PINK1 and Parkin models do not produce functional disruption of the nigrostriatal pathway or other PD-related pathology, thus their usefulness is questionable.

3.4. DJ-1

Missense DJ-1 mutations are linked to autosomal recessive and early-onset PD. DJ-1 KO mice showed no loss of SNpc dopaminergic neurons but reduced striatal DA release and decreased locomotor activity [148, 149]. Recently, a new DJ-1 KO mouse, backcrossed on a C57/BL6 background, displayed an early-onset unilateral loss of DA neurons in the SNpc, progressing to bilateral degeneration with aging. Also, these mice exhibit age-dependent bilateral degeneration in the locus coeruleus and mild motor behavioral deficits [150]. If confirmed, this model could provide a possible tool to study the progression of PD.

4. Concluding remarks

Our current understanding of PD pathology greatly benefited from the use of animal models. However, despite these accomplishments, current PD animal models still have to be improved a lot. It seems difficult that a single model can fully recapitulate the complexity of the human PD in the short term. Because there is no perfect model to date, it is very important to choose the correct animal model for each experiment. By providing an overview of the different animal models available to modeling PD, readers would find that there are a lot of options addressing a specific experimental need.

Acknowledgements

We acknowledge HM CINAC and many individuals and corporations that supported Parkinson Disease research at HM CINAC for financial support. The authors are supported by grants from CIBERNED and Plan Nacional from Spanish Ministry of Education.

Author details

Javier Blesa[1*], Ines Trigo-Damas[1], Ana Quiroga-Varela[2] and Natalia Lopez-Gonzalez del Rey[1]

*Address all correspondence to: jblesa.hmcinac@hmhospitales.com

1 Centre for Integrative Neuroscience A.C. (HM CINAC), Hospital HM Puerta del Sur, Mostoles, Madrid, Spain

2 Department of Neuroscience, Biodonostia Institute, San Sebastián, Spain

References

[1] Lees AJ, Hardy J, Revesz T. Parkinson's disease. Lancet. 2009 Jun 13;373(9680):2055–66.

[2] Blesa J, Przedborski S. Parkinson's disease: animal models and dopaminergic cell vulnerability. Front Neuroanat. 2014 Dec 15;8:155.

[3] Dawson TM, Ko HS, Dawson VL. Genetic animal models of Parkinson's disease. Neuron. 2010 Jun 10;66(5):646–61.

[4] Berg J, Roch M, Altschüler J, Winter C, Schwerk A, Kurtz A, et al. Human adipose-derived mesenchymal stem cells improve motor functions and are neuroprotective in the 6-hydroxydopamine-rat model for Parkinson's disease when cultured in monolayer cultures but suppress hippocampal neurogenesis and hippocampal memory Function when cultured in spheroids. Stem Cell Rev. 2015 Feb;11(1):133–49.

[5] Guo M. Drosophila as a model to study mitochondrial dysfunction in Parkinson's disease. Cold Spring Harb Perspect Med. 2012 Nov 1;2(11).

[6] Matsui H, Uemura N, Yamakado H, Takeda S, Takahashi R. Exploring the pathogenetic mechanisms underlying Parkinson's disease in medaka fish. J Parkinsons Dis. 2014 Jan;4(2):301–10.

[7] Chege PM, McColl G. Caenorhabditis elegans: a model to investigate oxidative stress and metal dyshomeostasis in Parkinson's disease. Front Aging Neurosci. 2014 Jan;6:89.

[8] Gonzalez-Reyes LE, Verbitsky M, Blesa J, Jackson-Lewis V, Paredes D, Tillack K, et al. Sonic hedgehog maintains cellular and neurochemical homeostasis in the adult nigrostriatal circuit. Neuron. 2012 Jul 26;75(2):306–19.

[9] Jankovic J, Chen S, Le WD. The role of Nurr1 in the development of dopaminergic neurons and Parkinson's disease. Prog Neurobiol. 2005 Sep–Oct;77(1–2):128–38.

[10] Li J, Dani JA, Le W. The role of transcription factor Pitx3 in dopamine neuron development and Parkinson's disease. Curr Top Med Chem. 2009 Jan;9(10):855–9.

[11] Nordström U, Beauvais G, Ghosh A, Pulikkaparambil Sasidharan BC, Lundblad M, Fuchs J, Joshi RL, Lipton JW, Roholt A, Medicetty S, Feinstein TN, Steiner JA, Escobar Galvis ML, Prochiantz A, Brundin P. Progressive nigrostriatal terminal dysfunction and degeneration in the engrailed1 heterozygous mouse model of Parkinson's disease. Neurobiol Dis. 2015 Jan;73:70–82.

[12] Chesselet M-F, Richter F. Modelling of Parkinson's disease in mice. Lancet Neurol. 2011 Dec;10(12):1108–18.

[13] Schwarting RK, Huston JP. Unilateral 6-hydroxydopamine lesions of meso-striatal dopamine neurons and their physiological sequelae. Prog Neurobiol. 1996;49(3):215–66.

[14] Schwarting RK, Huston JP. The unilateral 6-hydroxydopamine lesion model in behavioral brain research. Analysis of functional deficits, recovery and treatments. Prog Neurobiol. 1996;50(2–3):275–331.

[15] Valette H, Deleuze P, Syrota A, Delforge J, Crouzel C, Fuseau C, et al. Canine myocardial beta-adrenergic, muscarinic receptor densities after denervation: a PET study. J Nucl Med. 1995;36(1):140–6.

[16] Roeling TA, Docter GJ, Voorn P, Melchers BP, Wolters EC, Groenewegen HJ. Effects of unilateral 6-hydroxydopamine lesions on neuropeptide immunoreactivity in the basal ganglia of the common marmoset, *Callithrix jacchus*, a quantitative immunohistochemical analysis. J Chem Neuroanat. 1995;9(3):155–64.

[17] Blandini F, Armentero M-T, Martignoni E. The 6-hydroxydopamine model: news from the past. Parkinsonism Relat Disord. 2008 Jan;14 Suppl 2:S124–9.

[18] Porter CC, Totaro JA, Stone CA. Effect of 6-hydroxydopamine and some other compounds on the concentration of norepinephrine in the hearts of mice. J Pharmacol Exp Ther. 1963 Jun;140:308–16.

[19] Ungerstedt U. 6-Hydroxy-dopamine induced degeneration of central monoamine neurons. Eur J Pharmacol. 1968;5(1):107–10.

[20] Perese DA, Ulman J, Viola J, Ewing SE, Bankiewicz KS. A 6-hydroxydopamine-induced selective parkinsonian rat model. Brain Res. 1989;494(2):285–93.

[21] Przedborski S, Levivier M, Jiang H, Ferreira M, Jackson-Lewis V, Donaldson D, et al. Dose-dependent lesions of the dopaminergic nigrostriatal pathway induced by intrastriatal injection of 6-hydroxydopamine. Neuroscience. 1995;67(3):631–47.

[22] Rodríguez M, Barroso-Chinea P, Abdala P, Obeso J, González-Hernández T. Dopamine cell degeneration induced by intraventricular administration of 6-hydroxydopamine in the rat: similarities with cell loss in Parkinson's disease. Exp Neurol. 2001 May;169(1): 163–81.

[23] Ungerstedt U. Adipsia and aphagia after 6-hydroxydopamine induced degeneration of the nigro-striatal dopamine system. Acta Physiol Scand Suppl. 1971;367:95–122.

[24] Bourn WM, Chin L, Picchioni AL. Enhancement of audiogenic seizure by 6-hydroxy-dopamine. J Pharm Pharmacol. 1972;24(11):913–4.

[25] Sauer H, Oertel WH. Progressive degeneration of nigrostriatal dopamine neurons following intrastriatal terminal lesions with 6-hydroxydopamine: a combined retro-grade tracing and immunocytochemical study in the rat. Neuroscience. 1994;59(2):401–15.

[26] Alves da Costa C, Dunys J, Brau F, Wilk S, Cappai R, Checler F. 6-Hydroxydopamine but not 1-methyl-4-phenylpyridinium abolishes alpha-synuclein anti-apoptotic phenotype by inhibiting its proteasomal degradation and by promoting its aggrega-tion. J Biol Chem. 2006 Apr;281(14):9824–31.

[27] Glajch KE, Fleming SM, Surmeier DJ, Osten P. Sensorimotor assessment of the unilateral 6-hydroxydopamine mouse model of Parkinson's disease. Behav Brain Res. 2012 May 1;230(2):309–16.

[28] Lee CS, Sauer H, Bjorklund A. Dopaminergic neuronal degeneration and motor impairments following axon terminal lesion by instrastriatal 6-hydroxydopamine in the rat. Neuroscience. 1996;72(3):641–53.

[29] Langston JW, Ballard P, Tetrud JW, Irwin I. Chronic Parkinsonism in humans due to a product of meperidine-analog synthesis. Science. 1983 Feb 25;219(4587):979–80.

[30] Dauer W, Przedborski S. Parkinson's disease: mechanisms and models. Neuron. 2003 Sep 11;39(6):889–909.

[31] Forno LS, DeLanney LE, Irwin I, Langston JW. Similarities and differences between MPTP-induced parkinsonism and Parkinson's disease. Neuropathologic considera-tions. Adv Neurol. 1993;60:600–8.

[32] Halliday G, Herrero MT, Murphy K, McCann H, Ros-Bernal F, Barcia C, et al. No Lewy pathology in monkeys with over 10 years of severe MPTP Parkinsonism. Mov Disord. 2009 Jul 30;24(10):1519–23.

[33] Fornai F, Schlüter OM, Lenzi P, Gesi M, Ruffoli R, Ferrucci M, et al. Parkinson-like syndrome induced by continuous MPTP infusion: convergent roles of the ubiquitin-

proteasome system and alpha-synuclein. Proc Natl Acad Sci U S A. 2005 Mar;102(9): 3413–8.

[34] Kowall NW, Hantraye P, Brouillet E, Beal MF, McKee AC, Ferrante RJ. MPTP induces alpha-synuclein aggregation in the substantia nigra of baboons. Neuroreport. 2000 Jan 17;11(1):211–3.

[35] Guillot TS, Shepherd KR, Richardson JR, Wang MZ, Li Y, Emson PC, et al. Reduced vesicular storage of dopamine exacerbates methamphetamine-induced neurodegeneration and astrogliosis. J Neurochem. 2008 Sep;106(5):2205–17.

[36] Guillot TS, Miller GW. Protective actions of the vesicular monoamine transporter 2 (VMAT2) in monoaminergic neurons. Mol Neurobiol. 2009 Apr;39(2):149–70.

[37] Gainetdinov RR, Fumagalli F, Wang YM, Jones SR, Levey AI, Miller GW, et al. Increased MPTP neurotoxicity in vesicular monoamine transporter 2 heterozygote knockout mice. J Neurochem. 1998;70(5):1973–8.

[38] Bezard E, Gross CE, Fournier MC, Dovero S, Bloch B, Jaber M. Absence of MPTP-induced neuronal death in mice lacking the dopamine transporter. Exp Neurol. 1999;155(2):268–73.

[39] Panneton WM, Kumar VB, Gan Q, Burke WJ, Galvin JE. The neurotoxicity of DOPAL: behavioral and stereological evidence for its role in Parkinson disease pathogenesis. PLoS One. 2010;5(12):e15251.

[40] Chiueh CC, Markey SP, Burns RS, Johannessen JN, Pert A, Kopin IJ. Neurochemical and behavioral effects of systemic and intranigral administration of N-methyl-4-phenyl-1,2,3,6-tetrahydropyridine in the rat. Eur J Pharmacol. 1984;100(2):189–94.

[41] Tieu K. A guide to neurotoxic animal models of Parkinson's disease. Cold Spring Harb Perspect Med. 2011 Sep;1(1):a009316.

[42] Blesa J, Pifl C, Sánchez-González MA, Juri C, García-Cabezas MA, Adánez R, et al. The nigrostriatal system in the presymptomatic and symptomatic stages in the MPTP monkey model: a PET, histological and biochemical study. Neurobiol Dis. 2012 Oct; 48(1):79–91.

[43] Blesa J, Juri C, Collantes M, Peñuelas I, Prieto E, Iglesias E, et al. Progression of dopaminergic depletion in a model of MPTP-induced Parkinsonism in non-human primates. An (18)F-DOPA and (11)C-DTBZ PET study. Neurobiol Dis. 2010 Jun;38(3): 456–63.

[44] Przedborski S, Jackson-Lewis V, Naini AB, Jakowec M, Petzinger G, Miller R, et al. The parkinsonian toxin 1-methyl-4-phenyl-1,2,3,6-tetrahydropyridine (MPTP): a technical review of its utility and safety. J Neurochem. 2001 Mar;76(5):1265–74.

[45] Bankiewicz KS, Oldfield EH, Chiueh CC, Doppman JL, Jacobowitz DM, Kopin IJ. Hemiparkinsonism in monkeys after unilateral internal carotid artery infusion of 1-methyl-4-phenyl-1,2,3,6-tetrahydropyridine (MPTP). Life Sci. 1986;39(1):7–16.

[46] Hantraye P, Varastet M, Peschanski M, Riche D, Cesaro P, Willer JC, et al. Stable parkinsonian syndrome and uneven loss of striatal dopamine fibres following chronic MPTP administration in baboons. Neuroscience. 1993;53(1):169–78.

[47] Bezard E, Imbert C, Deloire X, Bioulac B, Gross CE. A chronic MPTP model reproducing the slow evolution of Parkinson's disease: evolution of motor symptoms in the monkey. Brain Res. 1997 Aug 22;766(1–2):107–12.

[48] Moratalla R, Quinn B, DeLanney LE, Irwin I, Langston JW, Graybiel AM. Differential vulnerability of primate caudate-putamen and striosome-matrix dopamine systems to the neurotoxic effects of 1-methyl-4-phenyl-1,2,3,6-tetrahydropyridine. Proc Natl Acad Sci U S A. 1992 May 1;89(9):3859–63.

[49] Ovadia A, Zhang Z, Gash DM. Increased susceptibility to MPTP toxicity in middle-aged rhesus monkeys. Neurobiol Aging. 1995;16(6):931–7.

[50] Pessiglione M, Guehl D, Hirsch EC, Féger J, Tremblay L. Disruption of self-organized actions in monkeys with progressive MPTP-induced parkinsonism. I. Effects of task complexity. Eur J Neurosci. 2004 Jan;19(2):426–36.

[51] Schneider JS. Modeling cognitive deficits associated with Parkinsonism in the chronic-low-dose MPTP-treated monkey. In: Levin ED, Buccafusco JJ, editors. Animal Models of Cognitive Impairment. Boca Raton (FL): CRC Press/Taylor & Francis; 2006. Chapter 9.

[52] Guridi J, Herrero MT, Luquin MR, Guillen J, Ruberg M, Laguna J, et al. Subthalamotomy in parkinsonian monkeys. Behavioural and biochemical analysis. Brain. 1996;119 (Pt 5):1717–27.

[53] Bergman H, Wichmann T, DeLong MR. Reversal of experimental parkinsonism by lesions of the subthalamic nucleus. Science 1990 Sep 21;249(4975):1436–8.

[54] Dauer W, Kholodilov N, Vila M, Trillat A-CC, Goodchild R, Larsen KE, et al. Resistance of alpha -synuclein null mice to the parkinsonian neurotoxin MPTP. Proc Natl Acad Sci U S A. 2002 Oct 29;99(22):14524–9.

[55] Vila M, Jackson-Lewis V, Vukosavic S, Djaldetti R, Liberatore G, Offen D, et al. Bax ablation prevents dopaminergic neurodegeneration in the 1-methyl- 4-phenyl-1,2,3,6-tetrahydropyridine mouse model of Parkinson's disease. Proc Natl Acad Sci U S A. 2001 Feb 27;98(5):2837–42.

[56] Hisata J. Lake and stream rehabilitation: rotenone use and health risks. 2002.

[57] Lake and Stream Rehabilitation: Rotenone Use and Health Risks, Final Supplemental Environmental Impact Statement (January 2002).

[58] Ferrante RJ, Schulz JB, Kowall NW, Beal MF. Systemic administration of rotenone produces selective damage in the striatum and globus pallidus, but not in the substantia nigra. Brain Res. 1997;753(1):157–62.

[59] Pan-Montojo F, Anichtchik O, Dening Y, Knels L, Pursche S, Jung R, et al. Progression of Parkinson's disease pathology is reproduced by intragastric administration of rotenone in mice. PLoS One. 2010 Jan;5(1):e8762.

[60] Alam M, Mayerhofer A, Schmidt WJ. The neurobehavioral changes induced by bilateral rotenone lesion in medial forebrain bundle of rats are reversed by L-DOPA. Behav Brain Res. 2004;151(1–2):117–24.

[61] Betarbet R, Sherer TB, MacKenzie G, Garcia-Osuna M, Panov A V, Greenamyre JT. Chronic systemic pesticide exposure reproduces features of Parkinson's disease. Nat Neurosci. 2000;3(12):1301–6.

[62] Inden M, Kitamura Y, Takeuchi H, Yanagida T, Takata K, Kobayashi Y, et al. Neurodegeneration of mouse nigrostriatal dopaminergic system induced by repeated oral administration of rotenone is prevented by 4-phenylbutyrate, a chemical chaperone. J Neurochem. 2007 Jun;101(6):1491–504.

[63] Cannon JR, Tapias V, Na HM, Honick AS, Drolet RE, Greenamyre JT. A highly reproducible rotenone model of Parkinson's disease. Neurobiol Dis. 2009 May;34(2): 279–90.

[64] Sherer TB, Kim JH, Betarbet R, Greenamyre JT. Subcutaneous rotenone exposure causes highly selective dopaminergic degeneration and alpha-synuclein aggregation. Exp Neurol. 2003 Jan;179(1):9–16.

[65] Höglinger GU, Féger J, Prigent A, Michel PP, Parain K, Champy P, et al. Chronic systemic complex I inhibition induces a hypokinetic multisystem degeneration in rats. J Neurochem. 2003 Feb;84(3):491–502.

[66] Wu Y-N, Johnson SW. Dopamine oxidation facilitates rotenone-dependent potentiation of N-methyl-D-aspartate currents in rat substantia nigra dopamine neurons. Neuroscience. 2011 Nov;195:138–44.

[67] Berry C, La Vecchia C, Nicotera P. Paraquat and Parkinson's disease. Cell Death Differ. 2010 Jul;17(7):1115–25.

[68] Day BJ, Patel M, Calavetta L, Chang LY, Stamler JS. A mechanism of paraquat toxicity involving nitric oxide synthase. Proc Natl Acad Sci U S A. 1999;96(22):12760–5.

[69] Przedborski S, Ischiropoulos H. Reactive oxygen and nitrogen species: weapons of neuronal destruction in models of Parkinson's disease. Antioxid Redox Signal. 2005 May–Jun;7(5–6):685–93

[70] Brooks AI, Chadwick CA, Gelbard HA, Cory-Slechta DA, Federoff HJ. Paraquat elicited neurobehavioral syndrome caused by dopaminergic neuron loss. Brain Res. 1999;823(1–2):1–10.

[71] McCormack AL, Thiruchelvam M, Manning-Bog AB, Thiffault C, Langston JW, Cory-Slechta DA, et al. Environmental risk factors and Parkinson's disease: selective degeneration of nigral dopaminergic neurons caused by the herbicide paraquat. Neurobiol Dis. 2002 Jul;10(2):119–27.

[72] Thiruchelvam M, Brockel BJ, Richfield EK, Baggs RB, Cory-Slechta DA. Potentiated and preferential effects of combined paraquat and maneb on nigrostriatal dopamine systems: environmental risk factors for Parkinson's disease? Brain Res. 2000;873(2):225–34.

[73] Rappold PM, Cui M, Chesser AS, Tibbett J, Grima JC, Duan L, et al. Paraquat neurotoxicity is mediated by the dopamine transporter and organic cation transporter-3. Proc Natl Acad Sci U S A. 2011 Dec 20;108(51):20766–71.

[74] Manning-Bog AB, McCormack AL, Li J, Uversky VN, Fink AL, Di Monte DA. The herbicide paraquat causes up-regulation and aggregation of alpha-synuclein in mice: paraquat and alpha-synuclein. J Biol Chem. 2002 Jan 18;277(3):1641–4.

[75] Tang CC, Poston KL, Dhawan V, Eidelberg D. Abnormalities in metabolic network activity precede the onset of motor symptoms in Parkinson's disease. J Neurosci. 2010 Jan;30(3):1049–56.

[76] Tanner CM, Kamel F, Ross GW, Hoppin JA, Goldman SM, Korell M, et al. Rotenone, paraquat, and Parkinson's disease. Environ Health Perspect. 2011 Jun;119(6):866–72.

[77] Butterfield PG, Valanis BG, Spencer PS, Lindeman CA, Nutt JG. Environmental antecedents of young-onset Parkinson's disease. Neurology. 1993;43(6):1150–8.

[78] Gorell JM, Johnson CC, Rybicki BA, Peterson EL, Richardson RJ. The risk of Parkinson's disease with exposure to pesticides, farming, well water, and rural living. Neurology. 1998;50(5):1346–50.

[79] Kalinderi K, Bostantjopoulou S, Fidani L. The genetic background of Parkinson's disease: current progress and future prospects. Acta Neurol Scand. 2016 Feb 12.

[80] Chesselet MF, Fleming S, Mortazavi F, Meurers B. Strengths and limitations of genetic mouse models of Parkinson's disease. Park Relat Disord. 2008;14 Suppl 2:S84–7.

[81] Goldberg MS, Fleming SM, Palacino JJ, Cepeda C, Lam HA, Bhatnagar A, et al. Parkin-deficient mice exhibit nigrostriatal deficits but not loss of dopaminergic neurons. J Biol Chem. 2003 Oct 31;278(44):43628–35.

[82] Hinkle KM, Yue M, Behrouz B, Dächsel JC, Lincoln SJ, Bowles EE, et al. LRRK2 knockout mice have an intact dopaminergic system but display alterations in exploratory and motor co-ordination behaviors. Mol Neurodegener. 2012 Jan;7:25.

[83] Sanchez G, Varaschin RK, Büeler H, Marcogliese PC, Park DS, Trudeau L-E. Unaltered striatal dopamine release levels in young Parkin knockout, Pink1 knockout, DJ-1 knockout and LRRK2 R1441G transgenic mice. PLoS One. 2014 Jan;9(4):e94826.

[84] Andres-Mateos E, Perier C, Zhang L, Blanchard-Fillion B, Greco TM, Thomas B, et al. DJ-1 gene deletion reveals that DJ-1 is an atypical peroxiredoxin-like peroxidase. Proc Natl Acad Sci U S A. 2007;104(37):14807–12.

[85] Goedert M, Spillantini MG, Del Tredici K, Braak H. 100 years of Lewy pathology. Nat Rev Neurol. 2013 Jan;9(1):13–24.

[86] Singleton AB, Farrer M, Johnson J, Singleton A, Hague S, Kachergus J, et al. alpha-Synuclein locus triplication causes Parkinson's disease. Science. 2003 Oct 31;302(5646):841.

[87] Schapira AH, Jenner P. Etiology and pathogenesis of Parkinson's disease. Mov Disord. 2011 May;26(6):1049–55.

[88] Vekrellis K, Xilouri M, Emmanouilidou E, Rideout HJ, Stefanis L. Pathological roles of α-synuclein in neurological disorders. Lancet Neurol. 2011 Nov;10(11):1015–25.

[89] Recasens A, Dehay B. Alpha-synuclein spreading in Parkinson's disease. Front Neuroanat. 2014 Jan;8:159.

[90] Oaks AW, Frankfurt M, Finkelstein DI, Sidhu A. Age-dependent effects of A53T alpha-synuclein on behavior and dopaminergic function. PLoS One. 2013 Jan;8(4):e60378.

[91] Sotiriou E, Vassilatis DK, Vila M, Stefanis L. Selective noradrenergic vulnerability in α-synuclein transgenic mice. Neurobiol Aging. 2010 Dec;31(12):2103–14.

[92] Paumier KL, Sukoff Rizzo SJ, Berger Z, Chen Y, Gonzales C, Kaftan E, et al. Behavioral characterization of A53T mice reveals early and late stage deficits related to Parkinson's disease. PLoS One. 2013 Jan;8(8):e70274.

[93] Masliah E, Rockenstein E, Veinbergs I, Mallory M, Hashimoto M, Takeda A, Sagara Y, Sisk A, Mucke L. Dopaminergic loss and inclusion body formation in alpha-synuclein mice: implications for neurodegenerative disorders. Science 2000 Feb 18;287(5456):1265–9. PubMed PMID: 10678833.

[94] van der Putten H, Wiederhold KH, Probst A, Barbieri S, Mistl C, Danner S, et al. Neuropathology in mice expressing human alpha-synuclein. J Neurosci. 2000 Aug 15;20(16):6021–9.

[95] Rockenstein E, Mallory M, Hashimoto M, Song D, Shults CW, Lang I, et al. Differential neuropathological alterations in transgenic mice expressing alpha-synuclein from the platelet-derived growth factor and Thy-1 promoters. J Neurosci Res. 2002 Jun 1;68(5):568–78.

[96] Ikeda M, Kawarabayashi T, Harigaya Y, Sasaki A, Yamada S, Matsubara E, et al. Motor impairment and aberrant production of neurochemicals in human alpha-synuclein

A30P+A53T transgenic mice with alpha-synuclein pathology. Brain Res. 2009 Jan 23;1250:232–41.

[97] Ono K, Ikemoto M, Kawarabayashi T, Ikeda M, Nishinakagawa T, Hosokawa M, et al. A chemical chaperone, sodium 4-phenylbutyric acid, attenuates the pathogenic potency in human alpha-synuclein A30P + A53T transgenic mice. Parkinsonism Relat Disord. 2009 Nov;15(9):649–54.

[98] Lam HA, Wu N, Cely I, Kelly RL, Hean S, Richter F, et al. Elevated tonic extracellular dopamine concentration and altered dopamine modulation of synaptic activity precede dopamine loss in the striatum of mice overexpressing human α-synuclein. J Neurosci Res. 2011 Jul;89(7):1091–102.

[99] Giasson BI, Duda JE, Quinn SM, Zhang B, Trojanowski JQ, Lee VM. Neuronal alpha-synucleinopathy with severe movement disorder in mice expressing A53T human alpha-synuclein. Neuron. 2002;34(4):521–33.

[100] Gispert S, Del Turco D, Garrett L, Chen A, Bernard DJ, Hamm-Clement J, et al. Transgenic mice expressing mutant A53T human alpha-synuclein show neuronal dysfunction in the absence of aggregate formation. Mol Cell Neurosci. 2003 Oct;24(2): 419–29.

[101] Gomez-Isla T, Irizarry MC, Mariash A, Cheung B, Soto O, Schrump S, et al. Motor dysfunction and gliosis with preserved dopaminergic markers in human alpha-synuclein A30P transgenic mice. Neurobiol Aging. 2003;24(2):245–58.

[102] Thiruchelvam MJ, Powers JM, Cory-Slechta DA, Richfield EK. Risk factors for dopaminergic neuron loss in human alpha-synuclein transgenic mice. Eur J Neurosci. 2004 Feb;19(4):845–54.

[103] Wakamatsu M, Ishii A, Iwata S, Sakagami J, Ukai Y, Ono M, et al. Selective loss of nigral dopamine neurons induced by overexpression of truncated human alpha-synuclein in mice. Neurobiol Aging. 2008 Apr;29(4):574–85.

[104] Janezic S, Threlfell S, Dodson PD, Dowie MJ, Taylor TN, Potgieter D, et al. Deficits in dopaminergic transmission precede neuron loss and dysfunction in a new Parkinson model. Proc Natl Acad Sci U S A. 2013 Oct 15;110(42):E4016–25.

[105] Kirik D, Rosenblad C, Burger C, Lundberg C, Johansen TE, Muzyczka N, et al. Parkinson-like neurodegeneration induced by targeted overexpression of alpha-synuclein in the nigrostriatal system. J Neurosci. 2002 Apr 1;22(7):2780–91.

[106] Lo Bianco C, Ridet J-L, Schneider BL, Deglon N, Aebischer P. alpha -Synucleinopathy and selective dopaminergic neuron loss in a rat lentiviral-based model of Parkinson's disease. Proc Natl Acad Sci U S A. 2002 Aug 6;99(16):10813–8.

[107] Klein RL, King MA, Hamby ME, Meyer EM. Dopaminergic cell loss induced by human A30P alpha-synuclein gene transfer to the rat substantia nigra. Hum Gene Ther. 2002 Mar 20;13(5):605–12.

[108] Lauwers E, Bequé D, Van Laere K, Nuyts J, Bormans G, Mortelmans L, et al. Non-invasive imaging of neuropathology in a rat model of alpha-synuclein overexpression. Neurobiol Aging. 2007 Feb;28(2):248–57.

[109] Lauwers E, Debyser Z, Van Dorpe J, De Strooper B, Nuttin B, Baekelandt V. Neuropathology and neurodegeneration in rodent brain induced by lentiviral vector-mediated overexpression of alpha-synuclein. Brain Pathol. 2003 Jul;13(3):364–72.

[110] Decressac M, Mattsson B, Lundblad M, Weikop P, Björklund A. Progressive neurodegenerative and behavioural changes induced by AAV-mediated overexpression of α-synuclein in midbrain dopamine neurons. Neurobiol Dis. 2012 Mar;45(3):939–53.

[111] Kirik D, Annett LE, Burger C, Muzyczka N, Mandel RJ, Björklund A. Nigrostriatal alpha-synucleinopathy induced by viral vector-mediated overexpression of human alpha-synuclein: a new primate model of Parkinson's disease. Proc Natl Acad Sci U S A. 2003 Mar 4;100(5):2884–9.

[112] Oliveras-Salvá M, Van der Perren A, Casadei N, Stroobants S, Nuber S, D'Hooge R, et al. rAAV2/7 vector-mediated overexpression of alpha-synuclein in mouse substantia nigra induces protein aggregation and progressive dose-dependent neurodegeneration. Mol Neurodegener. 2013 Jan;8:44.

[113] Luk KC, Lee VM-Y. Modeling Lewy pathology propagation in Parkinson's disease. Parkinsonism Relat Disord. 2014 Jan;20 Suppl 1:S85–7.

[114] Recasens A, Dehay B, Bové J, Carballo-Carbajal I, Dovero S, Pérez-Villalba A, et al. Lewy body extracts from Parkinson disease brains trigger α-synuclein pathology and neurodegeneration in mice and monkeys. Ann Neurol. 2014 Mar;75(3):351–62.

[115] Luk KC, Kehm V, Carroll J, Zhang B, O'Brien P, Trojanowski JQ, et al. Pathological α-synuclein transmission initiates Parkinson-like neurodegeneration in nontransgenic mice. Science. 2012 Nov 16;338(6109):949–53.

[116] Luk KC, Kehm VM, Zhang B, O'Brien P, Trojanowski JQ, Lee VMY. Intracerebral inoculation of pathological α-synuclein initiates a rapidly progressive neurodegenerative α-synucleinopathy in mice. J Exp Med. 2012 May 7;209(5):975–86.

[117] Masuda-Suzukake M, Nonaka T, Hosokawa M, Kubo M, Shimozawa A, Akiyama H, et al. Pathological alpha-synuclein propagates through neural networks. Acta Neuropathol Commun. 2014 Jan;2:88.

[118] Sacino AN, Brooks M, Thomas MA, McKinney AB, Lee S, Regenhardt RW, et al. Intramuscular injection of α-synuclein induces CNS α-synuclein pathology and a rapid-onset motor phenotype in transgenic mice. Proc Natl Acad Sci U S A. 2014 Jul 7;111(29):10732–7.

[119] Grofova I. The identification of striatal and pallidal neurons projecting to substantia nigra. An experimental study by means of retrograde axonal transport of horseradish peroxidase. Brain Res. 1975;91(2):286–91.

[120] Peelaerts W, Bousset L, Van der Perren A, Moskalyuk A, Pulizzi R, Giugliano M, et al. α-Synuclein strains cause distinct synucleinopathies after local and systemic administration. Nature. 2015 Jun 18;522(7556):340–4.

[121] Gubellini P, Kachidian P. Animal models of Parkinson's disease: an updated overview. Rev Neurol (Paris). 2015 Nov;171(11):750–61.

[122] Healy DG, Falchi M, O'Sullivan SS, Bonifati V, Durr A, Bressman S, et al. Phenotype, genotype, and worldwide genetic penetrance of LRRK2-associated Parkinson's disease: a case-control study. Lancet Neurol. 2008 Jul;7(7):583–90.

[123] Rudenko IN, Cookson MR. Heterogeneity of leucine-rich repeat kinase 2 mutations: genetics, mechanisms and therapeutic implications. Neurotherapeutics. 2014 Oct;11(4): 738-50. doi: 10.1007/s13311-014-0284-z.

[124] Andres-Mateos E, Mejias R, Sasaki M, Li X, Lin BM, Biskup S, et al. Unexpected lack of hypersensitivity in LRRK2 knock-out mice to MPTP (1-methyl-4-phenyl-1,2,3,6-tetrahydropyridine). J Neurosci. 2009 Dec 16;29(50):15846–50.

[125] Tong Y, Yamaguchi H, Giaime E, Boyle S, Kopan R, Kelleher RJ, et al. Loss of leucine-rich repeat kinase 2 causes impairment of protein degradation pathways, accumulation of alpha-synuclein, and apoptotic cell death in aged mice. Proc Natl Acad Sci U S A. 2010 May 25;107(21):9879–84.

[126] Lin X, Parisiadou L, Gu X-L, Wang L, Shim H, Sun L, et al. Leucine-rich repeat kinase 2 regulates the progression of neuropathology induced by Parkinson's-disease-related mutant alpha-synuclein. Neuron. 2009 Dec 24;64(6):807–27.

[127] Tong Y, Pisani A, Martella G, Karouani M, Yamaguchi H, Pothos EN, et al. R1441C mutation in LRRK2 impairs dopaminergic neurotransmission in mice. Proc Natl Acad Sci U S A. 2009 Aug 25;106(34):14622–7.

[128] Herzig MC, Kolly C, Persohn E, Theil D, Schweizer T, Hafner T, et al. LRRK2 protein levels are determined by kinase function and are crucial for kidney and lung homeostasis in mice. Hum Mol Genet. 2011 Nov 1;20(21):4209–23.

[129] Ramonet D, Daher JPL, Lin BM, Stafa K, Kim J, Banerjee R, et al. Dopaminergic neuronal loss, reduced neurite complexity and autophagic abnormalities in transgenic mice expressing G2019S mutant LRRK2. PLoS One. 2011 Jan;6(4):e18568.

[130] Chen C-Y, Weng Y-H, Chien K-Y, Lin K-J, Yeh T-H, Cheng Y-P, et al. (G2019S) LRRK2 activates MKK4-JNK pathway and causes degeneration of SN dopaminergic neurons in a transgenic mouse model of PD. Cell Death Differ. 2012 Oct;19(10):1623–33.

[131] Shaikh KT, Yang A, Youshin E, Schmid S. Transgenic LRRK2 (R1441G) rats-a model for Parkinson disease? PeerJ. 2015 Jan;3:e945.

[132] Li Y, Liu W, Oo TF, Wang L, Tang Y, Jackson-Lewis V, et al. Mutant LRRK2(R1441G) BAC transgenic mice recapitulate cardinal features of Parkinson's disease. Nat Neurosci. 2009 Jul;12(7):826–8.

[133] Winner B, Melrose HL, Zhao C, Hinkle KM, Yue M, Kent C, et al. Adult neurogenesis and neurite outgrowth are impaired in LRRK2 G2019S mice. Neurobiol Dis. 2011 Mar; 41(3):706–16.

[134] Tagliaferro P, Kareva T, Oo TF, Yarygina O, Kholodilov N, Burke RE. An early axonopathy in a hLRRK2(R1441G) transgenic model of Parkinson disease. Neurobiol Dis. 2015 Oct;82:359–71.

[135] Dusonchet J, Kochubey O, Stafa K, Young SM, Zufferey R, Moore DJ, et al. A rat model of progressive nigral neurodegeneration induced by the Parkinson's disease-associated G2019S mutation in LRRK2. J Neurosci. 2011 Jan 19;31(3):907–12.

[136] Lee BD, Shin J-H, VanKampen J, Petrucelli L, West AB, Ko HS, et al. Inhibitors of leucine-rich repeat kinase-2 protect against models of Parkinson's disease. Nat Med. 2010 Sep;16(9):998–1000.

[137] Kitada T, Asakawa S, Hattori N, Matsumine H, Yamamura Y, Minoshima S, et al. Mutations in the parkin gene cause autosomal recessive juvenile parkinsonism. Nature. 1998 Apr;392(6676):605–8.

[138] Gautier CA, Kitada T, Shen J. Loss of PINK1 causes mitochondrial functional defects and increased sensitivity to oxidative stress. Proc Natl Acad Sci U S A. 2008 Aug 12;105(32):11364–9.

[139] Gispert S, Ricciardi F, Kurz A, Azizov M, Hoepken H-H, Becker D, et al. Parkinson phenotype in aged PINK1-deficient mice is accompanied by progressive mitochondrial dysfunction in absence of neurodegeneration. PLoS One. 2009 Jan;4(6):e5777.

[140] Martella G, Platania P, Vita D, Sciamanna G, Cuomo D, Tassone A, et al. Enhanced sensitivity to group II mGlu receptor activation at corticostriatal synapses in mice lacking the familial parkinsonism-linked genes PINK1 or Parkin. Exp Neurol. 2009 Feb; 215(2):388–96.

[141] Palacino JJ, Sagi D, Goldberg MS, Krauss S, Motz C, Wacker M, et al. Mitochondrial dysfunction and oxidative damage in parkin-deficient mice. J Biol Chem. 2004 Apr 30;279(18):18614–22.

[142] Zhu X-R, Maskri L, Herold C, Bader V, Stichel CC, Güntürkün O, et al. Non-motor behavioural impairments in parkin-deficient mice. Eur J Neurosci. 2007 Oct;26(7):1902–11.

[143] Itier J-M, Ibanez P, Mena MA, Abbas N, Cohen-Salmon C, Bohme GA, et al. Parkin gene inactivation alters behaviour and dopamine neurotransmission in the mouse. Hum Mol Genet. 2003 Sep 15;12(18):2277–91.

[144] Von Coelln R, Thomas B, Savitt JM, Lim KL, Sasaki M, Hess EJ, et al. Loss of locus coeruleus neurons and reduced startle in parkin null mice. Proc Natl Acad Sci U S A. 2004 Jul 20;101(29):10744–9.

[145] Perez FA, Palmiter RD. Parkin-deficient mice are not a robust model of parkinsonism. Proc Natl Acad Sci U S A. 2005 Feb 8;102(6):2174–9.

[146] Van Rompuy A-S, Lobbestael E, Van der Perren A, Van den Haute C, Baekelandt V. Long-term overexpression of human wild-type and T240R mutant Parkin in rat substantia nigra induces progressive dopaminergic neurodegeneration. J Neuropathol Exp Neurol. 2014 Feb;73(2):159–74.

[147] Lu X-H, Fleming SM, Meurers B, Ackerson LC, Mortazavi F, Lo V, et al. Bacterial artificial chromosome transgenic mice expressing a truncated mutant parkin exhibit age-dependent hypokinetic motor deficits, dopaminergic neuron degeneration, and accumulation of proteinase K-resistant alpha-synuclein. J Neurosci. 2009 Feb 18;29(7): 1962–76.

[148] Goldberg MS, Pisani A, Haburcak M, Vortherms TA, Kitada T, Costa C, et al. Nigrostriatal dopaminergic deficits and hypokinesia caused by inactivation of the familial Parkinsonism-linked gene DJ-1. Neuron. 2005 Feb 17;45(4):489–96.

[149] Kim RH, Smith PD, Aleyasin H, Hayley S, Mount MP, Pownall S, et al. Hypersensitivity of DJ-1-deficient mice to 1-methyl-4-phenyl-1,2,3,6-tetrahydropyrindine (MPTP) and oxidative stress. Proc Natl Acad Sci U S A. 2005 Apr 5;102(14):5215–20.

[150] Rousseaux MWC, Marcogliese PC, Qu D, Hewitt SJ, Seang S, Kim RH, et al. Progressive dopaminergic cell loss with unilateral-to-bilateral progression in a genetic model of Parkinson disease. Proc Natl Acad Sci U S A. 2012 Sep 25;109(39):15918–23.

Chapter 11

Understanding Pathophysiology of Sporadic Parkinson's Disease in *Drosophila* Model: Potential Opportunities and Notable Limitations

Priyanka Modi, Ayajuddin Mohamad,
Limamanen Phom, Zevelou Koza,
Abhik Das, Rahul Chaurasia, Saikat Samadder,
Bovito Achumi, Muralidhara,
Rajesh Singh Pukhrambam and
Sarat Chandra Yenisetti

Additional information is available at the end of the chapter

http://dx.doi.org/10.5772/63767

Abstract

Parkinson's disease (PD) is the second most common neurodegenerative disorder affecting approximately 1% of the population over age 50. PD is widely accepted as a multifactorial disease with both genetic and environmental contributions. Despite extensive research conducted in the area the precise etiological factors responsible remain elusive. In about 95% Parkinsonism is considered to have a sporadic component. There are currently no established curative, preventative, or disease-modifying interventions, stemming from a poor understanding of the molecular mechanisms of pathogenesis. Here lies the importance of animal models. Pharmacological insults cause Parkinsonian like phenotypes in *Drosophila,* thereby modelling sporadic PD. The pesticides paraquat and rotenone induced oxidative damage causing cluster specific DA neuron loss together with motor deficits. Studies in fly PD model have deciphered that signaling pathways such as phosphatidylinositol 3-kinase (PI3K/Akt and target of rapamycin (TOR), c-Jun N-terminal kinase (JNK) have been defective. Further, these studies have demonstrated that fruit fly can be a potential model to screen chemical compounds for their neuroprotective efficacy.

This chapter overviews current knowledge on the pathophysiology of sporadic PD employing *Drosophila* model and discusses the future perspectives. Further we emphasize the importance of performing genome wide screens in fly model, which may lead to identification of novel pathways involved in PD, which may provide clues to develop therapeutic strategies that help to reduce the burden of PD.

Keywords: Parkinson's disease, *Drosophila*, dopaminergic neurons, neurotoxicants, genome-wide screens

---

1. Introduction

Parkinson's disease (PD) is the second most common neurodegenerative disorder after Alzheimer disease, affecting approximately 1% of the population over the age of 50. Frequency of PD increases with age, but an expected 4% of people with this disease are detected earlier the age of 50. It is assessed that 7–10 million people worldwide are suffering from PD. About one million Americans are surviving with PD, which is more than the collective number of sufferers diagnosed with muscular dystrophy, Lou Gehrig's disease, and multiple sclerosis. Further, about 60,000 Americans are diagnosed with PD each year and this number does not mirror thousands of unnoticed cases [1]. Studies illustrate that prevalence of PD in men is significantly higher (one and half times more) than in women. In poor and developing nations of Asia and Africa no systematic data are available about the number of sufferers. Painful truth is that in these regions, millions of elderly suffer in silence due to poverty and ignorance.

PD is widely accepted as a multifactorial disease with both genetic and environmental contributions. Clinical signs comprise bradykinesia, resting tremble, muscular rigidity, and postural unsteadiness. Supplementary symptoms are characteristic postural anomalies, dystonic spams, and dementia. PD is progressive and usually has a devious onset in mid to late adult life. Pathogenic characters of typical PD comprise loss of dopaminergic neurons in the *substantia nigra* (SN) and the manifestation of Lewy bodies, intracellular cytoplasmic inclusions, in enduring neurons in various areas of the brain, mainly the SN [2].

Despite intensive research conducted in the field of PD, the etiology of this neurodegenerative disease remains elusive. Although genetic elements and exposure to environmental toxins, such as pesticides, are thought to play a crucial role in disease onset, aging remains the predominant risk factor [3]. In about 95% patients, Parkinsonism is considered to have a sporadic component. Some findings suggest that environmental factors may be more important than genetic factors in familial aggregation of PD. In maximum PD cases the cause is environmental influence, probably toxic, overlaid on a background of slow, sustained neuronal loss due to progressing age [4]. Finding PD in 1-methyl-4-phenyl-1,2,3,6-tetrahydropyridine (MPTP) drug consumers rejuvenated curiosity in reassessing environmental influences [5]. Another theory of Parkinsonism suggests that genetic predisposition may be transmitted through mitochondrial inheritance.

Current therapeutic strategies for PD mitigate symptoms by the replacement of dopamine, with variable efficacy and considerable side effects. Levodopa (L-dopa), a dopamine precursor, the leading treatment of PD for over 40 years, improves motor impairment by increasing dopamine levels [6]. However, continued use of L-dopa leads to other motor dyskinesias that undermine the benefits of treatment. The development of effective treatment for PD is difficult because pathology is affected by several pathways that may act serially or in parallel. However, there are currently no established curative, preventative, or disease-modifying interventions, stemming from a poor understanding of the molecular mechanisms of pathogenesis.

This chapter primarily aims to present an overview of the sporadic PD, disease modeling in *Drosophila* and critically analyze the potential opportunities and the notable limitations associated with fly models. Further, we have also briefly discussed some of the current applications of the model to obtain insights into the underlying molecular mechanism/s related to PD.

2. Animal models of Parkinson's disease

Animal models have been invaluable tools for investigating the underlying mechanisms of the pathogenesis of PD. However, the usefulness of these models is dependent on how precisely they replicate the features of clinical PD. Nonmammalian models are a great cost-effective alternative to rodent and primate-based models, allowing rapid high-throughput screening of novel therapies and investigation of genetic and environmental risk factors. Thus far, the nonmammalian rotenone models have included worm (*Caenorhabditis elegans*), fly (*Drosophila*), zebrafish (*Danio rerio*), and pond snail (*Lymnea stagnalis*). A good model of PD should exhibit pathological and medical characteristics of PD including both dopaminergic and nondopaminergic systems, the central and peripheral nervous systems, also the motor and nonmotor symptoms associated with the disease. Furthermore, the age-reliant inception and progression of pathology should be reflected [7].

Contemporary knowledge on the potential pathogenic and pathophysiological mechanisms of PD derives from innumerable studies conducted, in the past four decades, on experimental models of PD. While animal models, in particular, have provided invaluable information, they also offer the opportunity of trying new therapeutic methods. These model systems have been traditionally grounded on the exposure of neurotoxins able to imitate *many* of the pathological and phenotypic characters of PD in mammals. Conversely in the previous decade, the dawn of the "genetic era" of PD has provided a significant growth in this field with a number of transgenic models for experimentation. It is well recognized that both these classes of animal PD models (genetic and neurotoxin) have their own specificities as well as limitations and employment of one model or the other depends on the specific questions that are being addressed.

Genetic models: Animal models are developed primarily based on identified target genes (i.e., by mutating or knocking out) associated with potential mechanisms known to cause PD in humans (**Table 1**) [8–21]. For example, the autosomal dominant transmission of LRRK2 mutations makes transgenic expression of pathogenic LRRK2 species suitable for modeling disease process in PD. The invertebrate transgenic models producing LRRK2 PD mutants phenotypes range from no change to apparent neuronal loss or deficits in DA systems and motor behavior [22] that were used to evaluate LRRK2 kinase inhibitors in neuroprotection, revealing the potential value of the invertebrate LRRK2 models in drug screening [23].

Symbol	Gene locus	Gene	*Drosophila* homolog	Inheritance	Disorder	Status and remarks
PARK1	4q21-22	SNCA [10]	No homolog	AD	Early-onset Parkinsonism	Confirmed
PARK2	6q25.2-q27	PARK2 encoding Parkin[11]	Parkin	AR	Early onset Parkinsonism	Confirmed
PARK3	2p13	Unknown	–	AD	Classical Parkinsonism	Unconfirmed
PARK4	4q21-q23	SNCA	No homolog	AD	Early-onset Parkinsonism	Erroneous locus (identical to PARK1)
PARK5	4p13	UCHL1	Uch	AD	Classical Parkinsonism	Unconfirmed
PARK6	1p35-p36	PINK1 [12]	Pink1	AR	Early onset Parkinsonism	Confirmed
PARK7	1p36	PARK7 encoding DJ-1[13]	Dj-1α and dj-1β	AR	Early onset Parkinsonism	Confirmed
PARK8	12q12	LRRK2 [14]	Lrrk	AD	Classical Parkinsonism	Confirmed
PARK9	1p36	ATP13A2 [15]	CG32000	AR	Kufor–Rakeb syndrome, a formof juvenile-onset atypical Parkinsonism with dementia, spasticity and supranuclear gaze palsy	Confirmed
PARK10	1p32	Unknown	–	Risk factor	Classical Parkinsonism	Confirmed susceptibility locus
PARK11	2q36-27	Unknown (maybe GIGYF2)	–	AD	Late onset Parkinsonism	Not independently confirmed
PARK12	Xq21-	Unknown	–	Risk factor	Classical Parkinsonism	Confirmed susceptibility

Symbol	Gene locus	Gene	*Drosophila* homolog	Inheritance	Disorder	Status and remarks
	q25					locus
PARK13	2p12	HTRA2	HtrA2	AD or risk factor	Classical Parkinsonism	Unconfirmed
PARK14	22q13.1	PLA2G6 [16]	iPLA2-VIA	AR	Early-onset dystonia-Parkinsonism	Confirmed
PARK15	22q12-q13	FBXO7 [17]	No homolog	AR	Early-onset Parkinsonian-pyramidal syndrome	Confirmed
PARK16	1q32	Unknown (maybe RAB7L1)	–	Risk factor	Classical Parkinsonism	Confirmed susceptibility locus
PARK17	16q11.2	VPS35	Vps35	AD	Classical Parkinsonism	Unconfirmed
PARK18	6p21.3	EIF4G1	eIF4G	AD	Late onset Parkinsonism	Unconfirmed
PARK19	1p31.3	DNAJC6 [18]	Auxillin	AR	Juvenile-onset Parkinsonism	Confirmed
PARK20	21q22.11	SYNJ1 [19, 20]	Synj	AR	Early-onset Parkinsonism	Confirmed

AD, autosomal dominant; AR, autosomal recessive (adapted from Marras *et al.* [21]).

Table 1. Monogenetic forms of PD and its fly homolog(s).

Neurotoxic models: Several studies have been performed to model PD-associated neuron loss by neurotoxin intoxication in animals, the most common Parkinsonian neurotoxins being 6-hydroxydopamine (6-OHDA), 1-methyl-4-phenyl-1,2,3,6-tetrahydropyridine (MPTP), rotenone, and paraquat [24, 25], and the common neurotoxic models of PD include that produced by the toxin 6-hydroxydopamine (6-OHDA) commonly used in rats, mice and marmosets, and 1-methyl-4- phenyl-1,2,3,6 tetrahydropyridine (MPTP), used in mice and also in nonhuman primates. Administration of MPTP to animals, such as monkeys, mice, cats, rats, guinea pigs, dogs, sheep and even frogs and goldfish, has been shown to cause Parkinsonian-like motor disturbances [26, 27].

3. Pathophysiology of Parkinson's disease

3.1. Sporadic Parkinson's disease: an overview

A sporadic disease can be explained as a disease occurring randomly in a population with no known cause. In sporadic PD, the cause is considered to be environmental though the genetic influence is also present and hence the pathogenesis of PD is likely to be multifactorial which may involve gene–environment interactions. The discovery of MPTP (1-methyl-4-phenyl-1,2,3,6-tetrahydropyridine), which reproduces pathological features of idiopathic Parkinsonism by targeting the nigrostriatal system [28] and pesticides (such as rotenone and paraquat), has implicated environmental toxins in the induction of sporadic PD [29, 30]. Both epidemiological and experimental data suggest the potential involvement of specific agents such as neurotoxicants (e.g., pesticides) or neuroprotective compounds (e.g., tobacco products) in the pathogenesis of nigrostriatal degeneration, further supporting a relationship between the environment and PD [28]. Further, the identification of the mutated α-synuclein (SCNA) gene causing familial PD [10] as a risk factor for sporadic disease [31] provides a genetic context for the disease. The finding of α-synuclein as a key component of the Lewy body [32] further links this gene to potential molecular mechanisms of PD.

3.2. Environmental basis of sporadic PD

The study of environmental risk factors for PD is difficult because environmental exposures and gene–environment interactions may occur well before the onset of clinical symptoms since it remains undetected for many years. Moreover, the severe neurodegenerative changes that underlie the symptoms of PD may be the result of synergistic effects of multiple exposures and these effects could have been compounded by increased vulnerability of the aging nigrostriatal system to toxic injury over the years. Epidemiological and case–control studies suggest that rural residence, well water consumption, pesticide use, and certain occupations (farming, mining, and welding) are associated with an increased risk of PD [33–36].

Epidemiological studies have suggested an association with environmental toxins, mainly mitochondrial complex I inhibitors like rotenone [37, 38]. The results are consistent with a dose-dependent effect in agricultural workers and the risk increased with duration of pesticide use [39, 40]. Data also suggest that exposure to specific pesticide such as bipyridyl, organochlorine, and carbamate derivatives could have a causal role in PD [39, 41]. Further, chronic exposure to metals/pesticides is also associated with a younger age at onset of PD among patients with no family history of the disease and that duration of exposure is a factor in the magnitude of this effect [42]. For instance, a study in Taiwan, where the herbicide paraquat (PQ) is commonly spurted on rice fields, a robust relationship was testified between paraquat contact and PD menace and the danger was amplified by more than six times in individuals who had been exposed to PQ chronically [43].

3.3. Environment toxins and their mechanisms of action

The accidental discovery of MPTP leading to Parkinsonian syndrome stimulated the search for environmental factors as potential causes of PD. Several epidemiological studies have suggested that environmental toxins are one of the major causes of sporadic PD [44]. Sporadic PD's main cause is the accumulation of alpha-synuclein but by an uncertain causative agent and uneven occurrence point in age of patients. The mechanisms by which the neurotoxins induce PD-like symptoms are briefly described below.

MPTP: MPTP is a metabolite of the drug heroin. It is transported through the blood–brain barrier (BBB) by the plasma membrane dopamine transporter (DAT) and once it crosses the blood–brain barrier, MPTP is metabolically activated to the fully oxidized 1-methyl-4-phenylpyridinium species (MPP+) which is then taken up into dopaminergic neurons via DAT [45, 46]. After MPP+ gains access into dopaminergic neurons, it is accumulated into synaptic vesicles via the vesicular monoamine transporter (VMAT2) [47]. The modulation of MPTP/MPP+ toxicity by DAT and VMAT2, where DAT enhances and VMAT2 protecting against toxicant injury, provides a paradigm linking environmental exposures to nigrostriatal degeneration. The ratio of DAT to VMAT2 indicates the sensitivity of dopaminergic neurons to toxic injury [48].

6-Hydroxy dopamine (6-OHDA)*:* 6-OHDA is the first catecholaminergic neurotoxin that was used to generate animal models of PD. Since this compound cannot cross BBB, it is needed to be injected and inserted systemically to aim dopamine pathways [49]. On injecting into *substantia nigra,* 6-OHDA causes severe loss of dopamine neurons within a day [50]. Inside neurons, 6-OHDA produces reactive oxygen species (ROS) and quinones that inactivate biological macromolecules. Till now, no Lewy body-like inclusion has been described in the 6-OHDA model. Owing to its inability to cross BBB, this model is less popular.

Rotenone (ROT): ROT is used as a broad-spectrum pesticide and belongs to the family of isoflavones naturally found in the roots and stems of several plants. Highly lipophilic, it easily crosses the BBB, and for cellular entry [51], it does not depend on the DAT. Within the cell rotenone mount up in mitochondria and inhibits complex I (where it impedes the transfer of electrons from iron–sulfur (Fe–S) centers to ubiquinone). It is opined that augmented ROS assembly is related with complex I inhibition, which may result in causing oxidative damage to DNA and proteins of neuronal cells. Further, nitric oxide may interact with ROS, particularly superoxide and hydroxyl radicals, resulting in peroxynitrite formation, eventually leading to cellular defects and impairment of dopaminergic neurons [52]. Further, ROT was shown to inhibit proteasome activity and dysfunction in proteasomes has been implicated in the pathogenesis of both genetic and sporadic forms of PD [53, 54].

Paraquat (PQ): PQ is one of the most widely used herbicides in the world. The structural similarity of PQ with 1-methyl-4-phenylpyridinium ion (MPP+) prompted the speculation that PQ might be dopaminergic neurotoxicant which may lead to PD. PQ is suspected to enter the brain by neutral amino acid transporters and subsequently the cells in a sodium-dependent fashion [55]. Once within cells of the CNS, PQ acts as a redox cycling compound at the cytosolic level, which potentially leads to indirect mitochondrial toxicity [56]. Recently, it has also been shown that PQ-induced apoptosis may involve Bak protein, a pro-apoptosis Bcl-2 family member [57].

Maneb (MB): MB, a commonly used fungicide, is an irritant to respiratory tracts and is capable of inducing sensitization by skin contact. Mechanistically, MB seems to cross the BBB. Although knowledge of the mechanisms of this toxin is very limited, MB preferentially inhibits mitochondrial complex III [58]. Further, MB was shown to induce apoptosis through Bak activation, whereas combination of PQ and MB inhibits the Bak-dependent pathway while potentiating apoptosis through Bak protein [59].

Metals: The potential role of metals due to prolonged exposure as risk factors for Parkinson's disease has been evaluated [60]. Chronic occupational exposure to high levels of manganese (Mn) in manganese miners causes accumulation of this metal in the basal ganglia, resulting in tremors, rigidity and psychosis that resemble PD [61]. The metal-induced Parkinsonian syndrome that results from Mn exposure differs significantly from idiopathic PD. The Parkinsonism caused by Mn does not respond to L-DOPA treatment and the primary target of Mn toxicity seems to be the globus pallidus rather than the nigrostriatal system [62]. The potential role of iron and other transition elements has also been studied. The level of ferritin (primary intracellular protein capable of keeping iron bound in a nonreactive status) in the nigral tissue of patients with PD was found to be decreased [63]. Thus, iron accumulation together with decreased binding capability may enhance the risk for iron-mediated toxic reactions in PD by generating the highly toxic hydroxyl radical in the presence of iron and hydrogen peroxide, thus leading to oxidative stress and ultimately neurodegeneration.

4. Molecular pathways in sporadic PD

Though Mendelian genes are responsible only for a small subset of PD patients, it is speculated that the same pathogenetic mechanisms could also play a relevant role in the development of more frequent sporadic PD [64]. With advancement in molecular biotechnological tools and techniques, a number of genes and proteins linked to PD have been identified, which reveal a complex network of molecular pathways involved in its etiology, suggesting that common mechanisms underlie both familial and sporadic forms of PD (**Table 2**) [65–79]. Three predominat pathways that can trigger the neurodegenerative process are as follows: (a) accumulation of aggregated and misfolded proteins, (b) impairment of the ubiquitin protein pathway (UPS) and the autophagy pathway, and (c) mitochondrial dysfunction [64]. Functional studies on the proteins encoded by PD-related genes supports these pathways and it is confirmed by both pathological and biochemical studies performed in patients with sporadic PD with no apparent genetic cause [80–82]. Further, critical cellular protective pathways, such as autophagy, UPS, and mitochondria dynamics, are shown to lose adeptness with increasing age and there is a progressive build-up of somatic mutations particularly in the mitochondrial DNA during aging process [64]. Recent studies have shown the role for chronic neuroinflammation and microglia activation in PD pathogenesis, suggesting that different molecular/cellular events may contribute to neurodegeneration by activating resident microglial populations in selected brain areas, with potential detrimental effects on vulnerable neuronal populations [83].

Compound treatment	*Drosophila* model	Modifies phenotype(s)	Pathway/ process	References
Sulforaphane and allyl Disulfide	*parkin*	DA neuron number	Oxidative stress	[65]
	α-synuclein	DA neuron number		[65]
S-Methyl-*L*-cysteine	*α-synuclein*	Locomotor activity		[66]
Polyphenols	*α-synuclein*	Lifespan, Locomotor activity		[67]
	Paraquat and Iron	Locomotor activity		[68]
α-Tocopherol	*DJ-1β*	Lifespan		[69]
	PINK1	Ommatidial degeneration		[70]
SOD	*PINK1*	Ommatidial degeneration		[70]
Melatonin	*DJ-1β*	Lifespan		[69]
	Paraquat	Locomotor activity		[71]
	Rotenone	Locomotor activity, Dopamine neuron number		[71]
Bacopa monieri leaf extract	Paraquat; Rotenone	Oxidative markers; Mitochondrial functions		[72, 73]
Minocycline	DJ-1α	DA neuron number, dopamine levels	Oxidative stress/ inflammatory process	[74]
Celestrol	DJ-1α	DA neuron number, dopamine levels, Locomotor activity and survival rate under oxidative stress conditions		[74]
Rapamycin	Parkin/PINK1	Thoracic indentations, Locomotor activity, DA neuron number, and muscle integrity.	TOR signaling	[75]

Compound treatment	*Drosophila* model	Modifies phenotype(s)	Pathway/ process	References
Geldanamycin	α-synuclein	DA neuron number	Removal of excess or toxic protein forms	[76, 77]
Zinc Chloride	Parkin	Life span, Locomotor activity, and percentage of adulthood survivors.	Zinc homeostasis	[78]

Modified from Munoz-Soriano and Paricio [79].

Table 2. Therapeutic compounds shown to modify phenotype(s) in the *Drosophila* PD model.

4.1. Genetic basis of sporadic PD

The use of genetically tractable organisms to model gene–environment interactions has become an efficient means of identifying genetic risk factors [84, 85]. Functional characterization of the genes involved in familial PD has shown significant comprehensions into the molecular mechanism(s) responsible to the pathogenesis of PD. Abnormal protein and mitochondrial homeostasis are the crucial factors behind the development of PD, with oxidative stress playing a vital connection between the two events. Genome-wide association studies (GWAS) showed variations in *α-synuclein* and *LRRK2* (well-known familial PD genes), i.e., as important risk causes for the sporadic PD [86]. The elevation of dopamine synthesis in response to a variety of stressors [87] may subject DA neurons to an increased risk for oxidative stress-mediated impairment [88]. Nevertheless, connotation studies of polymorphisms within these genes have not proved the hypothesis [89, 90].

The recent application of high throughput whole genome and exome analysis technologies along with bioinformatics has provided valuable inputs in the identification of novel susceptibility loci involved in apparent sporadic PD. It is predicted that many more variants remained to be discovered despite the success of GWAS in discovering novel genetic variants in PD. In this regard, genome-wide complex trait analysis [91, 92] may prove useful for a more exhaustive screening for PD risk variants [93]. Groundbreaking efforts have begun to establish the relationship between single nucleotide polymorphisms (SNPs) identified by GWAS and gene expression levels to describe their functional meaning. This approach has provided significant insights into various potential novel mechanisms underlying the observed SNP associations with PD etiology.

4.2. Interaction between genetics and environment

The concept that gene–environment interactions affect PD susceptibility was proposed more than a decade ago [94]. Although many studies have described positive associations between genetic polymorphisms and increased risk for PD, only a few human association studies have examined gene–environment interactions. Occupational pesticide exposure as well as high exposure to PQ and MB in carriers of DAT genetic variants was shown to increase the PD risk

[36, 95]. Further, SNP in *NOS1* (neuronal nitric oxide synthase 1) and *GSTP1* (glutathione S-transferase pi 1) have been linked to an increased risk for PD among pesticide-exposed individuals [96], although an association between *GSTP1* and pesticide exposure has not been supported by a large cohort study conducted subsequently [97]. However, European studies did not show noteworthy interaction between polymorphisms in 15 genes that impact metabolism of extraneous chemicals or dopamine and exposure to pesticides and metals [97].

Twin studies: Twin studies are particularly useful in distinguishing between the influence of genetics or the environment on the risks of a disease. If genetic factors predominate in etiology of a disease, it is expected that concordance in monozygotic (MZ) twins will be greater than dizygotic (DZ) twins. Using striatal ^{18}F[DOPA] positron emission tomography (PET) scan to detect dopaminergic dysfunction in asymptomatic cotwins of twin pairs with mostly sporadic and late onset PD, Piccini *et al.* [98] found a three-fold higher concordance rate of PD in MZ twins (55%) than in DZ twins (18%), suggesting a significant genetic contribution. Furthermore, when monitored over a period of 7 years, asymptomatic MZ cotwins all showed progressive loss of dopaminergic function and four developed clinical PD, while none of the DZ twin pairs became clinically concordant. Similarly, a recent longitudinal study carried out on Swedish twins with predominantly sporadic PD revealed concordance rates of 11% for MZ and 4% for same-sexed DZ twin pairs, with an overall heritability estimate of 34% [99].

Two-hit PD models: Present genetic PD models failed to reproduce nigrostriatal DA loss, hinting that a single genetic risk factor is not sufficient enough and an environmental factor may be required to initiate the process of neurodegeneration. To understand this paradigm and to decipher the interaction between genes and environment two hit animal models (animals with a genetic defect will be exposed to multiple environmental factors/toxicants to study if this synergy will lead to DA degeneration) will be of potential help.

5. Insights into sporadic PD pathophysiology through *Drosophila*

The fruit fly *Drosophila* has emerged as a suitable model for studying mechanisms of PD-related neurodegeneration in the past decade. Structural architecture and functional pathways involved in dopamine synthesis and degradation are well preserved between *Drosophila* and human. Transgenic flies (neuronal overexpression of *wt* or mutant (A53T or A50P) human alpha-synuclein) showed age-dependent and selective loss of dopaminergic neurons, formation of fibrillary inclusions containing alpha-synuclein, as well as a progressive loss of climbing activity, which could be alleviated by L-DOPA or DA agonists [100]. Mutational analyses of alpha-synuclein in *Drosophila* have permitted an extended evaluation of the protein domains involved and/or required for toxicity showing, for example, that truncated forms of alpha-synuclein have a central hydrophobic region, between residues 71 and 82, essential for the formation of oligomeric and fibrillary forms of the protein and toxicity. Importance of post-translational modification of alpha-synuclein (phosphorylation on serine 129 and tyrosine 125, on alpha-synuclein oligomerization and toxicity) was demonstrated using the *Drosophila* model. Using fly model it was also shown that early, soluble forms of aggregates of alpha-synuclein are more toxic.

Mutations that induce loss of function or inactivation of the fly homologs of mutations of fly homologs of PINK1, parkin, DJ-1, or LRKK2 lead to selective DA degeneration leading to mobility defects that can be characterized through behavioral assays. *Drosophila* parkin null mutants exhibit decreased life span, mitochondrial abnormalities, and flight muscle deterioration leading to mobility defects and diminished proteasome 26S activity. Overexpression of mutant but not with wild parkin (human gene) in *Drosophila* leads to dopaminergic deterioration and motor defects, signifying a dominant negative effect of the mutated protein in PD pathology. Further, PINK1 mutant flies also share PD characteristics with parkin mutants.

Drosophila models have been important to identify the role of both parkin and PINK1 in the regulation of mitochondrial physiology [101]. Unlike mammals, *Drosophila* expresses two DJ-1 homologs, viz., DJ-1 alpha, restricted to male germline, and DJ-1 beta that, similarly to mammals, is ubiquitously expressed. Different mutations of both genes have been induced. DJ-1beta KO flies showed enhanced susceptibility to cytotoxins, such as paraquat, H_2O_2, and rotenone, further supporting the protective redox function of DJ-1. Similarly, DJ-1beta mutations that cause loss of protein function lead to accumulation of ROS in fly's brain.

5.1. Induction of PD in *Drosophila*

Drosophila were first used to model PD, when Feany and Bender [100] produced transgenic flies that either expressed normal human α-synuclein or one of the mutant forms, A30P and A53T α-synuclein, which have both been linked to familial PD. This discovery revealed the potential of *Drosophila* system for modeling gain and loss-of-function genetic mutations that are associated with PD, thereby allowing the elucidation of the genes molecular functions and the pathways involved.

5.2. Toxin models of *Drosophila* for PD

Several environmental chemicals (neurotoxins) have been employed to recapitulate PD-like symptoms and pathology in *Drosophila* system [102]. *Drosophila* performs motor functions such as walking, climbing, and flying and has a well-developed nervous system which makes *Drosophila* a suitable model for understanding PD. These kinds of complex behavior phenotypes are similar from strain to strain and hence characterizing a toxin induced PD model for this organism becomes easy [100]. Extensively used chemical models with their salient features are briefly described below.

Rotenone (ROT) induced PD model in Drosophila: Inhibition of the mitochondrial respiratory chain by ROT has been widely used to study the role of the mitochondrial respiratory chain in apoptosis [103, 104]. The mitochondrial respiratory chain is the major site of ATP production in eukaryotes and it is well recognized that this organelle not only generates ATP, but also plays an important role in apoptosis [105–107]. It is now clear that upon apoptotic stimulation mitochondria can release several proapoptotic regulators, including cytochrome c [108], Smac/ Diablo [109, 110], endonuclease G [111], and apoptosis-inducing factor [112] to the cytosol. These proapoptotic regulators will then activate cellular apoptotic programs downstream [105–107]. The release of proapoptotic regulators is further regulated by the translocation of

Bcl-2 family proteins [113, 114]. Some of the salient pathophysiological features of the ROT fly model are: (a) being lipophilic, it can easily cross the blood–brain barrier but the final concentration of rotenone in the brain may probably be much lower than the initial because of these barriers and the powerful excretion system of flies. They have a tendency to stay at the bottom of vials and did not appear to coordinate their legs normally [37]. (b) Since neuronal dopaminergic clusters are normally present in each *Drosophila* adult brain hemisphere [115–117], abnormalities are characterized by the disappearance of part or the totality of dopaminergic cell clusters but this effect varies in intensity from one fly to another [37].

Paraquat (PQ) model of PD in Drosophila: Long-term exposure to environmental oxidative stressors, such as the herbicide PQ, has been linked to the development of PD. In view of this, PQ is frequently used in the *Drosophila system* and other animal models to study PD and the degeneration of dopaminergic neurons (DNs). Recently, it has been shown that expression of D_1 like dopaminergic receptor (DAMB receptor) was directly proportional to PQ induced toxicity in CNS of flies [118]. It is notable that a long-term neuronal DA synthesis decreases the DAMB expression and resists the PQ toxicity. Age-related decrement in PQ resistance is also observed with a significant increase in DAMB receptor. This evidence proves that there are more areas to be researched regarding DA related neurodegeneration in *Drosophila*. Some of the salient pathophysiological features of PQ fly model are: (a) flies exhibit rapid onset of movement disorders, including resting tremors, bradykinesis, rotational behaviors and postural instability which resemble Parkinsonian symptoms. Furthermore, the flies frequently freeze while attempting to climb vial walls and would often fall to the bottom of the vial. Males exhibit symptoms 12 hours earlier than females, but both males and females are strongly affected [71]; (b) PQ-dependent dopaminergic neuron loss is totally selective in a time-dependent loss of exposure where after 6 hours of exposure PPL1 and by 12 hours PPM2, PPM3 cluster will be affected whereas PPM1 and PPL2 clusters only get affected after 20–24 hour of exposure [71], and (c) changes in the neuronal cell are also a trait where cell bodies aggregate in a round shape, and fragment and then disappear [71].

6. Application of *Drosophila* model: screening platform for assessment of neuroprotective potential

Drosophila models are a great cost-effective alternative to rodent and primate-based models, allowing rapid high throughput screening of novel therapies. Studies done with *Drosophila* model coexposed to rotenone and melatonin (an antioxidant and free radical scavenger) showed that melatonin improved the movement behavior of rotenone-treated flies, even more evidently than L-dopa [119]. Quantification of the number of dopaminergic cells after 1 week of rotenone feeding revealed that the presence of melatonin significantly rescued the loss of neurons in all of the clusters [37]. Subsequently, the rotenone model of *Drosophila* has been extensively employed as a screening platform to assess the neuroprotective potential of various molecules and phytoconstituents. Over the last five years, numerous workers have employed the fly rotenone model (both wild type and genetically modified strains) to test potential neuroprotective treatments [72–73, 120, 121]. The majority of these studies used compounds that have multiple therapeutic properties such as antioxidant, anti-inflammatory, and anti-apoptotic properties, which largely yielded positive results such as reductions in ROS and inflammatory mediators, attenuation of TH-positive neuron loss and striatal dopamine loss as well as reversal of motor deficits [122].

6.1. Plant-derived neuroprotective agents in PD

The *Drosophila* model is extensively used due to the flies' rapid generation time, low cost, and amenability for genetic manipulation, and thus serves as an ideal model for identifying promising neuroprotective candidates that can then undergo further validation in mammalian models (**Table 2**) [65–79, 123]. Growing evidence indicate that the herbs used in traditional medicines contain neuroprotective compounds such as resveratol, curcumin or ginsenoside, green tea polyphenols or catechins, triptolide, etc. [124–128]. These compounds may help enhancing antioxidant activity, decrease loss of dopamine, inhibit activation of microglia, reduce the release of pro-inflammatory factors, prevent α-synuclein aggregation and fibrillation. These herbs also protect the dopaminergic neurons against neurotoxins like MTTP, 6-OHDA. Some of the major plant derived molecules suggested as therapeutic agents for PD are as follows.

Resveratol: This is a polyphenolic compound naturally found in grapes. This is able to cross the blood–brain barrier and is water soluble [129]. The numerous pharmacological functions include anti-inflammation, antiapoptosis, antioxidation, anticancer, etc.

Curcumin: In recent years curcumin has shown therapeutic potential for neurodegenerative diseases such as PD. It is a natural polyphenol found in the spice turmeric and is known for several biological and medicinal effects such as anti-inflammatory, antioxidant, anti-proliferative activities, etc. It is demonstrated to help in preventing the aggregation and fibrillation of α-synuclein [130]. Curcumin glucoside, a modified form, prevents the aggregation and enhances the solubility of α-synuclein [131]. Studies have shown that curcumin reduces the LRRK2 kinase activity and decreases the levels of oxidized proteins. Thus curcumin also acts as an inhibitor for LRRK2 kinase activity. Our laboratory has shown stage-specific neuroprotective efficacy of curcumin in *Drosophila* model of idiopathic PD [132].

Ginsenoside: There are two major categories of ginsenosides—protopanaxadiols and protopanaxatriols. In vitro and in vivo studies have shown ginsenosides to exert pharmacological effects against neuroinflammation, cerebral oxidative stress, radical formation, and apoptosis. It plays a neuroprotective role in regulation of synaptic plasticity, neurotransmitter release, and neuroinflammatory responses [126].

Blueberry extracts: Blueberry contains a large amount of polyphenols and has a greater antioxidant property than most fruits and vegetables. Consumption of blueberry has been reported to slow down the age-related functional and physiological deficits [133–135]. Peng *et al.* [136] were the first to show the anti-aging property of blueberry using *Drosophila* fly model. The study also showed that supplemented blueberry extracts increased the mRNA levels of SOD1, SOD2, and CAT in *Drosophila*. Blueberry extracts can partially reverse the chronic Paraquat exposure. Blueberry extracts in diet of flies could increase the mean life span, decrease Paraquat induced mortality, and partially reverse the locomotor deficiency.

7. Notable limitations

Animal models are absolutely necessary for reproducing physiologic and neurosystems aspects of neurodegenerative disorders. However, animal models are complicated by the differing expression levels and patterns of expression of target genes, with different promoters among other issues for genetic models, and complexities of drug administration, drug distribution, and metabolism for toxin models [79]. Rodent models have faced limitations due to lack of strong construct (i.e., genotype or intervention) and face validity (i.e., phenotype), as well as species and strain limitations. In general, toxin-induced PD models do not recapitulate the process of progressive neuron loss and the protein aggregation in LBs, due to the acute nature of the neurotoxin treatment [137, 138], but they have been useful to support the concept that alterations in mitochondrial biology are essential for the development of PD [139]. However, animal models allow studying a cellular process in the context of a whole organism and are thus more reliable.

Research on PD using cell cultures has many advantages in which they allow rapid screening for disease pathogenesis and drug candidates. Cellular models can be easily used for molecular, biochemical, and pharmacological approaches, but they can lead to misinterpretation and artifacts. *Vice versa* limitations include that the survival of neurons is dependent upon the culture conditions and the cells do not develop their natural neuronal networks. In most cases, neurons are deprived of the physiological afferent and efferent connections [140].

While there are many advantages of the fly PD model, the most common disadvantage is that the important pathogenetic factors which are vertebrate-specific may be ignored in invertebrate models. The differences between mammals and invertebrates represent potential drawbacks in modeling brain diseases such as PD [141].

8. Potential opportunities

Drosophila melanogaster was the first major complex organism to have its genome sequenced [142] and after the human genome was sequenced the homology between the two genomes greatly strengthened to understand human biology and the disease processes as a model [143]. More importantly, 75% of human disease-related loci have a *Drosophila* orthologue [144]. Fly model are less costly and time consuming to use when compared to mammals due to their rapid reproduction time and short lifespan [143, 145, 146]. In addition, flies are capable of performing complex motor behaviors such as walking, climbing, and flying and their brain is complex enough to make these behaviors relevant to humans [101, 147, 148].

Some of the unique features of the *Drosophila* model which have been identified are: (a) *Drosophila* models are instrumental in exploring the mechanisms of neurodegeneration, with several PD-related mutations eliciting related phenotypes including sensitivity to energy supply and vesicular deformities. These are leading to the identification of plausible cellular mechanisms, which may be specific to (dopaminergic) neurons and synapses rather than general cellular phenotypes. (b) Fly models show noncell autonomous signaling within the nervous system, offering the opportunity to develop our understanding of the way pathogenic signaling propagates, resembling Braak's scheme of spreading pathology in PD, (c) fly models link physiological deficits to changes in synaptic structure, and (d) the strong neuronal phenotypes observed in the fly models permit relevant *in vivo* drug testing [149]. Another key feature making *Drosophila* an attractive model is the range of genetic tools available to manipulate them and the ease of introducing human genes into the fly enables it to recapitulate the symptoms and progression of human disease in flies [150]. Two approaches employed are: the *reverse genetic approach* wherein a gene is tested for its potential functional role by using the GAL4/*UAS*-system and the *forward genetic approach* (function of a gene) for identification of genes based on phenotype, which is useful to understand diseases whose genetic basis is yet to determined [141]. The genomics era has played a crucial role in directing both the functional biology and the *in vitro*/*in vivo* modeling of neurodegenerative diseases in fly model.

9. Future perspectives

Drosophila has been used to model several aspects of neurodegenerative diseases, including aggregation toxicity of misfolding disease related proteins [151–156]. Ninety-five percent of the Parkinson's disease patients suffer from sporadic form. In those sporadic cases, no indication allows a decided inference about the underlying causes as well as the pathogenic mechanism involved [101]. The limitations of human genetics make it necessary to use model system to analyze affected genes and pathways knowledge of which is essential to develop therapeutic targets. During last three decades, genetically pliable fruit fly *Drosophila* has been a great model system to study human neurodegenerative disorders including PD human genetic screens, and pathological studies have been able to provide limited mechanistic insights into the molecular processes that determine disease susceptibility or age at onset of disease [157]. Genetic analysis has identified causative mutations for autosomal-dominant and recessive forms of familial PD. Functional studies of these genes have provided great insights into potential pathogenic mechanisms of inherited forms of PD; however it is unclear how these may relate to the more common sporadic forms of PD.

Identification of PD risk locus SREBF1 through GWAS (genome-wide association studies) analysis and substantiating its biological function as a regulator of mitophagy [158] remarkably emphasize the importance and potential to decipher the risk loci for idiopathic PD through genome-wide screens in animal models. However, no systematic genome-wide functional screens are performed in sporadic PD models. Here lies the importance and necessity to perform genome-wide screen to identify the risk locus for idiopathic PD. Comprehensive efforts in this direction will provide novel insights into the molecular mechanisms behind the dopaminergic neurodegeneration and also figure out genetic basis for sporadic PD. Here lies the potential relevance and advantage of fly genetics and available technologies such as UAS-

Gal4, fly deletion lines, and RNAi lines, which can be of great help to figure out novel players, pathways, and mechanistic interactions among neurodegenerative disorders. Hence, it is worth placing future endeavors in this direction.

10. Conclusion

In this chapter, we have provided an overview of current knowledge on the pathophysiology of sporadic PD employing *Drosophila* system. We also presented the future perspectives on the subject matter and emphasize the utmost importance for the need to generate comprehensive data employing genome-wide association studies in this model that may lead to identification of newer pathways. We also discussed the importance and necessity to reexamine the strategies/methods of screens to assess the potential of neuroprotective compounds/molecules employing *late life stages* that may provide us better answers on successful utilization of therapeutic compounds in late onset neurodegenerative disorders such as PD.

Acknowledgements

This work is partly supported by the Department of Biotechnology (DBT), Ministry of Science and Technology, India (R&D grant nos. BT/249/NE/TBP/2011, 25-4-2012, and BT/405/NE/U-Excel/2013, 11-12-2014), to the corresponding author. Dr Muralidhara is a recipient of DBT (Department of Biotechnology, India) Visiting Research Professorship under the North–East scheme.

Author details

Priyanka Modi[1,2], Ayajuddin Mohamad[1,2], Limamanen Phom[1,2], Zevelou Koza[1,2], Abhik Das, Rahul Chaurasia[1,2], Saikat Samadder[1,2], Bovito Achumi[1,2], Muralidhara[1,2], Rajesh Singh Pukhrambam[1,2] and Sarat Chandra Yenisetti[1,2*]

*Address all correspondence to: yschandrays@rediffmail.com, sarat@nagalanduniversity.ac.in

1 These authors contributed equally to this work

2 Drosophila Neurobiology Laboratory, Department of Zoology, Nagaland University (Central), Lumami, Nagaland, India

References

[1] http://www.pdf.org/en/parkinson_statistics (Accessed 2016:04:09)

[2] Polymeropoulos MH, Higgins JJ, Golbe LI, Johnson WG, et al: Mapping of a gene for Parkinson's disease to chromosome 4q21-q23. Science. 1996;274:1197–1199

[3] Reeve A, Simcox E, Turnbull D: Ageing and Parkinson's disease: why is advancing age the biggest risk factor? Ageing Res Rev. 2014; 14:19–30

[4] Calne DB, Langston JW: Aetiology of Parkinson's disease. Lancet. 1983;2(8365–8366): 1457–1459

[5] Langston JW, Ballard P, Tetrud JW, Irwin I: Chronic Parkinsonism in humans due to a product of melperidine-analog, synthesis. Science. 1983;219:979–980

[6] Poewe W, Antonini A, Zijlmans JCM, Burkhard PR: Levodopa in the treatment of Parkinson's disease: an old drug still going strong. Clin Interv Aging. 2010;5:229–238

[7] Tieu K: A guide to neurotoxic animal models of Parkinson's disease. Cold Spring Harb Perspect Med. 2011;1(1):a009316

[8] Meredith GE, Sonsalla PK, Chesselet M-F: Animal models of Parkinson's disease progression. Acta Neuropathol. 2008;115(4):385–398

[9] Bezard E, Przedborski S: A tale on animal models of Parkinson's disease. Mov Disord. 2011;26(6):993–1002. DOI:10.1002/mds.23696

[10] Polymeropoulos MH, Lavedan C, Leroy E, Ide SE, et al: Mutation in the alpha-synuclein gene identified in families with Parkinson's disease. Science. 1997;276:2045–2047

[11] Kitada T, Asakawa S, Hattori N, Matsumine H, Yamamura Y, et al: Mutations in the parkin gene cause autosomal recessive juvenile Parkinsonism. Nature. 1998;392:605–608

[12] Valente EM, Abou-Sleiman PM, Caputo V, Muqit MMK, et al: Hereditary early-onset Parkinson's disease caused by mutations in PINK1. Science. 2004;304:1158–1160

[13] Bonifati V, Rizzu P, van Baren MJ, Schaap O, Breedveld GJ et al: Mutations in the DJ-1 gene associated with autosomal recessive early-onset Parkinsonism. Science. 2003;299:256–259

[14] Paisán-Ruíz C, Jain S, Evans EW, Gilks WP, et al: Cloning of the gene containing mutations that cause PARK8-linked Parkinson's disease. Neuron. 2004;44:595–600

[15] Ramirez A, Heimbach A, Grundemann J, Stiller B, Hampshire D, et al: Hereditary Parkinsonism with dementia is caused by mutations in ATP13A2, encoding a lysosomal type 5 P-type ATPase. Nat Genet. 2006;38:1184–1191

[16] Paisan-Ruiz C, Bhatia KP, Li A, Hernandez D, Davis M, et al: Characterization of PLA2G6 as a locus for dystoniaparkinsonism. Ann Neurol. 2009;65:19–23

[17] Shojaee S, Sina F, Banihosseini SS, Kazemi MH, Kalhor R, et al: Genome-wide linkage analysis of a Parkinsonian-pyramidal syndrome pedigree by 500 K SNP arrays. Am J Hum Genet. 2008;82:1375–1384

[18] Edvardson S, Cinnamon Y, Ta-Shma A, Shaag A, et al: A deleterious mutation in DNAJC6 encoding the neuronal-specific clathrin-uncoating co-chaperone auxilin, is associated with juvenile Parkinsonism. PLoS One. 2012;7:e36458. DOI:10.1371/journal.pone.0036458

[19] Krebs CE, Karkheiran S, Powell JC, Cao M, Makarov V, et al: The Sac1 domain of SYNJ1 identified mutated in a family with early-onset progressive Parkinsonism with generalized seizures. Hum Mutat. 2013;34:1200–1207

[20] Quadri M, Fang M, Picillo M, Olgiati S, Breedveld GJ, et al: Mutation in the SYNJ1 gene associated with autosomal recessive, early-onset Parkinsonism. Hum Mutat. 2013;34:1208–1215

[21] Marras C, Lohmann K, Lang A, Klein C: Fixing the broken system of genetic locus symbols: Parkinson disease and dystonia as examples. Neurology. 2012;78:1016–1024

[22] Yue Z: LRRK2 in Parkinson's disease: in vivo models and approaches for understanding pathogenic roles. FEBS J. 2009;276(22):6445–6454

[23] Liu Z, Hamamichi S, Lee BD, et al: Inhibitors of LRRK2 kinase attenuate neurodegeneration and Parkinson-like phenotypes in Caenorhabditis elegans and Drosophila Parkinson's disease models. Hum Mol Genet. 2011;20(20):3933–3942

[24] Bove J, Prou D, Perier C, Przedborski S: Toxin induced models of Parkinson's disease. NeuroRx. 2005;2:484–494

[25] Betarbet R, Sherer TB, DiMonte DA, Greenamyre JT: Mechanistic approaches to Parkinson's disease pathogenesis. Brain Pathol. 2002;12:499–510

[26] Gerlach M, Desser H, Youdim MBH, Riederer P: New horizons in molecular mechanisms underlying Parkinson's disease and in our understanding of the neuroprotective effects of selegiline. J Neural Transm. 1996;48:7–21

[27] Zigmond MJ, Stricker EM: Animal models of Parkinsonism using selective neurotoxins: clinical and basic implications. Int Rev Neurobiol. 1989;31:1–79

[28] Di Monte DA, Mitra Lavasani, Manning-Bog AB: Environmental factors in Parkinson's disease. NeuroToxicology. 2002;23:487–502

[29] McCormack AL, Thiruchelvam M, Manning-Bog AB, Thiffault C, et al: Environmental risk factors and Parkinson's disease: selective degeneration of nigral dopaminergic neurons caused by the herbicide paraquat. Neurobiol Dis. 2002;10:119 –127

[30] Uversky VN: Neurotoxicant-induced animal models of Parkinson's disease: understanding the role of rotenone, Maneb and paraquat in neurodegeneration. Cell Tissue Res. 2004;318:225–241

[31] Simon-Sanchez J, Schulte C, Bras JM, Sharma M, et al: Genome-wide association study reveals genetic risk underlying Parkinson's disease. Nat Genet. 2009;41(12):1308–1312

[32] Spillantini MG, Schmidt ML, Lee VM, Trojanowski JQ, et al: Alpha-synuclein in Lewy bodies. Nature. 1997;388:839–840

[33] Dhillon AS, Tarbutton GL, Levin JL, Plotkin GM, et al: Pesticide/environmental exposures and Parkinson's disease in East Texas. J Agromedicine. 2008;13:37–48

[34] Elbaz A, Clavel J, Rathouz PJ, Moisan F, et al: Professional exposure to pesticides and Parkinson disease. Ann Neurol. 2009;66:494–504

[35] Kamel F, Tanner C, Umbach D, Hoppin J, et al: Pesticide exposure and self-reported Parkinson's disease in the agricultural health study. Am J Epidemiol. 2007;165:364–374

[36] Ritz BR, Manthripragada AD, Costello S, Lincoln SJ, et al: Dopamine transporter genetic variants and pesticides in Parkinson's disease. Environ Health Perspect. 2009;117:964–969

[37] Coulom H, Birman S: Chronic exposure to rotenone models sporadic Parkinson's disease in Drosophila melanogaster. J Neurosci. 2004;24(48):10993–10998

[38] Ascherio A, Chen H, Weisskopf MG, O'Reilly E, et al: Pesticide exposure and risk for Parkinson's disease. Ann Neurol. 2006;60:197–203

[39] Liou HH, Tsai MC, Chen CJ, et al: Environmental risk factors and Parkinson's disease: a case-control study in Taiwan. Neurology. 1997;48:1583–1588

[40] Petrovitch H, Ross GW, Abbott RD, Sanderson WT, et al: Plantation work and risk of Parkinson's disease in a population-based longitudinal study. Arch Neurol. 2002;59:1787–1792

[41] Seidler A, Hellenbrand W, Robra BP, Vieregge P, et al: Possible environmental, occupational, and other etiologic factors for Parkinson's disease: a case-control study in Germany. Neurology. 1996;46:1275–1284

[42] Ratner MH, David HF, Josef O, Robert GF, Raymon D: Younger age at onset of sporadic Parkinson's disease among subjects occupationally exposed to metals and pesticides. Interdiscip Toxicol. 2014;7(3):123–133

[43] Di Monte DA: The environment and Parkinson's disease: is the nigrostriatal system preferentially targeted by neurotoxins? Lancet Neurol. 2003;2(9):531–538

[44] Uversky VN, Li J, Bower K, Fink AL: Synergistic effects of pesticides and metals on the fibrillation of alpha-synuclein: implications for Parkinson's disease. Neurotoxicology. 2002;23(4–5):527–536

[45] Chiba K, Trevor AJ, Castagnoli Jr. N :Active uptake of MPP+, a metabolite of MPTP, by brain synaptosomes. Biochem Biophys. Res Commun. 1985;128:1228–1232

[46] Javitch JA, D'Amato RJ, Strittmatter SM, Snyder SH: Parkinsonism inducing neurotoxin, N-methyl-4-phenyl-1,2,3,6-tetrahydropyridine: uptake of the metabolite N-methyl-4-phenylpyridine by dopamine neurons explains selective toxicity. Proc Natl Acad Sci USA. 1985;82:2173–2177

[47] Daniels AJ, Reinhard Jr. JF: Energy-driven uptake of the neurotoxin 1-methyl-4-phenylpyridinium into chromaffin granules via the catecholamine transporter. J Biol Chem. 1988;263:5034–5036

[48] Miller GW, Gainetdinov RR, Levey AI, Caron MG: dopamine transporters and neuronal injury. Trends Pharmacol Sci. 1999;20:424–429

[49] Javoy F, Sotelo C, Herbet A, Agid Y: Specificity of dopaminergic neuronal degeneration induced by intracerebral injection of 6-hydroxydopamine in the nigrostriatal dopamine system. Brain Res. 1976;102:201–215

[50] Jeon BS, Jackson-Lewis V, Burke RE: 6-Hydroxydopamine lesion of the rat substantia nigra: time course and morphology of cell death. Neurodegeneration. 1995;4:131–137

[51] Dauer W, Przedborski S: Parkinson's disease: mechanisms and models. Neuron. 2003;39:889–909

[52] Cicchetti F, Drouin-Ouellet L, Gross RE: Environmental toxins and Parkinson's disease: what we have learned from pesticides-induced animal models? Trends Pharmacol Sci. 2009;30(9):475–483

[53] Wang XF, Li S, Chou AP, Bronstein JM: Inhibitory effects of pesticides on proteasome activity: implication in Parkinson's disease. Neurobiol Dis. 2006;23:198–205

[54] Olanow CW: The pathogenesis of cell death in Parkinson's disease. Mov Disord. 2007;22 (17):335–342

[55] Shimizu K, Ohtaki K, Matsubara K, Aoyama K, et al: Carrier-mediated processes in blood–brain barrier penetration and neural uptake of paraquat. Brain Res. 2001;906:135–142

[56] Miller GW: Paraquat: the red herring of Parkinson's disease research. Toxicol Sci. 2007;100:1–2

[57] Fei Q, McCormack AL, Di Monte DA, Ethell DW: Paraquat neurotoxicity is mediated by a Bak dependent mechanism. J Biol Chem. 2008;283:3357–3364

[58] Zhang J, Fitsanakis VA, Gu G, Jing D, et al: Manganese ethylene-bis-dithiocarbamate and selective dopaminergic neurodegeneration in rat: a link through mitochondrial dysfunction. J Neurochem. 2003;84:336–346

[59] Fei Q, Ethell DW: Maneb potentiates paraquat neurotoxicity by inducing key Bcl-2 family members. J Neurochem. 2008;105:2091–2097

[60] Gorell JM, Johnson CC, Rybicki BA, Peterson EL, et al: Occupational exposures to metals as risk factors for Parkinson's disease. Neurology. 1997;48:650–658

[61] Mergler D, Baldwin M: Early manifestations of manganese neurotoxicity in humans: an update. Environ Res. 1997;73:92–100

[62] Pal PK, Samii A, Calne DB: Manganese neurotoxicity: a review of clinical features. Neurotoxicology. 1999;20:227–238

[63] Dexter DT, Carayon A, Vidailhet M, Ruberg M, et al: Decreased ferritin levels in brain in Parkinson's disease. J Neurochem. 1990;55:16–20

[64] Valentea EM, Arenaa G, Torosantuccia L, Gelmettia V: Molecular pathways in sporadic PD. Parkinsonism Related Disorders. 2012;18(1):71–73

[65] Trinh K, Moore K, Wes PD, et al: Induction of the phase II detoxification pathway suppresses neuron loss in Drosophila models of Parkinson's disease, J Neurosci. 2008;28(2):465–472

[66] Wassef R, Haenold R, Hansel A, Brot N: Methionine sulfoxide reductase A and a dietary supplement S-methyl-L-cysteine prevent Parkinson's-like symptoms, J Neurosci. 2007;27(47):12808–12816

[67] Long JH, Gao L, Sun L, Liu J, Zhao-Wilson X: Grape extract protects mitochondria from oxidative damage and improves locomotor dysfunction and extends lifespan in a Drosophila Parkinson's disease model. Rejuvenation Res. 2009;12(5):321–331

[68] Jimenez-Del-Rio M, C Guzman-Martinez, C Velez-Pardo: The effects of polyphenols on survival and locomotor activity in Drosophila melanogaster exposed to iron and paraquat. Neurochem Res. 2010;35:227–238

[69] Lavara-Culebras E, Mu˜noz-Soriano V, G'omez-Pastor R, Matallana E, and Paricio N: Effects of pharmacological agents on the lifespan phenotype of Drosophila DJ-1β mutants. Gene. 2010;462(1–2):26–33

[70] Wang D, Qian L, Xiong H, et al: Antioxidants protect PINK1-dependent dopaminergic neurons in Drosophila. Proc Natl Acad Sci USA. 2006a;103(36):13520–13525

[71] Chaudhuri A, Bowling K, Funderburk C, Lawal H, et al: Interaction of genetic and environmental factors in a Drosophila Parkinsonism model. J Neurosci. 2007;27(10): 2457–2467

[72] Hosamani, R., Muralidhara: Neuroprotective efficacy of Bacopa monnieri against rotenone induced oxidative stress and neurotoxicity in Drosophila melanogaster. Neurotoxicology. 2009;30:977–985

[73] Hosamani R, Ramesh SR, Muralidhara: Attenuation of rotenone-induced mitochondrial oxidative damage and neurotoxicity in Drosophila melanogaster supplemented with creatine. Neurochem Res. 2010;35(9):1402–1412

[74] Faust K, Gehrke S, Yang Y, Yang L, et al: Neuroprotective effects of compounds with antioxidant and anti-inflammatory properties in a Drosophila model of Parkinson's disease. BMC Neurosci. 2009;10:109

[75] Tain LS, Chowdhury RB, Tao RN, et al: Drosophila HtrA2 is dispensable for apoptosis but acts downstream of PINK1 independently from Parkin. Cell Death Differentiation. 2009;16(8):1118–1125

[76] Auluck PK, Chan HY, Trojanowski JQ, Lee VM, Bonini NM: Chaperone suppression of alpha-synuclein toxicity in a Drosophila model for Parkinson's disease. Science. 2002;295:865–868.

[77] Auluck PK, Meulener MC, Bonini NM: Mechanisms of suppression of α-synuclein neurotoxicity by geldanamycin in Drosophila. J Biol Chem. 2005;280:2873–2878.

[78] Saini N, Schaffner W: Zinc supplement greatly improves the condition of parkin mutant Drosophila. BiolChem. 2010;391(5):513–518

[79] Munoz-Soriano V, Paricio N: Drosophila models of Parkinson's disease: discovering relevant pathways and novel therapeutic strategies. Parkinson's Disease. 2011;1–14. DOI:10.4061/2011/520640

[80] Burbulla LF, Kruger R: Converging environmental and genetic pathways in the pathogenesis of Parkinson's disease. J Neurol Sci. 2011;306:1–8

[81] Martin I, Dawson VL, Dawson TM: Recent advances in the genetics of Parkinson's disease. Annu Rev Genom Human Genet. 2011;12:301–325

[82] Cookson MR, Bandmann O: Parkinson's disease: insights from pathways. Hum Mol Genet. 2010;19:R1–R27

[83] Tansey MG, Goldberg MS: Neuroinflammation in Parkinson's disease: its role in neuronal death and implications for therapeutic intervention. Neurobiol Dis. 2010;37:510–518

[84] Bilen J, Bonini NM: Drosophila as a model for human neurodegenerative disease. Annu Rev Genet. 2005;39:153–171

[85] Cooper AA, Gitler AD, Cashikar A, Haynes CM, et al: α-Synuclein blocks ER-Golgi traffic and Rab1 rescues neuron loss in Parkinson's models. Science. 2006;313:324–328

[86] Chai C, Lim KL: Genetic insights into sporadic Parkinson's disease pathogenesis. Curr Genomics. 2013;14:486–501.

[87] De Bellis MD, Baum AS, Birmaher B, Keshavan MS, et al: Developmental traumatology, Part I: Biological stress systems. Biol Psychiatry. 1999;45:1259–1270

[88] Kim ST, Choi JH, Chang JW, Kim SW, Hwang O: Immobilization stress causes increase in tetrahydrobiopterin, dopamine, and neuromelanin and oxidative damage in the nigrostriatal system. J Neurochem. 2005;95:89–98

[89] Tan EK, Khajavi M, Thronby JI, Nagamitsu S, et al: Variability and validity of polymorphism association studies in Parkinson's disease. Neurology. 2000;5:533–538

[90] Warner TT, Schapira AHV: Genetic and environmental factors in the cause of Parkinson's disease. Ann Neurol. 2003;53(3):16–25

[91] Yang J, Benyamin B, McEvoy BP, Gordon S, Henders AK, et al: Common SNPs explain a large proportion of the heritability for human height. Nat Genet. 2010;42(7):565–569

[92] Yang J, Lee SH, Goddard ME, Visscher PM: GCTA: a tool for genome-wide complex trait. Am J Hum Genet. 2011;88(1):76–82

[93] Keller MF, Saad M, Bras J, Bettella F, et al: Using genomewide complex trait analysis to quantify 'missing heritability' in Parkinson's disease. Hum Mol Genet. 2012;21(22): 4996–5009

[94] Ross CA, Smith WW: Gene-environment interactions in Parkinson's disease. Parkinsonism Relat Disord. 2007;13(3):309–315.

[95] Kelada SN, Checkoway H, Kardia SL, Carlson CS, et al: 5′ and 3′ region variability in the dopamine transporter gene (SLC6A3), pesticide exposure and Parkinson's disease risk: a hypothesis-generating study. Hum Mol Genet. 2006;15:3055–3062

[96] Hancock DB, Martin ER, Vance JM, Scott WK: Nitric oxide synthase genes and their interactions with environmental factors in Parkinson's disease. Neurogenetics. 2008;9:249–262

[97] Dick FD, De Palma G, Ahmadi A, Osborne A, et al: Gene environment interactions in Parkinsonism and Parkinson's disease: the Geoparkinson study. Occup Environ Med. 2007;64:673–680

[98] Piccini P, Burn DJ, Ceravolo R, Maraganore D, Brooks DJ: The role of inheritance in sporadic Parkinson's disease: evidence from a longitudinal study of dopaminergic function in twins. Ann Neurol. 1999;45(5):577–582

[99] Wirdefeldt K, Gatz M, Reynolds CA, Prescott CA, Pedersen NL: Heritability of Parkinson disease in Swedish twins: a longitudinal study. Neurobiol Aging. 2011;32(10):1921–1928

[100] Feany MB, Bender WW: A Drosophila model of Parkinson's disease. Nature. 2000;404:394–398

[101] Hirth F: Drosophila melanogaster in the study of human neurodegeneration. CNS Neurological Disorders. 2010;9:504–523

[102] Bonini NM, Fortini ME: Human neurodegenerative disease modeling using Drosophila. Annu Rev Neurosc. 2003;26:627–656

[103] Barrientos A, Moraes CT: Titrating the effects of mitochondrial complex I impairment in the cell physiology. J Biol Chem. 1999;274:16188–1619

[104] Chauvin C, De Oliveira F, Ronot X, Mousseau M, et al: Ubiquinone analogs: a mitochondrial permeability transition pore-dependent pathway to selective cell Death J Biol Chem. 2001;276,41394–41398

[105] Green DR, Reed JC: Mitochondria and apoptosis. Science. 1998;281:1309–1312

[106] Kroemer G, Reed JC: Mitochondrial control of cell death. Nat Med. 2000;6:513–519

[107] Wang X: The expanding role of mitochondria in apoptosis. Genes Dev. 2001;15:2922–2933

[108] Liu X, Kim CN, Yang J, Jemmerson R, Wang X: Induction of apoptotic program in cell-free extracts: requirement for dATP and cytochrome c. Cell. 1996;86:147–157

[109] Du C, Fang M, Li Y, Li L, Wang X: Smac, a mitochondrial protein that promotes cytochrome c-dependent caspase activation by eliminating IAP inhibition. Cell. 2000;102:33–42

[110] Verhagen AM, Ekert PG, Pakusch M, Silke J, Connolly LM, et al: Identification of DIABLO, a mammalian protein that promotes apoptosis by binding to and antagonizing IAP proteins. Cell. 2000;102:43–53

[111] Li LY, Luo X, Wang X: Endonuclease G is an apoptotic DNase when released from mitochondria. Nature. 2001;412:95–99

[112] Susin SA, Lorenzo HK, Zamzami N, Marzo I, et al: Molecular characterization of mitochondrial apoptosis-inducing factor. Nature. 1999;397:441–446

[113] Reed JC: Bcl-2 and the regulation of programmed cell death. J Cell Biol. 1994;124:1–6

[114] Reed JC: Double identity for proteins of the Bcl-2 family. Nature. 1997;387:773–776

[115] Budnik V, White K: Catecholamine containing neurons in Drosophila melanogaster: distribution and development. J Comp Neurol. 1988;268:400–413

[116] Nassel DR, Elekes K: Aminergic neurons in the brain of blowflies and Drosophila: dopamine- and tyrosine hydroxylase-immunoreactive neurons and their relationship with putative histaminergic neurons. Cell Tissue Res. 1992;267:147–167

[117] Friggi-Grelin F, Coulom H, Meller M, Gomez D, et al: Targeted gene expression in Drosophila dopaminergic cells using regulatory sequences from tyrosine hydroxylase. J Neurobiol. 2003;54:618–627

[118] Cassar M, Issa AR, Riemensperger T, Petitgas C, et al: A dopamine receptor contributes to paraquat-induced neurotoxicity in Drosophila. Hum Mol Genet. 2015;24(1):197–212

[119] Reiter LT, Potocki L, Chien S, Gribskov M, et al: A systematic analysis of human disease-associated gene sequences in Drosophila melanogaster. Genome Res. 2001;11:1114–1125

[120] Girish C, Muralidhara: Propensity of Selaginella delicatula aqueous extract to offset rotenone-induced oxidative dysfunctions and neurotoxicity in Drosophila melanogaster: implications. NeuroToxicology. 2012;33:444–456

[121] Manjunath MJ, Muralidhara: Standardized extract of Withania somnifera (Aswagandha) markedly offsets Rotenone-Induced locomotor deficits, oxidative impairments and neurotoxicity in Drosophila melanogaster. J Food Sci Technol. 2015;52:1971–1981

[122] Johnson ME, Bobrovskaya L: An update on the rotenone models of Parkinson's disease: their ability to reproduce the features of clinical disease and model gene–environment interactions. NeuroToxicology. 2015;46:101–116

[123] Marsh JL, Thompson LM: Drosophila in the study of neurodegenerative disease. Neuron. 2006;52:169–178

[124] Virmani A, Pinto L, Binienda Z, Ali S: Food nutrigenomics and neurodegeneration-neuroprotection by what you eat! Mol Neurobiol. 2013;48:353–362

[125] Lee WH, Lee CY, Bebaway M, Luk F, et al: Curcumin and its derivatives:their application in neuropharmacology and neuroscience in the 21st century. Curr Neuropharmacol. 2013;11:338–378

[126] Kim HJ, Kim P, Shin CY: A comprehensive review of the therapeutic and pharmacological effects of ginseng and ginsenosides in central nervous system. J Ginseng Res. 2013;37:8–29

[127] Sun AY, Wang Q, Simonyi A, Sun GY: Resveratol as a therapeutic agent for neurodegenerative diseases. Mol Neurobiol. 2010;41:375–383

[128] Chen LW, Wang YQ, Wei LC, Shi M, Chan YS: Chinese herbs and herbal extracts for neuroprotection of dopaminergic neurons and potential therapeutic treatment of Parkinson's disease. CNS Neurol Disord Drug Targets. 2007;6:273–281

[129] Chao J, Yu MS, Ho YS, Wang M, Chang RC: Dietary oxyresveratrol prevents Parkinsonian mimetic 6-hydroxydopamine neurotoxicity. Free Radic Biol Med. 2008;45:1019–1026

[130] Ji HF, Shen L: The multiple pharmaceutical potential of curcumin in Parkinson's disease. CNS Neurol Disord Drug Targets. 2014;13:369–373

[131] Gadad BS, Subramanya PK, Pullabhatla S, Shantharam IS, Rao KS: Curcumin-glucoside, a novel synthetic derivative of curcumin, inhibits alpha-synuclein oligomer formation: relevance to Parkinson's disease. Curr Pharm Des. 2012;18:76–84

[132] Phom L, Achumi B, Alone DP, Muralidhara, Yenisetti SC: Curcumin's neuroprotective efficacy in Drosophila model of idiopathic Parkinson's disease is phase specific: implication of its therapeutic effectiveness. Rejuvenation Res. 2014;17(6):481–489

[133] Prior RI, Cao G, Martin A, Sofic A, et al: Antioxidant capacity as influenced by total phenolic and anthocyanine content maturity and variety of vaccinium species. J Agri Food Chem. 1998;46:2586–2593

[134] Joseph JA, Hale-Shukitt B, Casadesus G: Reversing the deleterious effect of aging on neuronal communications and behavior: beneficial properties of fruit polyphenol compounds. Am J Clin Nutr. 2005;81:313S–316S

[135] Krikorian K, Slider MD, Nash TA, Kalt W, et al: Blueberry supplementation improves memory in older patients. J Agri Food Chem. 2010;58:3996–4000

[136] Peng C, Yuanyun Z, KinMing K, Yintong L, et al: Blueberry extract prolongs lifespan of Drosophila melanogaster. Exper Gerontol. 2012;47:170–178

[137] Lim LM, Ng CH: Genetic models of Parkinson disease. Biochimica Biophysica Acta. 2009;1792(7):604–615

[138] Dawson TM, Ko HS, Dawson VL: Genetic animal models of Parkinson's disease. Neuron. 2010;66(5):646–661

[139] Dagda RK, Zhu J, Chu CT: Mitochondrial kinases in Parkinson's disease: converging insights from neurotoxin and genetic models. Mitochondrion. 2009;9:289–298

[140] Falkenburger BH, Schulz JB: Limitations of cellular models in Parkinson's disease research. J Neural Transm. 2006;70:261–268

[141] Jeibmann A, Paulus W: Drosophila melanogaster as a model organism of brain diseases. Int J Mol Sci. 2009;10:407–440

[142] Adams MD, Celniker SE, Holt RA, Evans CA, et al: The genome sequence of Drosophila melanogaster. Science. 2000;287:2185–2219

[143] Pandey UB, Nichols CD: Human disease models in Drosophila melanogaster and the role of the fly in therapeutic drug discovery. Pharmacol Rev. 2011;63:411–436

[144] Cauchi RJ, vanden Heuvel M: The fly as a model for neurodegenerative diseases: is it worth the jump? Neurodegener Dis. 2006;3:338–356

[145] Chan HY, Bonini NM: Drosophila models of human neurodegenerative disease. Cell Death Differ. 2000;7:1075–1080

[146] Kohler RE: Drosophila: a life in the laboratory. J Hist Biol. 1993;26:281–310

[147] Lu B, Vogel H: Drosophila models of neurodegenerative diseases. Annu Rev Pathol. 2009;4:315–342

[148] Ambegaokar SS, Roy B, Jackson GR: Neurodegenerative models in Drosophila: polyglutamine disorders, Parkinson disease, and amyotrophic lateral sclerosis. Neurobiol Disease. 2010;40:29–39

[149] West RJH, Furmston R, Williams CAC, Elliott CJH: Neurophysiology of Drosophila models of Parkinson's disease. Parkinson's Disease. 2015;ID381281:11. DOI: 10.1155/2015/381281

[150] Stephenson R, Metcalfe NH: Drosophila melanogaster: a fly through its history and current use. J R Coll Physicians Edinb. 2013;43:70–75

[151] Fernandez-Funez P, Nino-Rosales ML, de Gouyon B, She WC, et al: Identification of genes that modify ataxin-1-induced neurodegeneration. Nature. 2000;408:101–106

[152] Ghosh S, Feany MB: Comparison of pathways controlling toxicity in the eye and brain in Drosophila model of human neurodegenerative diseases. Hum Mol Genet. 2004;13:2011–2018

[153] Hamamichi S, Rivas RN, Knight AL, Cao S, et al: Hypothesis based RNAi screening identifies neuroprotective genes in a Parkinson's disease model. Proc Natl Acad Sci USA. 2008;105:728–733

[154] Kazemi-Esfarjani P, Benzer S: Genetic suppression of polyglutamine toxicity in Drosophila. Science. 2000;287:1837–1840

[155] Menzies FM, Yenisetti YS, Min KT: Roles of Drosophila DJ-1 in survival of dopaminergic neurons and oxidative stress. Curr Biol. 2005;15(17):1578–1582

[156] Merzetti EM, Staveley BE: Spargel, the PGC-1 alpha homologue, in models of Parkinson disease in Drosophila melanogaster. BMC Neuroscience. 2015; 16(70): 1–8. DOI:10.1186/s12868-015-0210-2.

[157] Van Ham TJ, Breitling R, Morris A Swertz MA, Nollen EAA: Neurodegenerative diseases: lessons from genome-wide screens in small model organisms. EMBO Mol Med. 2009;1(8–9):360–370. DOI:10.1002/emmm.200900051

[158] Ivatt RM, Sanchez-Martinez A, Godena VK, Brown S, et al: Genome wide RNAi screen identifies the Parkinson disease GWAS risk locus SREBF1 as a regulator of mitophagy. Proc Nat Acad Sci USA. 2014;111(23):8494–8499

Chapter 12

Pharmacotherapeutic Challenges in Parkinson's Disease Inpatients

Unax Lertxundi, Rafael Hernández,
Saioa Domingo-Echaburu,
Javier Peral-Aguirregoitia and Juan Medrano

Additional information is available at the end of the chapter

http://dx.doi.org/10.5772/62561

Abstract

During the natural history of Parkinson's disease (PD), many patients require hospital admission for medical or surgical problems other than the motor features of PD. Therefore, they are often admitted to non-neurological wards where the staff is unfamiliar with PD management. Among the issues related to hospitalization in patients with PD, drug-related problems such as inappropriate levodopa timing of administration, the use of contraindicated, centrally acting antidopaminergic drugs and anticholinergic burden remain among the most troublesome.

Keywords: Parkinson's disease, antidopaminergic, levodopa, inappropriate prescription, antipsychotic

1. Introduction

Parkinson's disease (PD) is a chronic, progressive neurodegenerative disease known to occur primarily from middle age to later in life [1]. The frequency of PD varies depending on the diagnostic criteria, study population, and is estimated to be 0.3% of the entire population, about 1–2% in people over 60–65 years [1] and 3–5% in people 85 years and older [2, 3]. It is a common progressive and disabling neurological disorder characterized by the degeneration of several different neuronal populations that lead to the cardinal features of PD, which are tremor, bradykinesia, rigidity and postural instability [4].

During the natural history of the disease, many patients require hospital admission for medical or surgical problems other than the motor features of PD. As a consequence, they are often admitted to non-neurological wards where staff is unfamiliar with PD management, as it is generally managed in the outpatient setting [5, 6]. The problems and complications faced by PD patients while in hospital have urged specialists to develop specific guidelines [7]. Among the issues related to hospitalization in PD patients, drug-related problems remain amongst the most troublesome [8, 9]. In this chapter we will review some of them, such as inappropriate levodopa timing administration, centrally acting antidopaminergic drug administration and anticholinergic burden.

2. Inappropriate inpatient levodopa administration

Management of medication regimens increases in complexity as PD progresses, frequently leading to prescriptions taken six or more times per day. Besides, dosing intervals are specific to each individual patient. Although adequate anti-PD medication management is essential during hospital admissions (regarding drugs, dosages and specific dosage schedules), its management is frequently described as suboptimal, leading to adverse clinical sequelae.

One of the first studies about the problem came from a retrospective study of patients with PD hospitalized in the United Kingdom [10]. In that report, an alarming percentage of patients admitted to the hospital had critical medications stopped or omitted. Even more worryingly, of these around 60% experienced significant adverse effects, including the need to transfer a patient to the intensive care unit. In another study carried out in surgical wards of a Scottish hospital, three out of four hospitalized patients with PD did not receive their medications on time or had had doses entirely omitted [11]. In the same line, in a small study we conducted in Alto Deba hospital (in the Basque Country, Spain) we found that chronic anti-PD prescription was omitted in 12/73 admissions [12].

In a survey of National Parkinson Foundation Center, the majority of the participating centers were not confident that medication schedules were adhered to during hospital stays, perhaps because the importance of medication timing in PD was not well understood by hospital staff [13]. Again, from a patient perspective, a survey carried out by a Dutch team showed that incorrect medication distribution contributed to intrahospital deterioration [14].

The same Dutch team published a prospective study that showed that medication error was the most important risk factor for deterioration [15]. More recently, a cross-sectional chart review carried out in 339 consecutive hospital encounters from 212 PD subjects in Florida has shown that patients who had delayed administration or missed at least one dose stayed longer [16].

Skelly et al. [17], in a study carried out in the Royal Derby Hospital in the United Kingdom (National Parkinson Foundation Centre of Excellence for Parkinson's Disease), reported that 2.5% of all doses were not administered because the drug was not available on time. It has to be remarked that this happened in a ward specially designed to treat patients with PD, with

http://dx.doi.org/10.5772/62561

an enhanced stock of anti-PD medications [17]. We consider that this problem is likely to be aggravated in other non-specialized wards and especially in smaller hospitals.

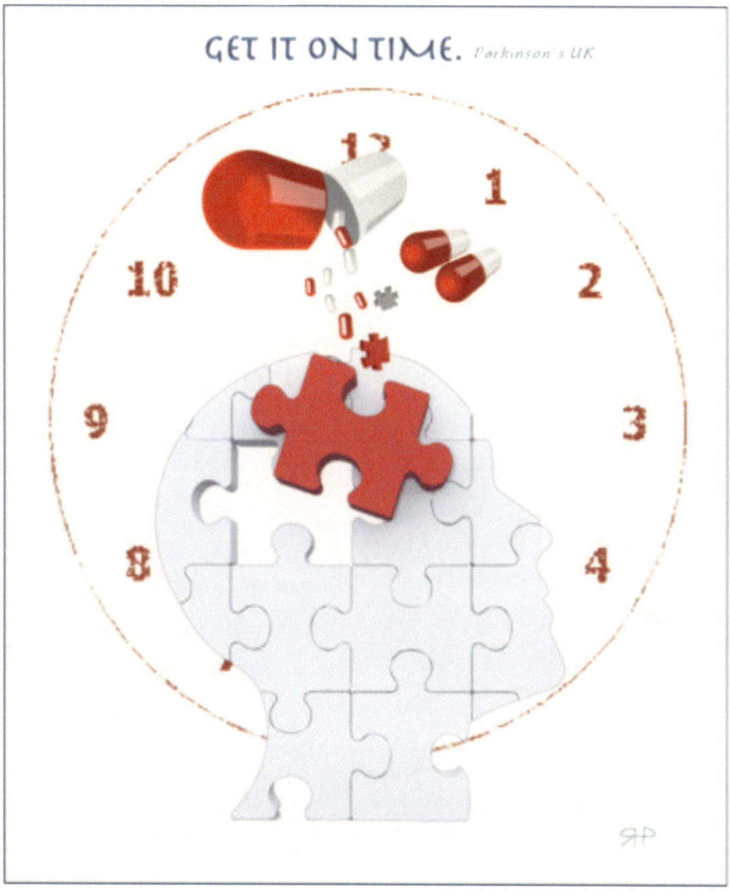

Figure 1. The importance of on-time levodopa administration.

To counteract this difficulty, Parkinson's United Kingdom "**Get it on time campaign**" [18], (**Figure 1**) among others [19], advices that all commercially available antiparkinsonian drugs should be timely available in all hospital wards. Given the data described previously, we find this unfeasible, especially in small hospitals where the availability of all the anti-PD drugs would certainly result in the expiration of many of these drugs before they could be used. May be a reasonable solution can be found in Skelly et al.'s own final considerations: *"The available stock was not used as flexibly as we had hoped: e.g. doses of modified release medications were omitted rather than a temporary switch to available standard release drugs."*

The Institute for Safe Medication Practices (ISMP) has recently issued a generic recommendation that, whereas undoubtedly helpful, will result insufficient. Their recommendation specifically states *"avoiding non-formulary delays ensuring that your formulary provides common*

PD medications and doses so that drug administration is not delayed while the pharmacy obtains non-formulary medications" [20]. Based on the available data, we have recently proposed an algorithm to prevent drug omissions and delays [21] using the equivalent dosages proposed by Tomlinson et al. [22] (**Table 1**).

Drug	Conversion Factor
Immediate release levodopa	1
Controlled release levodopa	0.75
Entacapone*	LD 0.33
Tolcapone*	LD 0.5
Duodopa®	1.11
Pramipexole	100
Ropirinole	20
Rotigotine	30
Selegiline	10
Rasagiline	100
Amantadine	1
Apomorphine	10
Bromocriptine	10

*To calculate the total LED for COMT inhibitors (entacapone and tolcapone), the total levodopa (including controlled release levodopa if COMT inhibitor is given simultaneously) amount should be calculated and then multiplied by the appropriate value. For Stalevo®, the levodopa and COMT inhibitor should be split and calculated separately.

Table 1. Conversion factors to calculate levodopa equivalent dose (LED) adapted from ref [22].

In **Figure 2**, we provide an example for how the algorithm could be applied to prevent an omission.

Nevertheless, if a PD patient must be kept *Nil per Os (NPO)*, thus interfering with the patient's unique schedule of medication administration, a neurologist or Neurology team should oversee the medication regimen change to avoid complications, using alternatives such as intradermal rotigotin or subcutaneous apomorphine [23]. In the same study mentioned above, 88% of admissions (227/257) were some dosage was not administered because of "oral intolerance" or NPO status, no alternative drug was used. In four hospitals, no patient received an alternative drug.

Paraphrasing Magdalinou *"PD medications should be regarded as important as insulin is for diabetics"* [10]. We completely agree. It is about time we take the appropriate measures to minimize the problem.

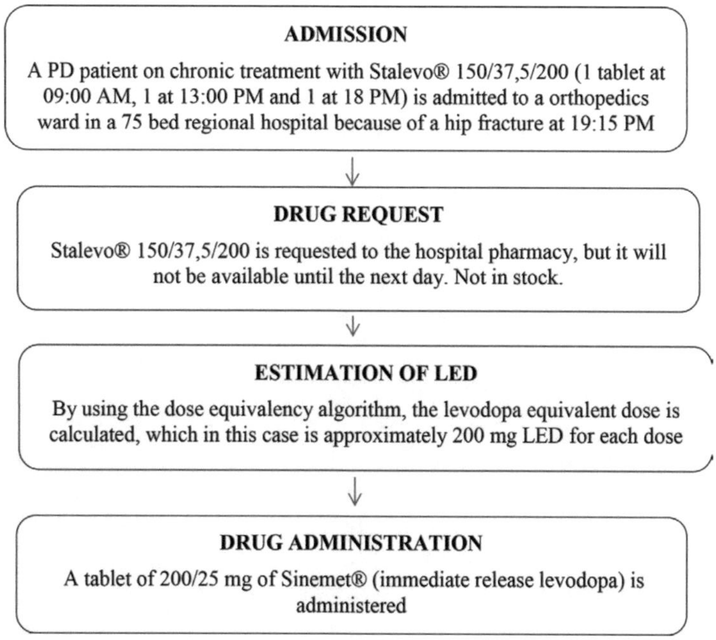

Figure 2. Theoretical example of the algorithm application.

3. Central-acting antidopaminergic administration

Not only anti-PD drugs like levodopa should be taken into account when patients are admitted to hospital. Some drugs are considered inappropriate in PD, since in the same way as dopaminergic drug omissions, they can worsen motor functioning. This is the case with central-acting dopamine antagonists.

While PD has traditionally been considered a motor system disorder, it is nowadays recognized to be a complex condition with diverse clinical features that include neuropsychiatric and many other non-motor symptoms. Researchers are increasingly attending to and characterizing the non-motor symptoms of the disease such as depression, apathy, dementia and psychosis.

3.1. Psychosis

Although patients with both parkinsonism and dementia commonly experience spontaneous visual hallucinations, delusions and paranoia even in the absence of medications for the motor dysfunction, the introduction of dopaminergic therapies frequently triggers or exacerbates the underlying propensity to psychosis in patients who have PD dementia. Correctable infectious, toxic and metabolic etiologies (delirium) must be ruled out. If symptoms persist, antiparkinsonian drugs should be slowly reduced, which usually results in a worsening of the parkinsonian features that may be poorly tolerated. When these measures fail, therapy with antipsychotic drugs might be needed [24–26].

Almost all antipsychotic drugs are known to produce PD exacerbation. Clozapine is the only antipsychotic that has level I evidence to support its use in these patients [26]. Nevertheless, quetiapine is frequently considered the first-line choice for treating psychotic symptoms in PD (e.g., by the American Academy of Neurology), and it is usually reported as the most frequently used [27]. The rest of antipsychotic agents, especially high potency drugs such as haloperidol, are considered inappropriate in PD. In the same line, and as PD disease usually affects old people (aged >65 years), the most frequently used tools employing explicit criteria to detect potentially inappropriate prescriptions in older patients (Beers and STOPP-START) criteria consider inappropriate all antipsychotics other than clozapine or quetiapine [28, 29]. We were surprised to find aripiprazole included as one of the least-problematic antipsychotic therapies for PD psychosis, at the same level as quetiapine and clozapine in the last version of the Beers criteria. Despite its promising receptorial profile, preliminary experience with aripiprazole shows a discouraging safety and efficacy profile in individuals with PD, who represent the most stringent test of a drug's potential for inducing parkinsonism. In this sense, severe worsening of motor function has been reported, with one individual requiring parenteral fluid substitution and another requiring nasogastric tube feeding [30]. In light of the evidence mentioned above and considering the widespread use of the Beers criteria, we believe including aripiprazole in the same category as clozapine and quetiapine for the treatment of PD psychosis could do more harm than good [31].

Delirium, or acute confusional state, has been reported as very prevalent in PD inpatients, and being involved in as many as a quarter of admissions [32, 33]. Dementia, which mainly affects patients with advanced disease, constitutes a known risk factor for delirium. As pointed out before, correctable infectious, toxic and metabolic etiologies should be ruled out before considering antipsychotic treatment. Sadly, many times haloperidol is prescribed in our setting to treat "agitation" in patients, either with PD or not.

3.2. Nausea and vomiting

Nausea and vomiting, which are common adverse effects of anti-PD medications (levodopa and dopamine agonists), might require treatment with antiemetic drugs. Metoclopramide and other centrally acting antiemetics are contraindicated in PD patients because they block dopaminergic receptors in the nigrostriatal area, generating deleterious motor effects [26]. Some cases of metoclopramide-associated encephalopathy have even been reported [34, 35].

On the other side, domperidone has traditionally been considered as the gold standard, since it does not readily cross the blood-brain barrier [26]. Nevertheless, its cardiac safety has been put into question recently [36, 37].

3.3. Hiccups

Hiccups are starting to be considered one more "non-motor" symptom of PD [38]. A study evaluated the presence of hiccups in 90 PD patients and 100 age-matched controls, finding that hiccups were more frequent in PD patients than in healthy controls. Interestingly, chlorpromazine (a "typical" antipsychotic formally contraindicated in PD) is usually used to treat incoercible hiccups.

Whatever the reason for they were prescribed, centrally acting antidopaminergic drugs have shown to generate deleterious effects in PD inpatients. The study carried out in Florida, which was mentioned above [16], showed that contraindicated dopamine blocking agent's administration (which occurred in 23% of the cases) was significantly related to an increased length of stay (8,2 vs 3,5 days)(**Figure 3**).

In conclusion, avoiding drugs known to exacerbate motor symptoms should be a priority. Clozapine and quetiapine should be preferred among antipsychotics [9]. Regarding antiemetic use, low dose of domperidone seems reasonable.

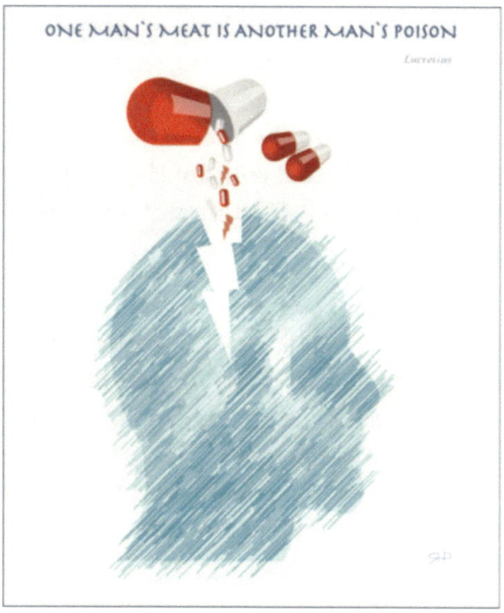

Figure 3. Deleterous effects of antidopaminergics in Parkinson's Disease.

4. Anticholinergic burden in PD inpatients

Anticholinergic toxicity is often the consequence of the cumulative burden of multiple medications and metabolites rather than a result of the action of a single drug [39]. Thus, treatment of comorbidities (e.g., bladder control problems, psychosis and depression) with drugs with anticholinergic properties could contribute to aggravate the problem. Indeed, the most frequently used tools employing explicit criteria to detect potentially inappropriate prescriptions in the elderly dedicate a specific section to anticholinergic drug use [28, 29]. Drugs with anticholinergic activity can lead to adverse reactions in the central nervous system such as cognitive disturbance, especially in elderly people, so extreme caution is required when using them in people with previously known cognitive dysfunction. In this sense, dementia has a prevalence of 80–90% in the most advanced phases of PD [25, 27]. Besides, using anticholinergics in patients on cholinesterase inhibitors (which are the treatment of dementia in PD) could limit their beneficial effect due to a pharmacodynamic interaction [28]. Further, peripheral anticholinergic side effects, including tachycardia, constipation, urinary retention and blurred vision, should also be considered because they may lead to serious morbidity, especially in PD patients who frequently present with autonomic dysfunction.

Anticholinergics like trihexyphenidil, biperiden and benztropine have remained one of the available antiparkinsonian drugs in the antiparkinsonian armamentarium. But considering the potential risks, it is easier to understand why nowadays anticholinergics are hardly used to treat PD, with the exception of severe tremor in younger patients without cognitive dysfunction [40].

In a recent study on PD patients admitted to acute care hospitals in the Basque Health care system, we found that anticholinergic burden was relatively high and arose from drugs prescribed to treat non-motor symptoms and other comorbidities rather than the motor symptoms of the disease [41]. Interestingly, the total number of drugs and cholinesterase drug prescriptions were independently associated with anticholinergic drug use whatever the scale administered (the study was performed using four different scales to measure anticholinergic burden).

As described above, anticholinergic toxicity is often the result of the cumulative burden of multiple medications. For that purpose, many drug lists have been designed to measure the total anticholinergic burden, but they substantially differ both in which drugs are included and in the anticholinergic activity assigned to each compound [42]. Moreover, some drugs with undoubted anticholinergic properties (such as biperiden, solifenacin, trospium and fesoterodine) that were prescribed to some inpatients had to be discarded in this study as these compounds do not appear in any of the published lists [43], including the list providing a systematic review of the literature, which in our opinion is the most complete so far [44]. Thus, developing a credible, consistent, periodically updated screening tool to measure anticholinergic burden should be a priority, in order to avoid confusion in the future [45].

In definitive, potential anticholinergic toxicity should be kept in mind by clinicians, especially in those elderly patients suffering from cognitive dysfunction. Alternative drugs that lack anticholinergic activity should be used when possible.

In conclusion, all professionals involved in healthcare should pay attention to the specific pharmacotherapeutic challenges faced by PD patients in acute care hospitals. Efforts should be made to administer each levodopa dose on time. Drugs with central antidopaminergic activity like haloperidol and metoclopramide should be avoided. And finally, using alternative drugs without antimuscarinic properties when possible seems a reasonable option.

http://dx.doi.org/10.5772/62561

Author details

Unax Lertxundi[1*], Rafael Hernández[2], Saioa Domingo-Echaburu[3], Javier Peral-Aguirregoitia[4] and Juan Medrano[5]

*Address all correspondence to: Unaxlertxundietxebarria@osakidetza.net

1 Pharmacy Service, Araba's Mental Health Network, Vitoria-Gasteiz, Spain

2 Internal Medicine, Araba's Mental Health Network, Vitoria-Gasteiz, Spain

3 Pharmacy Service, Alto Deba's Integrated Health Organization, Arrasate, Spain

4 Pharmacy Service, Galdakao-Usansolo Hospital, Galdakao, Spain

5 Psychiatry Service, Bizkaia's Mental Health Network, Portugalete, Spain

References

[1] De Lau LM, Breteler MM. Epidemiology of Parkinson's disease. Lancet Neurol. 2006; 5: 525-535.

[2] Alves G, Forsaa EB, Pedersen KF, et al. Epidemiology of Parkinson's disease. J Neurol. 2008; 255 (Suppl 5): 18-32.

[3] De Rijk MC, Tzourio C, Breteler MM, et al. Prevalence of parkinsonism and Parkinson's disease in Europe: the EUROPARKINSON Collaborative Study. European Community Concerted Action on the Epidemiology of Parkinson's disease. J Neurol Neurosurg Psychiatry. 1997; 62: 10.

[4] Chou KL. Clinical manifestations of Parkinson disease. Available from: http://www.uptodate.com/contents/clinical-manifestations-of-parkinson-disease?source=search_result&search=parkinson+disease&selectedTitle=1~150 [Accessed: 02/16/2016].

[5] Hassan A, Wu SS, Scmhidt P, et al, NPF-QII Investigators. High rates and the risk factors for emergency room visits and hospitalization in Parkinson's disease. Parkinsonism Relat Disord. 2013; 19: 949-954.

[6] Temlett JA, Thompson PD. Reasons for admission to hospital for Parkinson's disease. Intern Med J. 2006; 36: 524-526.

[7] Aminoff MJ, Christine CW, Friedman JH, et al. National Parkinson Foundation Working Group on Hospitalization in Parkinson's disease. Management of the

hospitalized patient with Parkinson's disease: current state of the field and need for guidelines. Parkinsonism Relat Disord. 2011; 17: 139-145.

[8] Wood LD, Neumiller JJ, Setter SM, et al. Clinical review of treatment options for select nonmotor symptoms of Parkinson's disease. Am J Geriatr Pharmacother. 2010; 8: 294-315.

[9] Lertxundi U, Domingo-Echaburu S, Irigoyen I, et al. Challenges in the pharmacotherapeutic management of the hospitalised patient with Parkinson's disease. Rev Neurol. 2014; 58: 353-364.

[10] Magdalinou KN, Martin A, Kessel B. Prescribing medications in Parkinson's disease (PD) patients during acute admissions to a District General Hospital. Parkinsonism Relat Disord. 2007; 13: 539-540.

[11] Derry CP, Shah KJ, Caie L, et al. Medication management in people with Parkinson's disease during surgical admissions. Postgrad Med J. 2010; 86: 334-337.

[12] Domingo-Echaburu S, Lertxundi U, Gonzalo-Olazabal E, et al. Inappropriate antidopaminergic drug use in Parkinson's disease inpatients. Cur Drug Ther. 2012; 7: 164-169.

[13] Chou KL, Zamudio J, Schmidt P, et al. Hospitalization in Parkinson's disease: a survey of National Parkinson Foundation Centers. Parkinsonism Relat Disord. 2011; 17: 440-445.

[14] Gerlach OH, Broen MP, van Domburg PH, et al. Deterioration of Parkinson's disease during hospitalization: survey of 684 patients. BMC Neurol. 2012; 12: 13.

[15] Gerlach OH, Broen MP, Weber WE. Motor outcomes during hospitalization in Parkinson's disease patients: a prospective study. Parkinsonism Relat Disord. 2013; 19: 737-741.

[16] Martínez-Ramírez D, Giugni JC, Little CS, et al. Missing dosages and neuroleptic usage may prolong length of stay in hospitalized Parkinson's disease patients. PLoS One. 2015;10: e0124356.

[17] Skelly R, Brown L, Fakis A, et al. Does a specialist unit improve outcomes for hospitalized patients with Parkinson's disease? Parkinsonism Relat Disord. 2014; 20: 1242-1247.

[18] Parkinson's UK. "Get It on Time" campaign. Available from: www.parkinsons.org.uk [Accessed 2015/04/28].

[19] Aware in Care Campaign. National Parkinson Foundation. Available from: http://www.awareincare.org. [Accessed 2015/04/28].

[20] Cohen M, Smetzer L. ISMP medication error report analysis delayed administration and contraindicated drugs place hospitalized Parkinson's disease patients at risk. Hosp Pharm. 2015; 50: 559-563.

[21] Lertxundi U, Isla A, Solinís MA, Domingo-Echaburu S, et al. A proposal to prevent omissions and delays of antiparkinsonian drug administration in hospitals. Neurohospitalist. 2015; 5: 53-54.

[22] Tomlinson CL, Stowe R, Patel S, et al. Systematic review of levodopa dose equivalency reporting in Parkinson's disease. Mov Disord. 2010; 25: 2649-2653.

[23] Brennan KA, Genever RW. Managing Parkinson's disease during surgery. BMJ. 2010; 341: c5718.

[24] Domingo-Echaburu S. Antipsychotic use in Parkinson's disease. In: Lertxundi U, Hernández R, Medrano J, eds. Psychopharmacolical Issues in Geriatrics. Bentham Science; 2015. pp. 273-286.

[25] Friedman JH. Parkinson disease psychosis: update. Behav Neurol. 2013; 27: 469-477.

[26] Lertxundi U, Peral J, Mora O, et al. Antidopaminergic therapy for managing comorbidities in patients with Parkinson's disease. Am J Health Syst Pharm. 2008; 65: 414-419.

[27] Weintraub D, Chen P, Ignacio RV, et al. Patterns and trends in antipsychotic prescribing for Parkinson's disease psychosis. Arch Neurol. 2011; 68: 899-904.

[28] American Geriatrics Society 2015. Beers Criteria Update Expert Panel. American Geriatrics Society 2015 updated beers criteria for potentially inappropriate medication use in older adults. J Am Geriatr Soc. 2015; 63: 2227-2246.

[29] O'Mahony D, O'Sullivan D, Byrne S, et al. STOPP/START criteria for potentially inappropriate prescribing in older people: version 2. Age Ageing. 2015; 44: 213-218.

[30] Lertxundi U, Isla A, Solinís MA, et al. Adverse reactions to antipsychotics in Parkinson's disease: an analysis of the Spanish Pharmacovigilance Database. Clin Neuropharmacol. 2015; 38: 69-84.

[31] Lertxundi U, Domingo-Echaburu R, Peral-Aguirregoitia J, et al. Beers 2015 criteria. Aripiprazole in Parkinson´s disease. J Am Geriatr Soc. 2016. in press.

[32] Lubomski M, Rushworth RL, Tisch S. Hospitalisation and comorbidities in Parkinson's disease: a large Australian retrospective study. J Neurol Neurosurg Psychiatry. 2015; 86: 324-330.

[33] Boorsma M, Joling KJ, Frijters DH, et al. The prevalence, incidence and risk factors for delirium in Dutch nursing homes and residential care homes. Int J Geriatr Psychiatry. 2012; 27: 709-15.

[34] Messerschmidt KA, Johnson BR, Khan MA. Encephalopathy associated with metoclopramide use in a patient with Parkinson's disease. Am J Health Syst Pharm. 2012; 69: 1303-1306.

[35] Robottom BJ, Shulman LM, Anderson KE, et al. Metoclopramide-induced encephalopathy in Parkinson's disease. South Med J. 2010; 103: 178-180.

[36] Spanish Agency for Medicines and Health Products. Domperidone and cardiac risk: restrictions on authorization conditions. 2014. Nota informativa 4-2014. Available from http://www.aemps.gob.es/informa/notasInformativas/medicamentosUsoHumano/seguridad/2014/docs/NI-MUH_FV_04-2014-domperidona.pdf [Accessed: 2015/10/29].

[37] Lertxundi U, Domingo-Echaburu S, Soraluce A, et al. Domperidone in Parkinson's disease: a perilous arrythmogenic or the gold standard? Curr Drug Saf. 2013; 8: 63-68.

[38] Miwa H, Kondo T. Hiccups in Parkinson's disease: an overlooked non-motor symptom? Parkinsonism Relat Disord. 2010; 16: 249-251.

[39] Hernández R, Gómez de Segura A, Medrano J, et al. Potentially inappropriate medication in elderly. In: Lertxundi U, Hernández R, Medrano J. eds. Psychopharmacological Issues in Geriatrics, Bentham Science; 2015, pp. 65-96.

[40] Goetz CG, Pal G. Initial management of Parkinson's disease. BMJ. 2014; 349: g6258.

[41] Lertxundi U, Isla A, Solinis MA, et al. Anticholinergic burden in Parkinson's disease inpatients. Eur J Clin Pharmacol. 2015; 71: 1271-1277.

[42] Lertxundi U, Domingo-Echaburu S, Hernandez R, et al. Expert-based drug lists to measure anticholinergic burden: similar names, different results. Psychogeriatrics. 2013; 13: 17-24.

[43] Lertxundi U, Domingo-Echaburu S, Ruiz-Osante B, et al. Comments on Duran et al.'s systematic review of anticholinergic risk scales (EJCP 2DOI 10.1007/s00228-013-1499-3). Eur J Clin Pharmacol. 2013; 69: 1729.

[44] Durán CE, Azermai M, Vander Stichele RH. Systematic review of anticholinergic risk scales in older adults. Eur J Clin Pharmacol. 2013; 69: 1485-1496.

[45] Lertxundi U, Domingo-Echaburu S, Hernandez R, et al. Confusion on anticholinergic burden measurement. J Am Geriatr Soc. 2015; 63: 1054.

Chapter 13

Clinical and Experimental Cell Therapy in Parkinson's Disease

Keun-A Chang and Seonghan Kim

Additional information is available at the end of the chapter

http://dx.doi.org/10.5772/63764

Abstract

Parkinson's disease (PD), a chronic neurodegenerative disorder, is characterized as a movement disorder with resting tremor, dyskinesia, gait disturbance, etc. The main pathology is based on the progressive loss of dopaminergic neurons in the substantia nigra of the midbrain. These motor symptoms can be treated by dopaminergic drugs, but over time, the drug's effect has less efficacy, and side effects develop such as involuntary movements. As there is no gold standard long-term treatment for this condition, there is a strong need to develop new drugs and therapies. The clinical and experimental findings of successful intrastriatal transplantation of fetal mesencephalic dopaminergic neurons into the brains of patients with PD have been well established. The development of human stem cell technology including embryonic stem (ES) cells or induced pluripotent stem (iPS) cells opened a new field called clinical cell therapy, especially for PD. In this chapter, we cover the scientific progress of the clinical and experimental trials of cell therapy for patients with PD. It also contains the recent advances in the clinical application of stem cells including neural stem cells, mesencephalic stem cell, ESC, and iPS cells and unsolved problems in the clinical setting. The combination of gene therapy and gene-manipulated stem cell application in PD therapy will be the most discussed in this area.

Keywords: Parkinson's disease, neurodegenerative disorder, dopaminergic neuron, stem cell, cell therapy

1. Introduction

The principal pathological features of Parkinson's disease (PD) is the progressive degeneration of dopaminergic (DA) neurons located in the substantia nigra in the midbrain and their projections to the striatum, leading to a major loss of striatal dopamine that controls motor functions [1]. The degeneration of DA neurons in many patients with PD also results in non-motor symptoms, such as mood problems and cognitive impairment [2]. The etiology of PD remains unknown in the vast majority of cases, and there are no disease-modifying treatments in the clinic. Characteristic motor symptoms, including rigidity, hypokinesia, tremor, and postural instability, can be treated effectively with the DA precursor L-dopa, DA agonists, monoamine oxidase-B inhibitors, and Catechol-O-methyl transferase inhibitors that reduce the breakdown of DA. The current pharmacologic treatments, including L-dopa, mostly target symptoms only. However, the effect of these drugs decreases over time, and patients may acquire side effects such as motor disturbances along with behavioral and neuropsychiatric problems. Deep brain stimulation (DBS), in the subthalamic nucleus or globus pallidus, has been introduced as an advanced surgical intervention that works electrically to enhance the motor output. However, none of these treatments reverse the progress of DA neuron degeneration. A new treatment is cell transplantation therapy to replace lost DA neurons and accompanied tissues in PD [3]. Treating PD with cell transplantation began over three decades ago [4]. Cell transplantation trials for DA cell replacement and restoration used a variety of different catecholaminergic cells, but the beneficial effect was minimal [5]. So, there have been many efforts to find an available source of nigral DA cells for grafting, including DA neurons from different species [6] and various types of stem cells. Neurorestorative approaches to PD, based on stem cell technology, have been improved to make a large number of nigral DA cells from a stem cell source safe. With two main features (i) the ability of self-renewal and (ii) the capacity to differentiate into specialized cell types, stem cell therapy is in the spotlight for PD treatment, and new studies are being developed recently. The advanced trials of stem cell-based DA cell production have also opened the possibility of developing novel reprogramming strategies [7]. In this chapter, we discuss how stem cells are currently used in research and are translated into clinical trial for the future treatment of PD.

2. Advent of cell transplantation for treatment of Parkinson's disease

The fundamental principle of cell replacement therapy is simple. The strategy is to restore brain function by replacing dead cells with new healthy cells through intracerebral transplantation. Until the late 1970s, it was believed that repairing the central nervous system might never be possible and then experimental trials showed that intracerebral grafts of fetal mesencephalic DA-rich tissue in rats could ameliorate the symptoms of experimental PD [8, 9]. These preclinical data raised the possibility of transplantation therapy for patients with PD using a human fetal mesencephalic tissue. Although there was much enthusiasm for human cell transplantation, the translation into clinical practice was hindered by three main issues. First, there are practical problems of collecting enough human fetal tissue and identifying the ventral mesencephalon, containing the dopaminergic neurons to graft into the brain of patients with PD. Second, there are ethical problems regarding whether it is morally justified to use human fetal tissues derived from dead, aborted human fetuses. Finally, there were inconsistent results of trials and development of graft-induced dyskinesias in some patients [10, 11]. The initial clinical transplantations in patients with PD were not performed with human fetal tissue.

Backlund and Lindval performed pioneering work to implant autologous adrenal medulla cells into the striatum of patients with PD as a local catecholamine source [4, 12]. However, there were adverse effects and low efficacy that led researchers to abandon this method. Clinical trials continued until the early 2000s. Even though there were some reports of improvements, overall there was no significant change in treated patients as compared to controls [13–15].

Clinical cell therapy for PD now has renewed interest due to recent scientific advances in the development of a method for producing dopaminergic neurons from stem cells and reprogrammed cells. In addition to human fetal mesencephalic tissue, human embryonic stem (ES) cells and human-induced pluripotent stem (iPS) cells are being planned for clinical application. These new cell sources have the potential to prepare dopaminergic neurons in large numbers for cell transplantation therapy for PD [16]. Local factors within the microenvironment of transplanted neural stem cells affect the fate of the transplanted cells, long-term survival, proliferation, and differentiation [17]. Further studies for cell delivery route, cell dose, and patient selection are also required and need to be evaluated in greater depth to establish Backlund pre-conditional evaluation system for the successful clinical application of cell-based therapies [18].

3. Application of stem cells in Parkinson's disease

There are several types of stem cells that are under consideration for therapeutic purposes, including embryonic stem cells (ES cells), neural stem cells (NSCs), mesenchymal stem cells (MSCs), and induced pluripotent stem cells (iPSCs).

3.1. Embryonic stem (ES) cells

ES cells are pluripotent cells which are derived from the inner cell mass (ICM) of blastocysts. The indefinite self-renewal ability and plasticity of ES cells allows for *in vitro* generation of an unlimited number of distinct cell types [19]. In neuronal systems, previous studies have found that functional neurons, astrocytes, and oligodendrocytes could be derived from ES cells *in vitro* [20, 21]. Therefore, ES cells are believed to be able to generate specialized cells to replace damaged tissue in patients suffering from various degenerative diseases [22].

ES cells are one of the promising sources that might differentiate into DA neurons. Rodent and human ES cell-derived DA neurons have been shown to repair brain circuitry and restore cerebral function after transplantation into the striatum of rats with PD [23, 24]. Primate ES cell-derived DA neurons were successfully placed into the putamen of 1-methyl-4-phenyl-1, 2, 3, 6-tetrahydropyridine (MPTP)-lesioned monkeys [25]. In that study, 14 weeks after transplantation, the uptake of [18F]-DOPA increased, suggesting the functional recovery of ES cell-derived DA neurons. However, the differentiation rate and the survival rate of these neurons after transplantation are still low [23, 26]; less than 300 tyrosine hydroxylase (TH)-positive cells survived after transplantation of $1 \sim 4 \times 10^5$ ES cells into the striatum [27, 28]. Furthermore, residual undifferentiated ES cells may potentially cause tumors, especially teratomas [29]. Ethical and political concerns regarding ES cell origin are another major limitation. Isolating ICM from blastocysts destroys embryos and increases moral concerns [30]. Therefore, non-ES cells have become the focus for cell-based therapies.

3.2. Neural stem cells (NSCs)

NSCs are multipotent stem cells that are isolated from either fetal brains or specific regions in adult brains [31]. In the adult brain, neural stem cells have been found in two major niches: the subgranular zone (SGZ) in the dentate gyrus of the hippocampus and the subventricular zone (SVZ) of the lateral ventricles [32]. NSCs might differentiate into neurons, astrocytes, and oligodendrocytes [33]. Due to the specific lineage restriction of NSGs, the risk of potential tumor formation is reduced, and NSCs retain their regional specificity [31].

Recent reports have shown the potential ability of NSCs to differentiate into DA neurons [34, 35]. Overexpression of several genes, such as Brn4, TH, glial cell line-derived neurotrophic factor (GDNF), and Lmx1a, may contribute to the maturation and survival of differentiated DA neurons from NSCs [35–37]. Transplantation of NSC-derived DA neurons or NSC-derived DA neurons overexpressing Wnt5a or Nurr1 has led to functional improvement in animal models of PD [38, 39]. However, the survival rate for TH-positive DA neurons after transplantation was very low, less than 4.3%, and the transfection of Wnt5a into NSCs increased 10-fold over TH-positive DA neurons [38]. The transplantation of NSCs from SVZ improved the symptoms of PD, but the survival rate of these cells was still low [40, 41]. Therefore, new methods to increase the cell number and survival rate of transplanted cells must be developed for successful NSC transplantation.

3.3. Mesenchymal stem cells (MSCs)

MSCs are typically defined as multipotent stromal cells that can differentiate into all cells of mesodermal origin [42]. MSCs are commonly sourced from the bone marrow, but there has been successful isolation of MSCs from the adipose tissue, umbilical cord blood, amniotic fluid, and synovial membranes [42]. MSCs have several advantages; first, these cells are easily collected from patients' own tissue. Second, ethical concerns for MSCs are decreased because they can be retrieved from adult tissues or umbilical cord blood donations. Third, MSCs are an immunologically favorable source for transplantation. MSCs have a property of immunomodulation to suppress inflammation and downregulate pathogenic immune responses to limit graft-versus-host disease [43]. This characteristic would be an important benefit for use in transplantation.

3.3.1. Bone marrow MSCs (BMSCs)

Bone marrow is the most common source of MSCs. Important features of BMSCs are that they are a resource with easy access for harvesting, and they have the ability to migrate into the brain across the blood-brain barrier [44]. This important advantage suggests the possibility that MSC transplantation may be applicable with noninvasive and peripheral delivery tools. Several reports promote the possible potentials of neuronal differentiation of BMSCs [45–47].

Although these results support the therapeutic potential of BMSCs for treating neurological disease, their rate of differentiation into neuronal cells is low, and these cells can be maintained for a few passages [48]. However, only 0.8% of grafted cells expressed TH immunoreactivity [48]. Transfection with Notch1 intracellular domain (NICD), basic fibroblast growth factor (bFGF), forskolin, ciliary neurotrophic factor (CNTF), or GDNF increased the proportion of tyrosine hydroxylase-positive and dopamine-producing cells [45]. In a clinical trial, advanced patients with PD unilaterally transplanted with bFGF-treated BMSCs in the SVZ showed clinical improvement after 12–18 months of follow-up without being teratogenic [49].

However, this result suggests that while BMSCs may be a good source for patient health and harvesting safely, their low differentiation rate limits the potency of BMSCs for transplantation.

3.3.2. Umbilical cord blood (UCB) cells

UCB cells are MSCs that are derived from umbilical cord blood attached to the placenta. The amount of cells that could be collected from cord blood is limited after delivery. However, UCB cells have many potencies for transplantation such as easy expandability and tolerance to human leukocyte antigen (HLA) disparities, which significantly decrease the risk of immune rejection [50].

Although several reports showed that UCB cells could be differentiated into neuronal and glial cells [51, 52], the differentiation potential of UCB cells is similar to that of BMSCs. To induce neuronal differentiation of UCB, UCB cells were cultured with sonic hedgehog (SHH) and fibroblast growth factor-8 (FGF-8), increasing the neuronal differentiation to 12.7%. However, transplantation of both undifferentiated MSCs and differentiated UCBs improved the symptoms of PD in 6-OHDA PD models [53, 54].

3.3.3. Adipose-derived stem cells (ASCs)

ASC has an advantage due to easy access to adipose tissue and abundance with proliferation and differentiation potential [55]. ASCs have a high proliferation capacity *in vitro* and differentiate into cells with several neuronal and glial characteristics [55]. The implantation of human ASCs leads to no adverse side effects such as tumorigenicity, chromosomal abnormalities, or immune rejection [56]. In an *in vitro* study, the LIM homeobox transcription factor 1, alpha (LMX1A)- and neurturin (NTN)-infected ASCs showed a dopaminergic differentiation by secreting the dopamine [57].

The therapeutic efficacy of ASCs has been assessed in various animal models with PD. The ASCs were intravenously injected into the tail vein of a PD mouse model induced by 6-hydroxydopamine (6-OHDA) [58]. After the injection of ASC, the behavioral performances were significantly improved, and dopaminergic neurons were rescued [58]. In a rotenone-induced PD rat model, transplantation with ASCs increased the serum level of BDNF and the brain levels of dopamine and TH [59]. This study suggests that ASC transplantation might be advantageous due to their immunomodulatory, anti-inflammatory, and neurotrophic effects. A recent study found that the transplantation of neuronal-primed ASCs derived from rhesus monkey tissue combined with adenovirus containing NTN and TH improved PD behavior including tremor recovery and motility in MPTP-lesioned hemi-parkinsonian rhesus monkeys [57]. In postmortem analysis, combined transplanted ASCs with NTN and TH could replace lost neurons and reconstruct the nigrostriatal pathway in the brain [57]. Overall, this study underscores that transplanted ASCs may have therapeutic potential for PD.

3.4. Induced pluripotent stem cells (iPSCs)

iPSCs were recently focused one as a potential cell source to repair neuronal networks in various neurological diseases. Since iPSCs are derived from adult tissues, complicated ethical issues and the risk of immune rejection can be avoided when used as a substrate for transplantation. For the production of iPSCs, retroviral transduction of four transcription factors Oct3/4, Sox2, Klf4, and c-Myc were needed [60]. Since c-Myc is well defined as an oncogene, and Oct4 and Sox2 are also overexpressed or activated in various types of cancer, reactivation of these genes increases the risk of tumor formation [60–62]. Therefore, one major weakness of the iPSC is an increased risk of tumor formation.

In a recent report, disease-specific iPSC derived from patients suffering from PD showed disease-specific cellular pathological phenotypes, such as abnormal pathological ;-synuclein protein and accumulation and alterations in autophagy [63]. The use of iPSC in patients suffering from sporadic or genetic forms of PD can offer a PD iPSC-based model for drug discovery, earlier diagnosis and development of individualized treatment in the preclinical phase of the disease [63].

DA neurons generated from mouse iPSCs were first transplanted into the striatum of a rat PD model, improving the symptoms of PD [64, 65]. DA neurons differentiated from iPSCs of patients with PD were transplanted into the striatum of a PD transgenic rat, and these neurons survived for several months and further improved the symptoms of PD [66]. Most importantly, these transplanted cells did not display signs of teratoma formation in the grafts [66].

4. Challenging points

The trials of cell transplantation to treat PD were first tested three decades ago [4]. Despite long time basic and clinical studies, there still is no cure of dopaminergic cell therapy for PD. Since the first trial of cell transplantation with autologous adrenal medulla cells into the striatum of patients with PD, cell sources of implants have been developed into fetal mesencephalic tissue, which was rich in dopaminergic neurons [67, 68]. However, the minimal beneficial effects of transplantation, lack of efficacy, and occurrence of troublesome graft-induced dyskinesia (GID) have halted the clinical application of cell therapy for a while [13, 69, 70]. The translational trial of fetal ventral mesencephalon (fVM) has raised arguments about ethical decisions to use human fetal tissue. In addition, collecting enough fetal tissue to graft has been a problem in practical aspects and not promising for PD therapy due to their low efficacy.

The development of human stem cell technology including human embryonic stem (hES) cells or induced pluripotent stem cells (iPSCs) opens a new era to the field of clinical cell therapy, especially for PD in the restoration and replacement of degenerated dopaminergic neurons and DA neural circuit. Scientists are investigating which stem cells (e.g., embryonic, neural stem cells, mesenchymal stem cells, induced pluripotent stem cells, umbilical cord blood cells, etc.) are best for developing a potential therapy for PD. Translating animal model results into human trials requires controlling many factors including the type of stem cells, culture conditions, the protocols for injecting cells into the brain, and the method of activation into DA neuronal differentiation. Although stem cells have the best potential to become a future treatment for PD, there are some challenging points to overcome before application into human trials.

Point 1: Ethical issue regarding their origin

ES cells are inner cell mass (ICM) of blastocyst-derived pluripotent cells. For the isolation of ICM, it is inevitable to destroy early embryos, which leads to a moral concern [30]. This moral concern has been overcome by the ability to harvest adult stem cells and iPSCs. Thus, the number of basic and clinical studies has been increased. Therefore, this inherent ethical issue needs to be solved before launching the practical application of hES cells in PD cell therapy. This is very complicated due to multiple concerns such as regional, religious, and social interests. That is why scientists keep trying to find a common ground for future research. Since the iPSCs may be derived directly from adult tissues, complicated ethical issues may be avoided when they are used as a potential cell source for cell therapy.

Point 2: Development of large numbers of dopaminergic neurons in standardized preparations

It is estimated that for successful implantation into the human brain, the number of dopaminergic neurons needed will be >100,000. The overexpression of transcription factors involved in DA neuron development has been used in hES cell-derived DA neurons in culture. Lmx1A, Nurr1, and Pitx3 have been shown to expand the number of DA neurons in culture [71, 72]. GSK3β inhibitor and FGF8 also showed reliable production of DA neurons [73]. iPSCs can be produced as patient-specific cells potentially used for transplantation. However, the reprogrammed dopaminergic neurons are still incomplete regarding their functional efficacy. The majority of generated neurons were glutaminergic and GABAergic. Several recent studies developed neuronal subtype-specific transcription factors that are involved in the direct conversion process into DA neurons [74, 75].

Point 3: Risk of tumor formation

The tumorigenicity of stem cell-derived cells should be assessed, and all cell types in the implants must be identified. The high capacity of self-renewing and pluripotency of ES cells increases the risk of tumor formation, especially teratoma [29]. The major drawback of the iPSCs is also tumor formation because of the reactivation of c-Myc, one of the major oncogenes [60]. With a modified reprogramming protocol that eliminates c-Myc, it can reduce the tumorigenicity and also significantly decrease iPSC formation [60]. Recently, poly(ADP-ribose) polymerase I (ParpI) reported significantly decreased tumor formation in iPSC production [76], but the teratoma formation after transplantation could not be completely excluded [16]. However, these trials are promising regarding the potential to overcome major drawbacks before clinical use. Tumor formation also reduces the efficacy of stem cell production in these patients. To generate better-defined stem cell populations free from tumor tumor cells, fluorescence-activated cell srting (FACS) and/or magnetic-activated cell sorting (MACS) techniques can be applied. The sorter can select transplantable safe stem cells, and thus deplete tumor cells simultaneously [77, 78].

Point 4: Improvement of efficacy of the graft

After reviewing all of the previous points, cell potency of stem cell-derived dopaminergic neurons must be analyzed and compared to fetal dopaminergic neurons before application in patients. This comparison can be considered as the gold standard and can be used to estimate the number of cells to be implanted. The growth capacity of the dopaminergic neurons needs to be analyzed to determine the distribution of implants required to reinnervate human striatum. The recovery after cell therapy also depends on patient selection. For successful transplantation, it will be advantageous if patients are in an early stage of the disease.

5. Perspectives

Stem cells are unique in that they can self-renew and differentiate into specialized cell types, especially all neural lineage cells. These two key features have drawn the interest to develop and apply these cells in basic and translational research for cell therapy strategies. Despite three decades of DA neuron cell replacement research, transplantation of DA neurons into striatum has not yet been established as a competitive therapy for patients with PD. However, there have been several scientific advances in clinical trials. The grafted neurons survive over time, and neuronal growth with functional connections in adult human brain has been established for potential clinical applications. Dopaminergic innervation by cell replacement therapy shows major relief of motor symptoms. However, the patients developed non-motor symptoms such as anxiety, mood fluctuations, and sleep problems and were detected with a progressive loss of serotonergic neurons that occur concomitantly with the graft-induced dopaminergic regeneration. There are still significant challenges for the successful clinical application of stem cells as a treatment for PD. The issue regarding the risk for tumorigenicity and graft-induced dyskinesias should be assessed seriously. In this evaluation, the determination of identity of all cell types in the implants will be essential. Theoretically, cell sorting can eliminate tumor-forming cells and serotonergic neurons to improve the safety of cell transplantation. Combined with recent development in stem cell fields, cell-replacement strategy provides optimistic options. Human ES and iPSC-derived DA neurons are in development for clinical applications. With these new sources of cells, there will be a great development of clinically competitive cell therapy for patients with PD. Many challenges still remain for successful clinical trials; many research groups provide scientific progress and significant clinical advances in these fields.

Author details

Keun-A Chang[1*] and Seonghan Kim[2]

*Address all correspondence to: keuna705@gachon.ac.kr

1 Department of Pharmacology, College of Medicine, Gachon University, Yeonsu-gu, Incheon, South Korea

2 Department of Anatomy, Inje University, College of Medicine, Busanjin-gu, Busan, South Korea

References

[1] P.C. Buttery, R.A. Barker, Treating Parkinson's disease in the 21st century: can stem cell transplantation compete? J Comp Neurol 522 (2014) 2802–2816.

[2] K.R. Chaudhuri, D.G. Healy, A.H. Schapira, E. National Institute for Clinical, Non-motor symptoms of Parkinson's disease: diagnosis and management, Lancet Neurol 5 (2006) 235–245.

[3] R. Savica, W.A. Rocca, J.E. Ahlskog, When does Parkinson disease start? Arch Neurol 67 (2010) 798–801.

[4] E.O. Backlund, P.O. Granberg, B. Hamberger, E. Knutsson, A. Martensson, G. Sedvall, A. Seiger, L. Olson, Transplantation of adrenal medullary tissue to striatum in parkinsonism. First clinical trials, J Neurosurg 62 (1985) 169–173.

[5] R.A. Barker, S.B. Dunnett, Functional integration of neural grafts in Parkinson's disease, Nat Neurosci 2 (1999) 1047–1048.

[6] R.A. Barker, Porcine neural xenografts: what are the issues? Novartis Found Symp 231 (2000) 184–196; discussion 196–201, 302–306.

[7] A. Shaltouki, R. Sivapatham, Y. Pei, A.A. Gerencser, O. Momcilovic, M.S. Rao, X. Zeng, Mitochondrial alterations by PARKIN in dopaminergic neurons using PARK2 patient-specific and PARK2 knockout isogenic iPSC lines, Stem Cell Reports 4 (2015) 847–859.

[8] A. Bjorklund, U. Stenevi, Reconstruction of the nigrostriatal dopamine pathway by intracerebral nigral transplants, Brain Res 177 (1979) 555–560.

[9] M.J. Perlow, W.J. Freed, B.J. Hoffer, A. Seiger, L. Olson, R.J. Wyatt, Brain grafts reduce motor abnormalities produced by destruction of nigrostriatal dopamine system, Science 204 (1979) 643–647.

[10] R.A. Barker, W.L. Kuan, Graft-induced dyskinesias in Parkinson's disease: what is it all about? Cell Stem Cell 7 (2010) 148–149.

[11] W.R. Galpern, J. Corrigan-Curay, A.E. Lang, J. Kahn, D. Tagle, R.A. Barker, T.B. Freeman, C.G. Goetz, K. Kieburtz, S.Y. Kim, S. Piantadosi, A. Comstock Rick, H.J. Federoff, Sham neurosurgical procedures in clinical trials for neurodegenerative diseases: scientific and ethical considerations, Lancet Neurol 11 (2012) 643–650.

[12] O. Lindvall, E.O. Backlund, L. Farde, G. Sedvall, R. Freedman, B. Hoffer, A. Nobin, A. Seiger, L. Olson, Transplantation in Parkinson's disease: two cases of adrenal medullary grafts to the putamen, Ann Neurol 22 (1987) 457–468.

[13] C.R. Freed, P.E. Greene, R.E. Breeze, W.Y. Tsai, W. DuMouchel, R. Kao, S. Dillon, H. Winfield, S. Culver, J.Q. Trojanowski, D. Eidelberg, S. Fahn, Transplantation of embryonic dopamine neurons for severe Parkinson's disease, N Engl J Med 344 (2001) 710–719.

[14] O. Lindvall, Developing dopaminergic cell therapy for Parkinson's disease—give up or move forward? Mov Disord 28 (2013) 268–273.

[15] C.W. Olanow, C.G. Goetz, J.H. Kordower, A.J. Stoessl, V. Sossi, M.F. Brin, K.M. Shannon, G.M. Nauert, D.P. Perl, J. Godbold, T.B. Freeman, A double-blind controlled trial of bilateral fetal nigral transplantation in Parkinson's disease, Ann Neurol 54 (2003) 403–414.

[16] G.H. Petit, T.T. Olsson, P. Brundin, The future of cell therapies and brain repair: Parkinson's disease leads the way, Neuropathol Appl Neurobiol 40 (2014) 60–70.

[17] H.C. Fan, S.J. Chen, H.J. Harn, S.Z. Lin, Parkinson's disease: from genetics to treatments, Cell Transplant 22 (2013) 639–652.

[18] V. Misra, M.M. Ritchie, L.L. Stone, W.C. Low, V. Janardhan, Stem cell therapy in ischemic stroke: role of IV and intra-arterial therapy, Neurology 79 (2012) S207–S212.

[19] J.A. Thomson, V.S. Marshall, Primate embryonic stem cells, Curr Top Dev Biol 38 (1998) 133–165.

[20] H. Wichterle, I. Lieberam, J.A. Porter, T.M. Jessell, Directed differentiation of embryonic stem cells into motor neurons, Cell 110 (2002) 385–397.

[21] S.C. Zhang, M. Wernig, I.D. Duncan, O. Brustle, J.A. Thomson, In vitro differentiation of transplantable neural precursors from human embryonic stem cells, Nat Biotechnol 19 (2001) 1129–1133.

[22] A. Aleynik, K.M. Gernavage, Y. Mourad, L.S. Sherman, K. Liu, Y.A. Gubenko, P. Rameshwar, Stem cell delivery of therapies for brain disorders, Clin Transl Med 3 (2014) 24.

[23] J.H. Kim, J.M. Auerbach, J.A. Rodriguez-Gomez, I. Velasco, D. Gavin, N. Lumelsky, S.H. Lee, J. Nguyen, R. Sanchez-Pernaute, K. Bankiewicz, R. McKay, Dopamine

neurons derived from embryonic stem cells function in an animal model of Parkinson's disease, Nature 418 (2002) 50–56.

[24] D. Yang, Z.J. Zhang, M. Oldenburg, M. Ayala, S.C. Zhang, Human embryonic stem cell-derived dopaminergic neurons reverse functional deficit in parkinsonian rats, Stem Cells 26 (2008) 55–63.

[25] Y. Takagi, J. Takahashi, H. Saiki, A. Morizane, T. Hayashi, Y. Kishi, H. Fukuda, Y. Okamoto, M. Koyanagi, M. Ideguchi, H. Hayashi, T. Imazato, H. Kawasaki, H. Suemori, S. Omachi, H. Iida, N. Itoh, N. Nakatsuji, Y. Sasai, N. Hashimoto, Dopaminergic neurons generated from monkey embryonic stem cells function in a Parkinson primate model, J Clin Invest 115 (2005) 102–109.

[26] J.A. Rodriguez-Gomez, J.Q. Lu, I. Velasco, S. Rivera, S.S. Zoghbi, J.S. Liow, J.L. Musachio, F.T. Chin, H. Toyama, J. Seidel, M.V. Green, P.K. Thanos, M. Ichise, V.W. Pike, R.B. Innis, R.D. McKay, Persistent dopamine functions of neurons derived from embryonic stem cells in a rodent model of Parkinson disease, Stem Cells 25 (2007) 918–928.

[27] T. Ben-Hur, M. Idelson, H. Khaner, M. Pera, E. Reinhartz, A. Itzik, B.E. Reubinoff, Transplantation of human embryonic stem cell-derived neural progenitors improves behavioral deficit in Parkinsonian rats, Stem Cells 22 (2004) 1246–1255.

[28] A. Brederlau, A.S. Correia, S.V. Anisimov, M. Elmi, G. Paul, L. Roybon, A. Morizane, F. Bergquist, I. Riebe, U. Nannmark, M. Carta, E. Hanse, J. Takahashi, Y. Sasai, K. Funa, P. Brundin, P.S. Eriksson, J.Y. Li, Transplantation of human embryonic stem cell-derived cells to a rat model of Parkinson's disease: effect of in vitro differentiation on graft survival and teratoma formation, Stem Cells 24 (2006) 1433–1440.

[29] O.F. Gordeeva, Pluripotent cells in embryogenesis and in teratoma formation, J Stem Cells 6 (2011) 51–63.

[30] A.S. Daar, L. Sheremeta, The science of stem cells: ethical, legal and social issues, Exp Clin Transplant 1 (2003) 139–146.

[31] S. Horiguchi, J. Takahashi, Y. Kishi, A. Morizane, Y. Okamoto, M. Koyanagi, M. Tsuji, K. Tashiro, T. Honjo, S. Fujii, N. Hashimoto, Neural precursor cells derived from human embryonic brain retain regional specificity, J Neurosci Res 75 (2004) 817–824.

[32] V.G. Kukekov, E.D. Laywell, O. Suslov, K. Davies, B. Scheffler, L.B. Thomas, T.F. O'Brien, M. Kusakabe, D.A. Steindler, Multipotent stem/progenitor cells with similar properties arise from two neurogenic regions of adult human brain, Exp Neurol 156 (1999) 333–344.

[33] S. Kelly, T.M. Bliss, A.K. Shah, G.H. Sun, M. Ma, W.C. Foo, J. Masel, M.A. Yenari, I.L. Weissman, N. Uchida, T. Palmer, G.K. Steinberg, Transplanted human fetal neural stem cells survive, migrate, and differentiate in ischemic rat cerebral cortex, Proc Natl Acad Sci U S A 101 (2004) 11839–11844.

[34] K.K. Tan, J.Y. Tann, S.R. Sathe, S.H. Goh, D. Ma, E.L. Goh, E.K. Yim, Enhanced differentiation of neural progenitor cells into neurons of the mesencephalic dopaminergic subtype on topographical patterns, Biomaterials 43 (2015) 32–43.

[35] X. Tan, L. Zhang, H. Zhu, J. Qin, M. Tian, C. Dong, H. Li, G. Jin, Brn4 and TH synergistically promote the differentiation of neural stem cells into dopaminergic neurons, Neurosci Lett 571 (2014) 23–28.

[36] D.R. Wakeman, D.E. Redmond, Jr., H.B. Dodiya, J.R. Sladek, Jr., C. Leranth, Y.D. Teng, R.J. Samulski, E.Y. Snyder, Human neural stem cells survive long term in the midbrain of dopamine-depleted monkeys after GDNF overexpression and project neurites toward an appropriate target, Stem Cells Transl Med 3 (2014) 692–701.

[37] J. Wu, C. Sheng, Z. Liu, W. Jia, B. Wang, M. Li, L. Fu, Z. Ren, J. An, L. Sang, G. Song, Y. Wu, Y. Xu, S. Wang, Z. Chen, Q. Zhou, Y.A. Zhang, Lmx1a enhances the effect of iNSCs in a PD model, Stem Cell Res 14 (2015) 1–9.

[38] C.L. Parish, G. Castelo-Branco, N. Rawal, J. Tonnesen, A.T. Sorensen, C. Salto, M. Kokaia, O. Lindvall, E. Arenas, Wnt5a-treated midbrain neural stem cells improve dopamine cell replacement therapy in parkinsonian mice, J Clin Invest 118 (2008) 149–160.

[39] C.H. Park, J.S. Kang, Y.H. Shin, M.Y. Chang, S. Chung, H.C. Koh, M.H. Zhu, S.B. Oh, Y.S. Lee, G. Panagiotakos, V. Tabar, L. Studer, S.H. Lee, Acquisition of in vitro and in vivo functionality of Nurr1-induced dopamine neurons, FASEB J 20 (2006) 2553–2555.

[40] K.K. Meissner, D.L. Kirkham, L.C. Doering, Transplants of neurosphere cell suspensions from aged mice are functional in the mouse model of Parkinson's, Brain Res 1057 (2005) 105–112.

[41] R.M. Richardson, W.C. Broaddus, K.L. Holloway, H.L. Fillmore, Grafts of adult subependymal zone neuronal progenitor cells rescue hemiparkinsonian behavioral decline, Brain Res 1032 (2005) 11–22.

[42] J.J. Minguell, A. Erices, P. Conget, Mesenchymal stem cells, Exp Biol Med (Maywood) 226 (2001) 507–520.

[43] J.D. Glenn, K.A. Whartenby, Mesenchymal stem cells: emerging mechanisms of immunomodulation and therapy, World J Stem Cells 6 (2014) 526–539.

[44] Y. Li, J. Chen, L. Wang, M. Lu, M. Chopp, Treatment of stroke in rat with intracarotid administration of marrow stromal cells, Neurology 56 (2001) 1666–1672.

[45] M. Dezawa, H. Kanno, M. Hoshino, H. Cho, N. Matsumoto, Y. Itokazu, N. Tajima, H. Yamada, H. Sawada, H. Ishikawa, T. Mimura, M. Kitada, Y. Suzuki, C. Ide, Specific induction of neuronal cells from bone marrow stromal cells and application for autologous transplantation, J Clin Invest 113 (2004) 1701–1710.

[46] H. Haragopal, D. Yu, X. Zeng, S.W. Kim, I.B. Han, A.E. Ropper, J.E. Anderson, Y.D. Teng, Stemness enhancement of human neural stem cells following bone marrow MSC coculture, Cell Transplant 24 (2015) 645–659.

[47] Y. Zhao, H. Jiang, X.W. Liu, L.B. Xiang, D.P. Zhou, J.T. Chen, MiR-124 promotes bone marrow mesenchymal stem cells differentiation into neurogenic cells for accelerating recovery in the spinal cord injury, Tissue Cell 47 (2015) 140–146.

[48] J.Y. Li, E. Englund, J.L. Holton, D. Soulet, P. Hagell, A.J. Lees, T. Lashley, N.P. Quinn, S. Rehncrona, A. Bjorklund, H. Widner, T. Revesz, O. Lindvall, P. Brundin, Lewy bodies in grafted neurons in subjects with Parkinson's disease suggest host-to-graft disease propagation, Nat Med 14 (2008) 501–503.

[49] N.K. Venkataramana, S.K. Kumar, S. Balaraju, R.C. Radhakrishnan, A. Bansal, A. Dixit, D.K. Rao, M. Das, M. Jan, P.K. Gupta, S.M. Totey, Open-labeled study of unilateral autologous bone-marrow-derived mesenchymal stem cell transplantation in Parkinson's disease, Transl Res 155 (2010) 62–70.

[50] R. Danby, V. Rocha, Improving engraftment and immune reconstitution in umbilical cord blood transplantation, Front Immunol 5 (2014) 68.

[51] L. Buzanska, M. Jurga, K. Domanska-Janik, Neuronal differentiation of human umbilical cord blood neural stem-like cell line, Neurodegener Dis 3 (2006) 19–26.

[52] Y.K. Jang, J.J. Park, M.C. Lee, B.H. Yoon, Y.S. Yang, S.E. Yang, S.U. Kim, Retinoic acid-mediated induction of neurons and glial cells from human umbilical cord-derived hematopoietic stem cells, J Neurosci Res 75 (2004) 573–584.

[53] P. Mathieu, V. Roca, C. Gamba, A. Del Pozo, F. Pitossi, Neuroprotective effects of human umbilical cord mesenchymal stromal cells in an immunocompetent animal model of Parkinson's disease, J Neuroimmunol 246 (2012) 43–50.

[54] M.L. Weiss, S. Medicetty, A.R. Bledsoe, R.S. Rachakatla, M. Choi, S. Merchav, Y. Luo, M.S. Rao, G. Velagaleti, D. Troyer, Human umbilical cord matrix stem cells: preliminary characterization and effect of transplantation in a rodent model of Parkinson's disease, Stem Cells 24 (2006) 781–792.

[55] B. Zavan, V. Vindigni, C. Gardin, D. D'Avella, A. Della Puppa, G. Abatangelo, R. Cortivo, Neural potential of adipose stem cells, Discov Med 10 (2010) 37–43.

[56] J.C. Ra, I.S. Shin, S.H. Kim, S.K. Kang, B.C. Kang, H.Y. Lee, Y.J. Kim, J.Y. Jo, E.J. Yoon, H.J. Choi, E. Kwon, Safety of intravenous infusion of human adipose tissue-derived mesenchymal stem cells in animals and humans, Stem Cells Dev (2011) 1297–1308.

[57] Y. Zhou, M. Sun, H. Li, M. Yan, Z. He, W. Wang, W. Wang, S. Lu, Recovery of behavioral symptoms in hemi-parkinsonian rhesus monkeys through combined gene and stem cell therapy, Cytotherapy 15 (2013) 467–480.

[58] H.S. Choi, H.J. Kim, J.H. Oh, H.G. Park, J.C. Ra, K.A. Chang, Y.H. Suh, Therapeutic potentials of human adipose-derived stem cells on the mouse model of Parkinson's disease, Neurobiol Aging 36 (2015) 2885–2892.

[59] H. Ahmed, A. Salem, H. Atta, M. Ghazy, H. Aglan, Do adipose tissue-derived mesenchymal stem cells ameliorate Parkinson's disease in rat model? Hum Exp Toxicol 33 (2014) 1217–1231.

[60] M. Nakagawa, M. Koyanagi, K. Tanabe, K. Takahashi, T. Ichisaka, T. Aoi, K. Okita, Y. Mochiduki, N. Takizawa, S. Yamanaka, Generation of induced pluripotent stem cells without Myc from mouse and human fibroblasts, Nat Biotechnol 26 (2008) 101–106.

[61] S. Peng, N.J. Maihle, Y. Huang, Pluripotency factors Lin28 and Oct4 identify a subpopulation of stem cell-like cells in ovarian cancer, Oncogene 29 (2010) 2153–2159.

[62] L.M. Sholl, J.A. Barletta, B.Y. Yeap, L.R. Chirieac, J.L. Hornick, Sox2 protein expression is an independent poor prognostic indicator in stage I lung adenocarcinoma, Am J Surg Pathol 34 (2010) 1193–1198.

[63] R. Torrent, F. De Angelis Rigotti, P. Dell'Era, M. Memo, A. Raya, A. Consiglio, Using iPS cells toward the understanding of Parkinson's disease, J Clin Med 4 (2015) 548–566.

[64] S.P. Peng, S. Copray, Comparison of human primary with human iPS cell-derived dopaminergic neuron grafts in the Rat model for Parkinson's disease, Stem Cell Rev 12 (2016) 105–120.

[65] M. Wernig, J.P. Zhao, J. Pruszak, E. Hedlund, D. Fu, F. Soldner, V. Broccoli, M. Constantine-Paton, O. Isacson, R. Jaenisch, Neurons derived from reprogrammed fibroblasts functionally integrate into the fetal brain and improve symptoms of rats with Parkinson's disease, Proc Natl Acad Sci U S A 105 (2008) 5856–5861.

[66] G. Hargus, O. Cooper, M. Deleidi, A. Levy, K. Lee, E. Marlow, A. Yow, F. Soldner, D. Hockemeyer, P.J. Hallett, T. Osborn, R. Jaenisch, O. Isacson, Differentiated Parkinson patient-derived induced pluripotent stem cells grow in the adult rodent brain and reduce motor asymmetry in Parkinsonian rats, Proc Natl Acad Sci U S A 107 (2010) 15921–15926.

[67] P. Brundin, O. Pogarell, P. Hagell, P. Piccini, H. Widner, A. Schrag, A. Kupsch, L. Crabb, P. Odin, B. Gustavii, A. Bjorklund, D.J. Brooks, C.D. Marsden, W.H. Oertel, N.P. Quinn, S. Rehncrona, O. Lindvall, Bilateral caudate and putamen grafts of embryonic mesencephalic tissue treated with lazaroids in Parkinson's disease, Brain 123 (Pt 7) (2000) 1380–1390.

[68] O. Lindvall, P. Brundin, H. Widner, S. Rehncrona, B. Gustavii, R. Frackowiak, K.L. Leenders, G. Sawle, J.C. Rothwell, C.D. Marsden, et al., Grafts of fetal dopamine neurons survive and improve motor function in Parkinson's disease, Science 247 (1990) 574–577.

[69] P. Hagell, P. Piccini, A. Bjorklund, P. Brundin, S. Rehncrona, H. Widner, L. Crabb, N. Pavese, W.H. Oertel, N. Quinn, D.J. Brooks, O. Lindvall, Dyskinesias following neural transplantation in Parkinson's disease, Nat Neurosci 5 (2002) 627–628.

[70] C.W. Olanow, J.M. Gracies, C.G. Goetz, A.J. Stoessl, T. Freeman, J.H. Kordower, J. Godbold, J.A. Obeso, Clinical pattern and risk factors for dyskinesias following fetal nigral transplantation in Parkinson's disease: a double blind video-based analysis, Mov Disord 24 (2009) 336–343.

[71] S. Friling, E. Andersson, L.H. Thompson, M.E. Jonsson, J.B. Hebsgaard, E. Nanou, Z. Alekseenko, U. Marklund, S. Kjellander, N. Volakakis, O. Hovatta, A. El Manira, A. Bjorklund, T. Perlmann, J. Ericson, Efficient production of mesencephalic dopamine neurons by Lmx1a expression in embryonic stem cells, Proc Natl Acad Sci U S A 106 (2009) 7613–7618.

[72] C. Martinat, J.J. Bacci, T. Leete, J. Kim, W.B. Vanti, A.H. Newman, J.H. Cha, U. Gether, H. Wang, A. Abeliovich, Cooperative transcription activation by Nurr1 and Pitx3 induces embryonic stem cell maturation to the midbrain dopamine neuron phenotype, Proc Natl Acad Sci U S A 103 (2006) 2874–2879.

[73] S. Kriks, J.W. Shim, J. Piao, Y.M. Ganat, D.R. Wakeman, Z. Xie, L. Carrillo-Reid, G. Auyeung, C. Antonacci, A. Buch, L. Yang, M.F. Beal, D.J. Surmeier, J.H. Kordower, V. Tabar, L. Studer, Dopamine neurons derived from human ES cells efficiently engraft in animal models of Parkinson's disease, Nature 480 (2011) 547–551.

[74] R.C. Addis, F.C. Hsu, R.L. Wright, M.A. Dichter, D.A. Coulter, J.D. Gearhart, Efficient conversion of astrocytes to functional midbrain dopaminergic neurons using a single polycistronic vector, PLoS One 6 (2011) e28719.

[75] M. Caiazzo, M.T. Dell'Anno, E. Dvoretskova, D. Lazarevic, S. Taverna, D. Leo, T.D. Sotnikova, A. Menegon, P. Roncaglia, G. Colciago, G. Russo, P. Carninci, G. Pezzoli, R.R. Gainetdinov, S. Gustincich, A. Dityatev, V. Broccoli, Direct generation of functional dopaminergic neurons from mouse and human fibroblasts, Nature 476 (2011) 224–227.

[76] S.H. Chiou, B.H. Jiang, Y.L. Yu, S.J. Chou, P.H. Tsai, W.C. Chang, L.K. Chen, L.H. Chen, Y. Chien, G.Y. Chiou, Poly(ADP-ribose) polymerase 1 regulates nuclear reprogramming and promotes iPSC generation without c-Myc, J Exp Med 210 (2013) 85–98.

[77] H. Fukuda, J. Takahashi, K. Watanabe, H. Hayashi, A. Morizne, M.Koyanagi, Y. Sasai, N. Hasgimoto, Fluorescence-activated cell sorting-based purification of embryonic stem cell-derived neural precursors averts tumor formation after transplantation, Stem Cells 24 (2006) 763–771.

[78] M. Geens, H.V. Velde, G.D. Block, E. Goossens, A.V. Steirteghem, H. Tournaye, The efficiency of magnetic-activated cell sorting in the decontamination of testicular cell suspension in cancer patients, Human Repro 22 (2007) 733–742.

Chapter 14

Cell-Based Therapies for Parkinson's Disease: Preclinical and Clinical Perspectives

Andrea R. Di Sebastiano, Michael D. Staudt,
Simon M. Benoit, Hu Xu, Matthew O. Hebb and
Susanne Schmid

Additional information is available at the end of the chapter

http://dx.doi.org/10.5772/63747

Abstract

Parkinson's Disease (PD) is a highly prevalent neurodegenerative disease that affects millions of people globally and remains without definitive treatment. There have been many recent advances in cell-based therapy to replace lost neural circuitry and provide chronic biological sources of therapeutic agents to disease-affected brain regions. Early neural transplantation studies highlighted the challenges of immune rejection, graft integration, and the need for renewable, autologous graft sources. Neurotrophic factors (NTFs) offer a potential class of cytoprotective agents that may complement dopamine (DA) replacement and cell-based therapies in PD. In fact, chronic NTF delivery may be an integral goal of cell transplantation in PD, with ideal grafts consisting of autologous drug (e.g., DA, NTF)-producing cells capable of integration and function in the host brain. This chapter outlines the past and recent preclinical and clinical advances in cell-based and NTF therapies as promising and integrated approaches for the treatment of PD.

Keywords: transplantation, tissue graft, stem cells, pluripotent cells, autologous cells, dopamine replacement, neurotrophic factors

1. Introduction

Parkinson's disease (PD) is the second most common neurodegenerative disorder, following Alzheimer's disease. In the developed world, the prevalence of PD is approximately 0.3% of the population and 1% of those over 60 years of age [1]. Hallmarks of PD include degeneration of dopamine (DA) neurons in the substantia nigra (SN) and of dopaminergic nerve terminals in the striatum, as well as the formation of Lewy bodies containing alpha-synuclein [2–4]. However, PD also has widespread effects on neurons and nonneuronal cells throughout the nervous system [4].

Motor symptoms of PD include bradykinesia (i.e. slowness of movement), rigidity, and rest tremor. These motor symptoms are often seen with postural and gait instability, sleep disorders, sensory dysfunction, neuropsychiatric conditions, and dysautonomia [5]. Nonmotor symptoms of PD include dementia, depression, gastrointestinal, or sexual dysfunction and are managed accordingly. Current therapies for PD aim to improve symptomology, but unfortunately there are no disease modifying treatments. Recent preclinical studies have provided promising leads for the development of potential new therapies to restore or preserve neurological function in patients with PD. As the pathophysiology of PD has become better understood, efforts are expanding to augment or replace the degenerated neural circuitry using cell-based therapies. The goal of this chapter is to discuss past and current approaches to cell-based therapies in PD, including studies to replace lost dopaminergic cells through neural grafting, and the potential of neurotrophic factors (NTFs) to promote DA neuron survival.

2. Current therapies

2.1. Medical therapies

The use of levodopa is the mainstay of PD treatment, and it is usually administered together with a decarboxylase inhibitor, carbidopa. Levodopa can cross the blood-brain barrier, whereas DA and carbidopa cannot. Carbidopa therefore prevents the peripheral conversion of levodopa to DA, allowing for higher doses in the central nervous system. Identified in the 1960s, levodopa was the first medication demonstrated to provide a significant clinical and mortality benefit in the treatment of PD [6]. However, long-term use of levodopa can lead to loss of therapeutic effect, dyskinesia, and neuropsychiatric complications, likely due to the progressive loss of DA neurons and increasing off-target effects of DA ([7], for review see [8]). Levodopa is converted by catechol-O-methyl transferase (COMT) to an inert metabolite [9]; as such, COMT inhibitors may be administered to prevent peripheral metabolism and increase levodopa availability to the brain. The use of selective monoamine oxidase B (MAO-B) inhibitors was initially thought to be neuroprotective and has since been used in symptom control [10] as monotherapy in early PD, as well as an adjunct treatment to levodopa [11]. Cholinergic, adrenergic, glutamatergic, and serotonergic drugs are also being used for treating PD symptoms that do not respond to DA treatment or for treating levodopa-induced side effects. All medical therapies only provide partial and temporal relief of symptoms and are not disease modifying [8].

2.2. Standard surgical therapies

Prior to the advent of levodopa therapy, ablative therapies were used in the control of motor symptoms. Pallidotomy and thalamotomy were used in the symptomatic control of rigidity and tremor, respectively [12,13]. Pallidotomy has been demonstrated to provide sustained improvement for tremor, rigidity, bradykinesia, and drug-induced dyskinesias, compared with medical therapy [14]. In the past decades, deep brain stimulation (DBS) has become the standard of surgical care for PD owing to the versatility of stimulator programming, and the avoidance of creating a permanent surgical lesion [15]. The two primary targets of DBS are the internal globus pallidus (GPi) and subthalamic nucleus (STN). DBS improves motor symptoms and often permits a reduction of medication dose and associated side effects, but does not slow or halt progression of the disease [16].

3. Burgeoning therapies for PD

3.1. Cell-based therapies

As PD is characterized by the loss of dopaminergic nigrostriatal neurons, cell-based therapies initially focused on the potential to replace these neurons and replenish DA supply in the striatum using fetal mesencephalic neural grafts. More recently, studies have included the transplantation of induced pluripotent stem cells (iPSCs), reprogrammed somatic cells or induced neural progenitor cells (iNPCs).

3.2. Fetal transplantation

3.2.1. Preclinical studies

Early PD transplantation studies involved grafting of fetal ventral mesencephalic (fVM) tissue into the anterior chamber of the rat eye [17]. These studies identified the optimal developmental stage of the neural tissue to be used to promote DA neuron survival and outgrowth [17]. The first graft transplantation studies in a unilaterally lesioned 6-hydroxydopamine (6-OHDA) PD rat model examined the effects of solid grafts of fetal adrenal medullary or fVM tissue implanted into the lateral ventricle or preformed cavities adjacent to the striatum and reported reduced amphetamine-induced rotation behavior [18]. Subsequent studies showed that grafting cell suspensions of fVM tissue from 14- to 15-day-old rat fetuses into the striatum of 6-OHDA rats also reduced amphetamine-induced rotation behavior [19]. Follow-up studies used fVM tissue from 9- to 19-week-old human fetuses. These implants reduced and even reversed motor asymmetry in unilaterally lesioned 6-OHDA rats [20].

3.2.2. Clinical studies

In 1987, solid graft adrenal medullary transplants were implanted in the head of the caudate in two patients and produced significant clinical improvement, including reduced tremor [21]. Unfortunately, follow-up studies showed only modest clinical effect, with concerns regarding efficacy and safety of this technique. Many patients suffered major postsurgical complications and psychiatric problems, thus this transplant approach was abandoned. Subsequent open label studies in six human patients utilized human fVM tissue from 6- to 8-week-old fetuses grafted into the caudate and putamen, demonstrating overall clinical improvement and normal DA signaling seen by ^{18}F-Fluorodopa (^{18}F-FDOPA) uptake in Positron Emission Tomography (PET) imaging [22–24]. Two patients in this study continued to demonstrate clinical improvement 20 years later [25]. In a subsequent open label study nigral grafts from 6- to 7-week-old embryos were implanted into the caudate and putamen of seven PD patients [26,27]. Significant improvement in the activities of daily living was noted after 12 months, in both "on" and "off" states. The dose of levodopa could be reduced by an average of 39%. Four patients reported an "important difference in their daily lives," two patients reported improvement in "some respects," and one patient did not improve. Other open label studies with a small number of patients also showed mostly beneficial effects ([28–31], reviewed in [32]).

A randomized double-blind controlled trial (RDBCT) enlisted 34 patients that underwent transplantation of fetal mesencephalic tissue into the putamen or sham surgery. The patients showed limited clinical improvement, despite graft survival and significant reinnervation of the striatum as confirmed by PET and at autopsy. Interestingly, patients with less severe motor dysfunction showed significant clinical improvement, suggesting this technique may have produced some degree of neuroprotection. Furthermore, graft-induced dyskinesias were observed in over half of the patients [33]. Interestingly, these patients underwent a 2- and 4-year follow-up RDBCT that demonstrated clinical improvement regardless of the age of the patient, which was accompanied by significantly increased ^{18}F-FDOPA uptake in the putamen [34]. Another RDBCT had 40 patients with advanced PD undergo transplantation. When results were normalized according to age, patients under the age of 60 showed significant clinical improvement, as measured with the Unified Parkinson's Disease Rating Scale (UPDRS) and Schwab and England score, while those over the age of 60 did not [35]. Clinical improvement was correlated with increased ^{18}F-FDOPA uptake in 85% of patients with a transplant and postmortem examination confirmed dopaminergic cell survival and fibre outgrowth; however, 15% of patients developed graft-induced dyskinesias or dystonia [35].

To more accurately assess the potential of fetal grafts, a new European study has been designed to optimize and control for patient selection, tissue composition, tissue placement, and trial design. TRANSEURO is an open label multicenter trial to define the feasibility and efficacy of human fetal ventral mesencephalic grafts in patients with PD (https://clinicaltrials.gov/ct2/show/NCT01898390). The primary outcome measure of this study is the change in motor UPDRS scores in the absence of PD medications at 3 years posttransplantation. It is hoped that this new trial will shed light on the true potential of dopaminergic allografts for PD treatment.

The use of human fVM tissue, however, is complicated by ethical issues and difficulty in obtaining human tissue. Strategies are being developed that involve expansion of fVM tissue and its dopaminergic neuroblasts [36], and other cell sources are also being investigated for cell-based treatment of PD.

3.3. Native human stem cells

3.3.1. Preclinical studies

Human embryonic stem cells (hESCs) were first isolated from the inner cell mass of blastocysts. These cells demonstrate pluripotency and have been shown to differentiate into neural cells, including neurons, astrocytes, and oligodendrocytes [37,38]. hESCs may prove useful to avoid the technical concerns associated with the use of fetal tissue. hESCs have been shown to differentiate into midbrain DA neurons, and injection of these cells in 6-OHDA lesioned rats [39] and 1-methyl-4-phenyl-1,2,3,6-tetrahydropyridine (MPTP)-lesioned monkeys [40] leads to significantly improved motor function in both models. However, the development of clinical applications using these cells has been slowed by various biological and social factors, including the potential for immune rejection and tumor formation, as well as ethical and political opposition [41].

Alternative stem cell sources have been investigated for differentiation into a neural lineage, in particular mesenchymal stem cells (MSCs) from bone marrow, umbilical cord blood, dental pulp, and adipose tissue [42]. Autologous MSCs are favorable due to their availability, potential for differentiation, and the absence of ethical issues associated with hESCs. In addition, MSCs have been demonstrated to exert regenerative and neuroprotective effects in a number of animal PD models potentially, due to endogenous NTF expression. MSCs have been shown to differentiate into dopaminergic cells that express tyrosine hydroxylase [43]. Implantation of these differentiated MSCs into the striatum of 6-OHDA mice led to significant behavioral improvement, with striatal graft cells confirmed at postmortem analysis [43].

3.3.2. Clinical studies

There is currently very limited clinical data on the efficacy of hESCs in PD. An initial clinical study in seven PD patients demonstrated that transplantation of autologous bone-marrow-derived MSCs was safe and feasible with no serious adverse side effects. Unfortunately, no clinical efficacy was observed, potentially due to the small number of patients and uncontrolled nature of the trial [44].

3.4. Induced pluripotent stem cells

3.4.1. Preclinical studies

With the discovery that somatic cells, such as fibroblasts, can be reprogrammed to a pluripotent state by viral delivery of four transcription factors, Oct4, Sox2, Klf4, and cMyc [45,46], studies have focused on the potential of these induced pluripotent stem cells (iPSCs) to improve current cell-based therapies for treatment of many degenerative medical conditions, including PD. Compared with fetal grafting and hESC cells, iPSCs provide increased accessibility as well as ethical advantages. These cells can differentiate into many different cell types including cardiomyocytes [47], hepatocytes [48], oligodendrocytes [49], glia, and neuronal subtypes [50]. Murine iPSCs have also been shown to be reprogrammed into dopaminergic neurons that express the transcription factors Nurr1, Pitx3 and tyrosine hydroxylase and demonstrate electrophysiological properties of DA neurons [51]. Subsequent studies demonstrated successful differentiation of dopaminergic neurons from both established human iPSC lines and patient-derived somatic cells [52,53].

In all of these studies, iPSC-derived DA cells demonstrated expression of key dopaminergic markers and electrophysiological properties of DA neurons. Furthermore, these DA cells were successfully incorporated into a 6-OHDA rat model of PD, leading to significantly reduced motor asymmetry [52]. Most recently, primate-derived iPSCs were successfully transplanted back into the putamen of MPTP lesioned monkeys; these autografts led to significant motor improvements, and postmortem analysis showed graft survival and outgrowth into the transplanted putamen [54]. Despite promising results in preclinical studies, several factors have provided road blocks to utilization of these cells in humans, including use of viruses to modify cells and risk of tumorigenicity [55].

3.4.2. Clinical studies

The first pilot study in humans was performed in Japan in 2014, and utilized iPSC-derived autologous pigmented retinal epithelial cells for treatment of macular degeneration. Transplantation in the first patient was completed without adverse effects; however, long-term follow-up is necessary [56]. Unfortunately, iPSCs derived from fibroblasts of a second patient were discovered to have genetic mutations, including three single-nucleotide variations and three copy-number variants, prompting suspension of the trial [57]. Studies are now focusing on use of allogenic partially matched donor cells from the Center for iPS Cell Research and Application, an iPSC bank, for treatment of macular degeneration [57]. There is also potential to transform fibroblasts directly into neurons (iN cells) or dopamine cells (iDA cells) using specific transcription factors: Ascl1, Brn2, Mrt1l, without or with Lmx1a and FoxA2, respectively [58–60]; however, this technology still needs to be tested in preclinical models.

3.5. Autologous brain-derived progenitor cells (BDPCs)

Recently, the safety and feasibility of performing small volume brain biopsies has been demonstrated in PD patients undergoing DBS surgery [61]. These tissue specimens yield an expandable cell population that expresses several NTFs known to be highly protective against PD neurodegeneration, including glial-derived neurotrophic factor (GDNF), brain-derived neurotrophic factor (BDNF), and cerebral dopamine neurotrophic factor (CDNF) [61]. The cultures yield large numbers (i.e. 10^7) of cells with limited capacity for self-renewal. These cells, called BDPCs, also show expression of progenitor and neural markers including nestin, Olig1, and GalC. Colocalization of neural and oligodendroglial markers suggests these BDPCs may be grafted into the host brain to integrate as autologous glia [61]. A patient-derived cellular source of neuroprotective agents, reimplanted into the host brain, may confer long-lasting therapeutic benefit in PD patients. Preclinical studies on the potential for these BDPCs to be used as an autologous cell-based therapy for PD are currently underway.

4. Neurotrophic factors

Neurotrophic factors (NTFs) are being intensively evaluated as therapeutic agents for PD owing to their known roles in neuronal survival, differentiation, and plasticity. Additionally, NTF deficiency has been associated with PD and replacement or enhancement of NTF signaling confers neuronal protection in both in vitro and in vivo preclinical PD models [62]. These secreted proteins regulate vital biological programs in the developing and adult nervous systems and are currently the most potent cytoprotective agents known against PD-related degeneration in the brain [63]. The NTF families include (1) glial-derived neurotrophic factor (GDNF) family of ligands (GFL), (2) neurotrophins, (3) neuropoietic cytokines (neurokines), and (4) cerebral DA neurotrophic factor (CDNF)/mesencephalic astrocyte-derived neurotrophic factor family (MANF). To date, GDNF and other GFL members have received the most attention in development of potential new clinical therapies for PD [64].

4.1. GDNF family of ligands

GDNF was the first member of the GDNF family of ligands (GFL) to be discovered. Other members include neurturin (NRTN), persephin (PSPN), and artemin (ARTN). GFLs are important for cell survival, neurite outgrowth, cell differentiation, and cell migration [65].

4.1.1. Preclinical studies

Application of GDNF to rat ventral mesencephalic cultures increased survival, neurite length, and differentiation of DA neurons [66]. GDNF also reduced apoptosis and enhanced cell survival in cultures derived from monkey, porcine, and human mesencephalic tissues [67]. These effects extend to promote differentiation and protection of dopaminergic neurons against 6-OHDA and MPTP neurotoxins [65]. Numerous in vivo studies have demonstrated therapeutic effects of GDNF in the 6-OHDA rat model of PD; the infusion of recombinant GDNF significantly increased DA neuron survival in both the SN and ventral tegmental area and improved parkinsonian symptomology, including motor impairments and amphetamine-induced rotational behavior [68–71]. GDNF has also been shown to be neuroprotective in the MPTP mouse model of PD [72,73]. Studies in nonhuman primates have demonstrated that intracerebral administration of GDNF in MPTP-treated rhesus monkeys results in significant improvements in bradykinesia, rigidity, and postural instability, as well as increased DA levels in the midbrain, globus pallidus, and SN [74].

4.1.2. Clinical studies

Based on the success of using GDNF in preclinical models of PD, GDNF has now been studied in four clinical trials via infusion into the ventricular system or putamen [75]. The first RDBCT compared effects of intracerebroventricular administration of recombinant methionyl human GDNF (r-metHuGDNF, Liatermin®; Amgen) in escalating doses or placebo in 50 PD patients over a period of 8 months. No significant improvement in "on" and "off" total and motor UPDRS was seen in patients treated with GDNF. Adverse effects included paresthesias, nausea, and vomiting. A follow-up open label study in 16 of these patients for 20 months showed no additional improvement in PD symptomology. It was felt that the adverse effects resulted from off-target GDNF influence and the lack of therapeutic benefit from an inability of GDNF to diffuse into the parenchyma from the ventricular source [76].

A subsequent open label study that enrolled 5 PD patients investigated the effects of intraparenchymal delivery of GDNF via implanted catheters in the dorsal putamen (unilateral in one patient; bilaterally in four patients) and connected to an extracranial pump system [77]. After one year, there were no serious clinical side effects, a 39% improvement in the off-medication UPDRS motor scores and a 61% improvement in the activities of daily living (ADL) subscore. Medication-induced dyskinesias were considerably reduced and (PET) scans of ^{18}F-FDOPA uptake showed a significant 28% increase in putamen DA storage after 18 months [78]. In a follow-up report, the group described one of the patients with bilateral GDNF infusions who had received treatment for 39 months, then was followed clinically and with PET for another 36 months. The UPDRS motor and ADL scores "off" medication remained improved by 74% and 76%, respectively, levodopa usage ceased after a year, and at 36 months post-GDNF cessation, the ^{18}F-FDOPA uptake remained 29% higher in the posterior putamen [79]. Another group led a second open label study that enrolled 10 patients treated unilaterally with intraputamenal GDNF [80]. A significant increase in total and motor UPDRS scores was observed after 24 weeks, but benefit was lost with cessation of treatment. These positive outcomes spurred a second multicenter, placebo-controlled trial in which 34 PD patients were randomized to receive bilateral intraputamenal GDNF (15 μg/putamen/day; a dose lower than that of the previous studies) or placebo via continuous infusion. At 6 months, there was no significant treatment benefit reflected in the "off" UPDRS motor scores; however, a 32.5% increase in putamenal ^{18}F-FDOPA uptake was observed in the GDNF-treated cohort [81]. The disparate outcomes of these studies may reflect differences in study design, cohort size, drug dosage, and/or delivery systems. The r-metHuGDNF manufacturing company subsequently withdrew the agent on the grounds of safety concerns regarding production of neutralizing antibodies in several patients and related cerebellar injuries in animal studies, although no such injuries were reported in human trials. Efforts are now underway to evaluate adeno-associated virus (AAV)-mediated GDNF in an open label phase I for patients with advanced PD (https://www.clinicaltrials.gov/ct2/show/NCT01621581).

4.2. Neurturin

4.2.1. Preclinical studies

Neurturin (NTRN) shares 40% sequence homology with GDNF [82] and has been shown to promote survival of DA neurons in the nigrostriatal system [82–84]. In vitro, NTRN leads to neurite outgrowth in cultured spinal motor neurons and protects against glutamate toxicity. Early studies infusing NTRN directly into the SN was shown to be neuroprotective against 6-OHDA toxicity, while striatal infusion improved behavioral parameters of DA neuronal function in rats [83,85]. In MPTP-lesioned monkeys, intraputamenal infusion of NTRN led to significant improvement in parkinsonian deficits as well as increased DA metabolite levels in the globus pallidus [86]. CERE-120, an (AAV) vector expressing NTRN, has also shown potential therapeutic benefit in preclinical studies [87]. When MPTP-lesioned monkeys were given CERE-120 into the striatum, motor symptoms were improved and loss of DA neurons was reduced [88]. After one year follow-up, no toxic adverse effects were observed [89].

4.2.2. Clinical studies

A Phase 1 open-label clinical trial demonstrated safety, tolerability, and potential therapeutic benefit in PD patients after one year [90]. A subsequent RDBCT enrolled 58 patients to receive AAV2-NTRN bilaterally into the putamen or sham surgery. The primary endpoint was change from baseline to 12 months in the UPDRS motor score in the off state, and no significant difference was found between patients treated with AAV2-NTRN compared with control individuals. Three of 38 patients in the AAV2-NTRN group and two of 20 in the sham surgery group developed tumors, with uncertain relations to the actual treatment [91]. Postmortem analysis of two patients revealed that, unlike the animal studies, putamenal AAV-NTRN injections did not confer adequate retrograde labeling of neurons in the SN [92]. This deficiency in axonal transport of AAV-NTRN to the SN was addressed in a phase 1 safety study that enrolled six patients who received bilateral dual injections into the putamen and SN [93]. Two-year follow-up suggested that the procedures were well-tolerated and no serious adverse effects were reported. A second phase 2 RDBCT was then conducted, enrolling 51 patients to receive bilateral putamen and SN AAV-NTRN (https://clinicaltrials.gov/ct2/show/NCT00985517). In 2013, it was announced that the trial did not demonstrate statistically significant improvement in patient UPDRS scores after 15–24 months of follow-up. However, a more robust response to CERE-120 was observed in PD patients treated within 5 years of diagnosis, and no safety concerns were raised. There was a marked placebo effect as the control patients and the CERE-120 treated patients both improved significantly following surgery. Long-term observational studies of the participants are planned to assess delayed clinical effect (http://www.prnewswire.com/news-releases/ceregene-reports-data-from-parkinsons-disease-phase-2b-study-203803541.html).

4.3. Preclinical studies with other neurotrophic factors

4.3.1. Persephin/artemin

Persephin (PSPN) shows approximately 40% sequence homology to GDNF and NTRN [94]. PSPN promotes survival of cultured ventral midbrain dopaminergic neurons as well as motor neurons and prevents their degeneration after 6-OHDA toxicity [94]. PSPN-overexpressing neural stem cells grafted into the striatum prevented loss of DA neurons and led to behavioral improvements in 6-OHDA lesioned rats [95]. Artemin (ARTN) promotes survival of DA neurons in culture [96] and also protects against DA neuron degeneration in the striatum following neurotoxic doses of methamphetamine [97]. Although early preclinical studies have shown therapeutic benefit of both PSPN and ARTN, more studies are necessary before these NTFs can be tested in a clinical setting.

4.3.2. BDNF

Brain-derived neurotrophic factor (BDNF) is an essential regulator of neuronal differentiation and plasticity. It has been suggested that alterations in BDNF expression may be responsible for the development of neurodegenerative disorders [98]. Postmortem studies of PD patients have demonstrated that BDNF levels are reduced in the substantia nigra pars compacta as a result of decreased transcription of the BDNF gene [99]. Another study reported that only 10% of melanized neurons in the substantia nigra of PD patients were immunoreactive for BDNF expression, compared with 65% in healthy controls [100]. Serum BDNF levels have also been shown to correlate with a loss of striatal DA transporter binding in PD patients, suggesting an influence on striatal neurodegeneration [101]. Animal studies have demonstrated that BDNF antisense oligonucleotide infusion in rats produces a Parkinsonian phenotype [102], and BDNF knockout mice have reduced dopaminergic neurons in the substantia nigra [103]. BDNF promotes *in vitro* survival and differentiation of human and rat embryonic dopaminergic neurons, and it has protective effects against various toxins including 6-OHDA and MPTP [99]. In a nonhuman primate model of PD, intrathecal BDNF infusion resulted in milder PD symptoms and less neuronal cell loss in the substantia nigra [104]. To date, there are no clinical studies evaluating the efficacy of BDNF therapy in human PD, likely due to the logistical challenges of CNS drug delivery and dosing, as BDNF has poor blood-brain barrier penetration if administered parenterally, and intrathecal or intraventricular delivery results in poor penetration of the brain parenchyma [105].

4.3.3. CDNF/MANF

Mesencephalic astrocyte-derived neurotrophic factor (MANF) was first discovered in 2003 and was shown to be selectively neuroprotective for dopaminergic neurons [106]. Later, cerebral DA neurotrophic factor (CDNF) was discovered as a homologue of MANF with 59% sequence homology [107]. CDNF has been shown to be neuroprotective to DA neurons and intrastriatal injection of CDNF or AAV-CDNF reduces degeneration of DA neurons and parkinsonian behavior in rats and increases TH levels in the striatum and SN [107–110]. Interestingly, intranigral infusion of a combination of both CDNF and MANF via lentiviral mediated delivery reduced amphetamine-induced rotational behavior and increased striatal TH-fibers and TH-positive neurons in the substantia nigra [111]. Intranigral CDNF alone also improved behavior and increased TH fibers in the striatum, but both to a lesser extent than with CDNF/MANF together, and did not protect against TH neuronal loss in the SN [111]. Intra-nigral MANF alone did not affect behavior or striatal TH fibers, but did protect against SN neuronal loss [111]. Results of these studies suggest that combined delivery of CDNF/MANF may be more effective than single NTFs and may be a more effective potential therapeutic treatment for PD, although neither NTF has been tested in a clinical setting.

5. Conclusions

There remains a critical need for new therapies to delay or prevent the progression of PD. As discussed in this chapter, cell-based therapies may provide a promising therapeutic benefit to

http://dx.doi.org/10.5772/63747

PD patients. NTFs offer a potential class of cytoprotective agents that complement DA replacement and cell-based therapies in PD, with ideal grafts consisting of immunologically inert cells that continuously produce and release these agents in the host brain. Further development and refinement of these potential therapies is essential to develop personalized care for PD patients.

Author details

Andrea R. Di Sebastiano[1], Michael D. Staudt[1], Simon M. Benoit[1], Hu Xu[1], Matthew O. Hebb[1,2] and Susanne Schmid[2*]

*Address all correspondence to: Susanne.schmid@schulich.uwo.ca

1 Clinical Neurological Sciences, Schulich School of Medicine & Dentistry, University of Western Ontario, London, ON, Canada

2 Anatomy & Cell Biology, Schulich School of Medicine & Dentistry, University of Western Ontario, London, ON, Canada

References

[1] de Lau, L.M. and M.M. Breteler, Epidemiology of Parkinson's disease. Lancet Neurol, 2006. 5(6): pp. 525–35.

[2] Spillantini, M.G., et al., Alpha-synuclein in Lewy bodies. Nature, 1997. 388(6645): pp. 839–40.

[3] Damier, P., New aspects in the pathophysiology of dyskinesia. Salpetriere Deep Brain Stimulation Group. Adv Neurol, 1999. 80: pp. 611–7.

[4] Dickson, D.W., Parkinson's disease and parkinsonism: neuropathology. Cold Spring Harb Perspect Med, 2012. 2(8).

[5] Massano, J. and K.P. Bhatia, Clinical approach to Parkinson's disease: features, diagnosis, and principles of management. Cold Spring Harb Perspect Med, 2012. 2(6): p. a008870.

[6] Cotzias, G.C., M.H. Van Woert, and L.M. Schiffer, Aromatic amino acids and modification of parkinsonism. N Engl J Med, 1967. 276(7): pp. 374–9.

[7] Marsden, C.D. and J.D. Parkes, "On-off" effects in patients with Parkinson's disease on chronic levodopa therapy. Lancet, 1976. 1(7954): pp. 292–6.

[8] Lotia, M. and J. Jankovic, New and emerging medical therapies in Parkinson's disease. Expert Opin Pharmacother, 2016: pp. 1–15.

[9] Nutt, J.G. and J.H. Fellman, Pharmacokinetics of levodopa. Clin Neuropharmacol, 1984. 7(1): pp. 35–49.

[10] Parkinson Study, G., Effects of tocopherol and deprenyl on the progression of disability in early Parkinson's disease. N Engl J Med, 1993. 328(3): pp. 176–83.

[11] Stern, M.B., et al., Double-blind, randomized, controlled trial of rasagiline as monotherapy in early Parkinson's disease patients. Mov Disord, 2004. 19(8): pp. 916–23.

[12] Spiegel, E.A., H.T. Wycis, and H.W. Baird, 3rd, Long-range effects of electropallidoansotomy in extrapyramidal and convulsive disorders. Neurology, 1958. 8(10): pp. 734–40.

[13] Hassler, R. and T. Riechert, [Indications and localization of stereotactic brain operations]. Nervenarzt, 1954. 25(11): pp. 441–7.

[14] Vitek, J.L., et al., Randomized trial of pallidotomy versus medical therapy for Parkinson's disease. Ann Neurol, 2003. 53(5): pp. 558–69.

[15] Munhoz, R.P., A. Cerasa, and M.S. Okun, Surgical treatment of dyskinesia in Parkinson's disease. Front Neurol, 2014. 5: pp. 65.

[16] Deep-Brain Stimulation for Parkinson's Disease Study, G., Deep-brain stimulation of the subthalamic nucleus or the pars interna of the globus pallidus in Parkinson's disease. N Engl J Med, 2001. 345(13): pp. 956–63.

[17] Olson, L. and A. Seiger, Development and growth of immature monoamine neurons in rat and man in situ and following intraocular transplantation in the rat. Brain Res, 1973. 62(2): pp. 353–60.

[18] Freed, W.J., et al., Transplanted adrenal chromaffin cells in rat brain reduce lesion-induced rotational behaviour. Nature, 1981. 292(5821): pp. 351–2.

[19] Brundin, P., et al., The rotating 6-hydroxydopamine-lesioned mouse as a model for assessing functional effects of neuronal grafting. Brain Res, 1986. 366(1–2): pp. 346–9.

[20] Brundin, P., et al., Behavioural effects of human fetal dopamine neurons grafted in a rat model of Parkinson's disease. Exp Brain Res, 1986. 65(1): pp. 235–40.

[21] Madrazo, I., et al., Open microsurgical autograft of adrenal medulla to the right caudate nucleus in two patients with intractable Parkinson's disease. N Engl J Med, 1987. 316(14): pp. 831–4.

[22] Lindvall, O., et al., Grafts of fetal dopamine neurons survive and improve motor function in Parkinson's disease. Science, 1990. 247(4942): pp. 574–7.

http://dx.doi.org/10.5772/63747

[23] Lindvall, O., et al., Human fetal dopamine neurons grafted into the striatum in two patients with severe Parkinson's disease. A detailed account of methodology and a 6-month follow-up. Arch Neurol, 1989. 46(6): pp. 615–31.

[24] Lindvall, O., et al., Transplantation of fetal dopamine neurons in Parkinson's disease: one-year clinical and neurophysiological observations in two patients with putaminal implants. Ann Neurol, 1992. 31(2): pp. 155–65.

[25] Kefalopoulou, Z., et al., Long-term clinical outcome of fetal cell transplantation for Parkinson disease: two case reports. JAMA Neurol, 2014. 71(1): pp. 83–7.

[26] Freed, C.R., et al., Survival of implanted fetal dopamine cells and neurologic improvement 12 to 46 months after transplantation for Parkinson's disease. N Engl J Med, 1992. 327(22): pp. 1549–55.

[27] Freed, C.R., et al., Transplantation of human fetal dopamine cells for Parkinson's disease. Results at 1 year. Arch Neurol, 1990. 47(5): pp. 505–12.

[28] Spencer, D.D., et al., Unilateral transplantation of human fetal mesencephalic tissue into the caudate nucleus of patients with Parkinson's disease. N Engl J Med, 1992. 327(22): pp. 1541–8.

[29] Peschanski, M., et al., Bilateral motor improvement and alteration of L-dopa effect in two patients with Parkinson's disease following intrastriatal transplantation of foetal ventral mesencephalon. Brain, 1994. 117 (Pt 3): pp. 487–99.

[30] Widner, H., et al., Bilateral fetal mesencephalic grafting in two patients with parkinsonism induced by 1-methyl-4-phenyl-1,2,3,6-tetrahydropyridine (MPTP). N Engl J Med, 1992. 327(22): pp. 1556–63.

[31] Freeman, T.B., et al., Bilateral fetal nigral transplantation into the postcommissural putamen in Parkinson's disease. Ann Neurol, 1995. 38(3): pp. 379–88.

[32] Olanow, C.W., J.H. Kordower, and T.B. Freeman, Fetal nigral transplantation as a therapy for Parkinson's disease. Trends Neurosci, 1996. 19(3): pp. 102–9.

[33] Olanow, C.W., et al., A double-blind controlled trial of bilateral fetal nigral transplantation in Parkinson's disease. Ann Neurol, 2003. 54(3): pp. 403–14.

[34] Ma, Y., et al., Dopamine cell implantation in Parkinson's disease: long-term clinical and (18)F-FDOPA PET outcomes. J Nucl Med, 2010. 51(1): pp. 7–15.

[35] Freed, C.R., et al., Transplantation of embryonic dopamine neurons for severe Parkinson's disease. N Engl J Med, 2001. 344(10): pp. 710–9.

[36] Ribeiro, D., et al., Efficient expansion and dopaminergic differentiation of human fetal ventral midbrain neural stem cells by midbrain morphogens. Neurobiol Dis, 2013. 49: pp. 118–27.

[37] Thomson, J.A., et al., Embryonic stem cell lines derived from human blastocysts. Science, 1998. 282(5391): pp. 1145–7.

[38] Barberi, T., et al., Neural subtype specification of fertilization and nuclear transfer embryonic stem cells and application in parkinsonian mice. Nat Biotechnol, 2003. 21(10): pp. 1200–7.

[39] Roy, N.S., et al., Functional engraftment of human ES cell-derived dopaminergic neurons enriched by coculture with telomerase-immortalized midbrain astrocytes. Nat Med, 2006. 12(11): pp. 1259–68.

[40] Takagi, Y., et al., Dopaminergic neurons generated from monkey embryonic stem cells function in a Parkinson primate model. J Clin Invest, 2005. 115(1): pp. 102–9.

[41] Cooper, O., M. Parmar, and O. Isacson, Characterization and criteria of embryonic stem and induced pluripotent stem cells for a dopamine replacement therapy. Prog Brain Res, 2012. 200: pp. 265–76.

[42] Glavaski-Joksimovic, A. and M.C. Bohn, Mesenchymal stem cells and neuroregeneration in Parkinson's disease. Exp Neurol, 2013. 247: pp. 25–38.

[43] Offen, D., et al., Intrastriatal transplantation of mouse bone marrow-derived stem cells improves motor behavior in a mouse model of Parkinson's disease. J Neural Transm Suppl, 2007(72): pp. 133–43.

[44] Venkataramana, N.K., et al., Open-labeled study of unilateral autologous bone-marrow-derived mesenchymal stem cell transplantation in Parkinson's disease. Transl Res, 2010. 155(2): pp. 62–70.

[45] Takahashi, K. and S. Yamanaka, Induction of pluripotent stem cells from mouse embryonic and adult fibroblast cultures by defined factors. Cell, 2006. 126(4): pp. 663–76.

[46] Takahashi, K., et al., Induction of pluripotent stem cells from adult human fibroblasts by defined factors. Cell, 2007. 131(5): pp. 861–72.

[47] Kuzmenkin, A., et al., Functional characterization of cardiomyocytes derived from murine induced pluripotent stem cells in vitro. FASEB J, 2009. 23(12): pp. 4168–80.

[48] Espejel, S., et al., Induced pluripotent stem cell-derived hepatocytes have the functional and proliferative capabilities needed for liver regeneration in mice. J Clin Invest, 2010. 120(9): pp. 3120–6.

[49] Czepiel, M., et al., Differentiation of induced pluripotent stem cells into functional oligodendrocytes. Glia, 2011. 59(6): pp. 882–92.

[50] Hu, B.Y., et al., Neural differentiation of human induced pluripotent stem cells follows developmental principles but with variable potency. Proc Natl Acad Sci U S A, 2010. 107(9): pp. 4335–40.

[51] Wernig, M., et al., Neurons derived from reprogrammed fibroblasts functionally integrate into the fetal brain and improve symptoms of rats with Parkinson's disease. Proc Natl Acad Sci U S A, 2008. 105(15): pp. 5856–61.

[52] Hargus, G., et al., Differentiated Parkinson patient-derived induced pluripotent stem cells grow in the adult rodent brain and reduce motor asymmetry in Parkinsonian rats. Proc Natl Acad Sci U S A, 2010. 107(36): pp. 15921–6.

[53] Swistowski, A., et al., Efficient generation of functional dopaminergic neurons from human induced pluripotent stem cells under defined conditions. Stem Cells, 2010. 28(10): pp. 1893–904.

[54] Hallett, P.J., et al., Successful function of autologous iPSC-derived dopamine neurons following transplantation in a non-human primate model of Parkinson's disease. Cell Stem Cell, 2015. 16(3): pp. 269–74.

[55] Momcilovic, O., et al., Genome wide profiling of dopaminergic neurons derived from human embryonic and induced pluripotent stem cells. Stem Cells Dev, 2014. 23(4): pp. 406–20.

[56] Reardon, S. and D. Cyranoski, Japan stem-cell trial stirs envy. Nature, 2014. 513(7518): pp. 287–8.

[57] Garber, K., RIKEN suspends first clinical trial involving induced pluripotent stem cells. Nat Biotechnol, 2015. 33(9): pp. 890–1.

[58] Pang, Z.P., et al., Induction of human neuronal cells by defined transcription factors. Nature, 2011. 476(7359): pp. 220–3.

[59] Pfisterer, U., et al., Direct conversion of human fibroblasts to dopaminergic neurons. Proc Natl Acad Sci U S A, 2011. 108(25): pp. 10343–8.

[60] Chanda, S., et al., Generation of induced neuronal cells by the single reprogramming factor ASCL1. Stem Cell Rep, 2014. 3(2): pp. 282–96.

[61] Xu, H., et al., Neurotrophic factor expression in expandable cell populations from brain samples in living patients with Parkinson's disease. FASEB J, 2013. 27(10): pp. 4157–68.

[62] Rangasamy, S.B., et al., Neurotrophic factor therapy for Parkinson's disease. Prog Brain Res, 2010. 184: pp. 237–64.

[63] Kordower, J.H. and A. Bjorklund, Trophic factor gene therapy for Parkinson's disease. Mov Disord, 2013. 28(1): pp. 96–109.

[64] Rodrigues, T.M., et al., Challenges and promises in the development of neurotrophic factor-based therapies for Parkinson's disease. Drugs Aging, 2014. 31(4): pp. 239–61.

[65] Airaksinen, M.S. and M. Saarma, The GDNF family: signalling, biological functions and therapeutic value. Nat Rev Neurosci, 2002. 3(5): pp. 383–94.

[66] Lin, L.F., et al., GDNF: a glial cell line-derived neurotrophic factor for midbrain dopaminergic neurons. Science, 1993. 260(5111): pp. 1130–2.

[67] Meyer, M., et al., Improved survival of embryonic porcine dopaminergic neurons in coculture with a conditionally immortalized GDNF-producing hippocampal cell line. Exp Neurol, 2000. 164(1): pp. 82–93.

[68] Beck, K.D., et al., GDNF induces a dystonia-like state in neonatal rats and stimulates dopamine and serotonin synthesis. Neuron, 1996. 16(3): pp. 665–73.

[69] Bowenkamp, K.E., et al., Glial cell line-derived neurotrophic factor supports survival of injured midbrain dopaminergic neurons. J Comp Neurol, 1995. 355(4): pp. 479–89.

[70] Winkler, C., et al., Short-term GDNF treatment provides long-term rescue of lesioned nigral dopaminergic neurons in a rat model of Parkinson's disease. J Neurosci, 1996. 16(22): pp. 7206–15.

[71] Clarkson, E.D., W.M. Zawada, and C.R. Freed, GDNF improves survival and reduces apoptosis in human embryonic dopaminergic neurons in vitro. Cell Tissue Res, 1997. 289(2): pp. 207–10.

[72] Schober, A., et al., GDNF applied to the MPTP-lesioned nigrostriatal system requires TGF-beta for its neuroprotective action. Neurobiol Dis, 2007. 25(2): pp. 378–91.

[73] Chen, Y.H., et al., MPTP-induced deficits in striatal synaptic plasticity are prevented by glial cell line-derived neurotrophic factor expressed via an adeno-associated viral vector. FASEB J, 2008. 22(1): pp. 261–75.

[74] Gash, D.M., et al., Functional recovery in parkinsonian monkeys treated with GDNF. Nature, 1996. 380(6571): pp. 252–5.

[75] Aron, L. and R. Klein, Repairing the parkinsonian brain with neurotrophic factors. Trends Neurosci, 2011. 34(2): pp. 88–100.

[76] Nutt, J.G., et al., Randomized, double-blind trial of glial cell line-derived neurotrophic factor (GDNF) in PD. Neurology, 2003. 60(1): pp. 69–73.

[77] Gill, S.S., et al., Direct brain infusion of glial cell line-derived neurotrophic factor in Parkinson disease. Nat Med, 2003. 9(5): pp. 589–95.

[78] Patel, N.K., et al., Intraputamenal infusion of glial cell line-derived neurotrophic factor in PD: a two-year outcome study. Ann Neurol, 2005. 57(2): pp. 298–302.

[79] Patel, N.K., et al., Benefits of putaminal GDNF infusion in Parkinson disease are maintained after GDNF cessation. Neurology, 2013. 81(13): pp. 1176–8.

[80] Slevin, J.T., et al., Improvement of bilateral motor functions in patients with Parkinson disease through the unilateral intraputaminal infusion of glial cell line-derived neurotrophic factor. J Neurosurg, 2005. 102(2):pp. 216–22.

[81] Lang, A.E., et al., Randomized controlled trial of intraputamenal glial cell line-derived neurotrophic factor infusion in Parkinson disease. Ann Neurol, 2006. 59(3): pp. 459–66.

[82] Kotzbauer, P.T., et al., Neurturin, a relative of glial-cell-line-derived neurotrophic factor. Nature, 1996. 384(6608): pp. 467–70.

[83] Horger, B.A., et al., Neurturin exerts potent actions on survival and function of midbrain dopaminergic neurons. J Neurosci, 1998. 18(13): pp. 4929–37.

[84] Akerud, P., et al., Differential effects of glial cell line-derived neurotrophic factor and neurturin on developing and adult substantia nigra dopaminergic neurons. J Neurochem, 1999. 73(1): pp. 70–8.

[85] Oiwa, Y., et al., Dopaminergic neuroprotection and regeneration by neurturin assessed by using behavioral, biochemical and histochemical measurements in a model of progressive Parkinson's disease. Brain Res, 2002. 947(2): pp. 271–83.

[86] Grondin, R., et al., Intraputamenal infusion of exogenous neurturin protein restores motor and dopaminergic function in the globus pallidus of MPTP-lesioned rhesus monkeys. Cell Transplant, 2008. 17(4): pp. 373–81.

[87] Gasmi, M., et al., AAV2-mediated delivery of human neurturin to the rat nigrostriatal system: long-term efficacy and tolerability of CERE-120 for Parkinson's disease. Neurobiol Dis, 2007. 27(1): pp. 67–76.

[88] Kordower, J.H., et al., Delivery of neurturin by AAV2 (CERE-120)-mediated gene transfer provides structural and functional neuroprotection and neurorestoration in MPTP-treated monkeys. Ann Neurol, 2006. 60(6): pp. 706–15.

[89] Herzog, C.D., et al., Expression, bioactivity, and safety 1 year after adeno-associated viral vector type 2-mediated delivery of neurturin to the monkey nigrostriatal system support cere-120 for Parkinson's disease. Neurosurgery, 2009. 64(4): pp. 602–12; discussion 612–3.

[90] Marks, W.J., Jr., et al., Safety and tolerability of intraputaminal delivery of CERE-120 (adeno-associated virus serotype 2-neurturin) to patients with idiopathic Parkinson's disease: an open-label, phase I trial. Lancet Neurol, 2008. 7(5): pp. 400–8.

[91] Marks, W.J., Jr., et al., Gene delivery of AAV2-neurturin for Parkinson's disease: a double-blind, randomised, controlled trial. Lancet Neurol, 2010. 9(12): pp. 1164–72.

[92] Bartus, R.T., et al., Bioactivity of AAV2-neurturin gene therapy (CERE-120): differences between Parkinson's disease and nonhuman primate brains. Mov Disord, 2011. 26(1): pp. 27–36.

[93] Bartus, R.T., et al., Safety/feasibility of targeting the substantia nigra with AAV2-neurturin in Parkinson patients. Neurology, 2013. 80(18): pp. 1698–701.

[94] Milbrandt, J., et al., Persephin, a novel neurotrophic factor related to GDNF and neurturin. Neuron, 1998. 20(2): pp. 245–53.

[95] Akerud, P., et al., Persephin-overexpressing neural stem cells regulate the function of nigral dopaminergic neurons and prevent their degeneration in a model of Parkinson's disease. Mol Cell Neurosci, 2002. 21(2): pp. 205–22.

[96] Baloh, R.H., et al., Artemin, a novel member of the GDNF ligand family, supports peripheral and central neurons and signals through the GFRalpha3-RET receptor complex. Neuron, 1998. 21(6): pp. 1291–302.

[97] Cass, W.A., et al., Protection by GDNF and other trophic factors against the dopamine-depleting effects of neurotoxic doses of methamphetamine. Ann N Y Acad Sci, 2006. 1074: pp. 272–81.

[98] Zuccato, C. and E. Cattaneo, Brain-derived neurotrophic factor in neurodegenerative diseases. Nat Rev Neurol, 2009. 5(6): pp. 311–22.

[99] Murer, M.G., Q. Yan, and R. Raisman-Vozari, Brain-derived neurotrophic factor in the control human brain, and in Alzheimer's disease and Parkinson's disease. Prog Neurobiol, 2001. 63(1): pp. 71–124.

[100] Parain, K., et al., Reduced expression of brain-derived neurotrophic factor protein in Parkinson's disease substantia nigra. Neuroreport, 1999. 10(3): pp. 557–61.

[101] Ziebell, M., et al., Striatal dopamine transporter binding correlates with serum BDNF levels in patients with striatal dopaminergic neurodegeneration. Neurobiol Aging, 2012. 33(2): pp. 428 e1–5.

[102] Porritt, M.J., P.E. Batchelor, and D.W. Howells, Inhibiting BDNF expression by antisense oligonucleotide infusion causes loss of nigral dopaminergic neurons. Exp Neurol, 2005. 192(1): pp. 226–34.

[103] Baquet, Z.C., P.C. Bickford, and K.R. Jones, Brain-derived neurotrophic factor is required for the establishment of the proper number of dopaminergic neurons in the substantia nigra pars compacta. J Neurosci, 2005. 25(26): pp. 6251–9.

[104] Tsukahara, T., et al., Effects of brain-derived neurotrophic factor on 1-methyl-4-phenyl-1,2,3,6-tetrahydropyridine-induced parkinsonism in monkeys. Neurosurgery, 1995. 37(4): pp. 733–9; discussion 739–41.

[105] Nagahara, A.H. and M.H. Tuszynski, Potential therapeutic uses of BDNF in neurological and psychiatric disorders. Nat Rev Drug Discov, 2011. 10(3): pp. 209–19.

[106] Petrova, P., et al., MANF: a new mesencephalic, astrocyte-derived neurotrophic factor with selectivity for dopaminergic neurons. J Mol Neurosci, 2003. 20(2): pp. 173–88.

[107] Lindholm, P., et al., Novel neurotrophic factor CDNF protects and rescues midbrain dopamine neurons in vivo. Nature, 2007. 448(7149): pp. 73–7.

[108] Voutilainen, M.H., et al., Chronic infusion of CDNF prevents 6-OHDA-induced deficits in a rat model of Parkinson's disease. Exp Neurol, 2011. 228(1): pp. 99–108.

[109] Back, S., et al., Gene therapy with AAV2-CDNF provides functional benefits in a rat model of Parkinson's disease. Brain Behav, 2013. 3(2): pp. 75–88.

[110] Ren, X., et al., AAV2-mediated striatum delivery of human CDNF prevents the deterioration of midbrain dopamine neurons in a 6-hydroxydopamine induced parkinsonian rat model. Exp Neurol, 2013. 248: pp. 148–56.

[111] Cordero-Llana, O., et al., Enhanced efficacy of the CDNF/MANF family by combined intranigral overexpression in the 6-OHDA rat model of Parkinson's disease. Mol Ther, 2015. 23(2): pp. 244–54.

Chapter 15

Stem Cell Therapy for Parkinson's Disease

Fabin Han

Additional information is available at the end of the chapter

http://dx.doi.org/10.5772/63340

Abstract

Parkinson's disease (PD) is the second most common neurodegenerative disorder of aging after Alzheimer's disease (AD). Pathologically, it is characterized by a degeneration of dopamine (DA) neurons in substantia nigra of middle brain, which causes the motor symptoms and nonmotor symptoms of PD. The dopamine replacement therapy using levodopa and surgical treatment of deep brain stimulation (DBS) can only improve the symptoms of PD, but cannot stop the disease progression. Because of the selective loss of DA neurons, cell transplantation provides an exciting potential for the treatment of Parkinson's disease. The available cell sources include mesenchymal stem cells (MSCs) from bone marrow, neural stem cells (NSCs) from fetal brain tissues, embryonic stem cells (ESCs) from blastocysts, and induced pluripotent stem cells (iPSCs) reprogrammed from somatic cells transfected with stem cell transcription factors of OCT4, SOX2, KLF4, and c-MYC. Here, we first review the research advance conducted in animal models and patients of PD with these cells, then moving forward to recent development of iPSCs as a future source for the treatment of PD, and highlight the current challenges to make good manufacturing practice (GMP) standard cells suitable for large-scale production to move the cell-based therapy from dish to clinic as soon as possible.

Keywords: cell-based therapy, dopamine neuron, embryonic stem cell, induced pluripotent stem cell, neural stem cell, Parkinson's disease

1. Introduction

Parkinson's disease (PD) is affecting 1–2% of the population over the age of 60 years old and 3–5% of the population above the age of 85. Clinically, PD patients are characterized with four cardinal symptoms of resting tremors, muscle rigidity, bradykinesia, and postural instability. These motor symptoms appear when 60–80% of dopamine (DA) neurons in the substantia nigra are degenerated and are used as diagnostic criteria. The nonmotor symptoms have recently been highlighted as some of these symptoms including depression, constipation, pain, genitourinary problems, and sleep disorders may precede the motor dysfunction and can be used as early diagnosis and treatment of PD [1].

Because of the decrease of dopamine release in brains of PD patients, either increasing dopamine levels using drugs such as levodopa or reducing the dopamine degradation by dopamine inhibitor carbidopa can play therapeutic effects on PD patients [2]. A surgical treatment called deep brain stimulation (DBS) using electrodes to stimulate to the nucleus subthalamicus is also effective. However, surgical DBS is only suitable for a small portion of the patients and has unclear long-term benefits, while the medications have been found to decline in effectiveness over time and moreover cause the side-effect of dyskinesias (involuntary muscle movements). Recently, great treatment potential has been provided through replacing lost DA neurons using embryonic stem cells (ESCs), induced pluripotent stem cells (iPSCs) reprogrammed from patients' somatic fibroblasts or blood cells, neural stem cells (NSCs), or fully differentiated DA neurons from fetal brain tissue and mesenchymal stem cells (MSCs) sourced from fetuses or adults [3]. A lot of efforts have been done to find suitable cells to improve treatments not just of PD, but of all neurodegenerative diseases.

2. Etiology and molecular genetics

The causes of PD can be divided into genetic susceptible genes and environmental toxic environmental substances such as the pesticide rotenone and manganese, which integrate to damage the DA neurons through oxidative stress and mitochondrial impairment to induce PD. The majority of PD cases are sporadic or idiopathic with unknown causes (80–90%); the remained cases (10–20%) are familial and can be associated with PD-related genes or linked to a particular monogenic mutation [4–6]. Genetic factors play a minor role in causing typical PD, particularly for the patients having PD after 50 years of age [7]. This suggested that genetic factors are an important factor when the disease begins at or before the age of 50.

Genetic linkage analysis has great power to identify the disease genes for inherited monogenic diseases. By now more than 200 genes or loci have been characterized for neurological diseases and more than 100 genes or loci were reported for neuromuscular diseases including PD. The public available database for the genes or loci can be found in online catalog of human inherited genes and disorders (http://www.ncbi.nlm.nih.gov/omim/). The first gene for PD is the α-synuclein gene that was identified in 1997 [8]. Afterward more genes or loci were found to be responsible for familial PD. The characterized mutated genes for the autosomal dominant form of PD are SNCA and LRRK2 whereas the early-onset autosomal recessive genes for PD are PARK2 (Parkin), PINK1, and PARK7, ATP13A2. Some susceptible genes were also reported to be associated with PD such as Tau, Nurr1, and β-glucocerebrosidase (GBA). SNCA, which codes for α-synuclein, has been particularly well-studied and different point mutations (A53T, A30P, and E46K) in SNCA were found in different families with PD. It seems that the missense mutations of the SNCA gene are rare and the genomic rearrangements including the duplication and triplications of SNCA are more common to induce the aggregation of α-synuclein in the dopamine neurons.

Leucine-rich repeat kinase 2 (LRRK2) is another disease gene for autosomal dominant form of PD. It contains more than 50 exons and codes an 832-amino acid protein, which plays GTPase and kinase functions. Mutations can occur in any exons of LRRK2 gene, but the most common missense mutations are R1441C, Y1699C, G2019A, and I2020T. The G2019S mutation in LRRK2 is worldly prevalent, constituting 4% of familial PD cases and 1% of sporadic PD cases. Identification of mutations in the enzymatic GTPase and kinase domains suggests change of these enzymatic activities leads to disease development. Studies have shown that R1441 and Y1699 mutations decrease GTPase activity of LRRK2 whereas G2019S and I2020T mutations increase kinase activity [9, 10].

The second locus for PD is PARK2 for parkin gene. Parkin mutations were first reported in the autosomal recessive families of PD. The total genomic size of parkin covered 1.4 Mb. It contains 12 exons, and the gene product is a protein with 462 amino acids. The parkin has 30% homology to ubiquitin in the amino terminal domain and has two RING-finger-like motifs in the carboxyl part of the protein. It was reported that the RING-like structures in parkin have some ubiquitin-ligase activity. By now, more than 100 different mutations of *parkin* were found in familial and sporadic cases of PD. Most of the Parkin mutations are exonic deletions but missense, nonsense mutations, and genomic rearrangements were also found in PD families.

In addition to the autosomal dominant or recessive genes, some other genes are also reported to be associated with PD. NURR1 is one of the important transcription factors to regulate the development and maturation of the dopamine neurons. We had ever screened 202 familial and sporadic patients with PD and identified one patient has missense mutation of the NURR1 gene. This mutation produced a truncated NURR1 protein that loses the important functional domain to bind the promoter region of the tyrosine hydroxylase (TH), the key kinase to control the synthesis of the dopamine neurotransmitter [11]. GBA is another susceptible gene involved with PD. This gene encodes the lysosomal hydrolase β-glucocerebrosidase in which mutations are associated with neurodegenerative diseases, such as PD and GD (Gaucher's disease). We have performed a case–control study in a Chinese Cohort with PD and a Chinese control cohort by sequencing all the 12 exons of the GBA gene and found that the PD patients have significantly higher frequency of mutations in the GBA gene. Totally, we found nine reported and three novel GBA mutations in 184 Chinese patients. These known GBA mutations are R163Q, F213I, E326K, S364S, F347L, V375L, L444P, RecNciI, and Q497R and the novel mutations are 5-bp deletion (c.334_338delCAGAA), L264I and L314V. Importantly, we identified the novel 5-bp deletion (CAGAA) that produces a nonfunctional GBA protein of 142 amino acids, which loses major enzymatic function domains of the full GBA protein [12].

3. Pathological mechanisms

The mainly pathological mechanism of PD is the degeneration and loss of dopamine (DA) neurons in the substantia nigra of the mesencephalon. These DA neurons project to the basal ganglia (the striatum), which is responsible for motor control and function. The loss of DA neurons is accompanied by Lewy neuritis and Lewy bodies, which cause motor dysfunctions accompanied by an intensification of the disease, including cognitive impairment which encompasses hallucinations, dementia, and speech difficulties. The Lewy neurites might hamper the survival and dendritic development of neurons and glial cells through forming insoluble aggregates of α-synuclein (coded by *SCNA*), ubiquitin, and other misfolded proteins [13].

To understand the molecular mechanism and replicate the phenotypic features of PD, different animal models have been studied to explore dopaminergic neurotoxicity mainly using transgenic models of the familial PD-causing genes such as SNCA and LRRK2. The transgenic mice expressing human SNCA showed pathological inclusions in some neurons and glial cells, motor behavior deficits, and loss of dopaminergic neuron terminals in the basal ganglia. Overexpression of SNCA in drosophila leads to age-dependent dopaminergic neuron degeneration. Furthermore, the slowness of movement in LRRK2-G2019S transgenic mouse models was shown to be associated with diminished dopamine release and axonal pathology. These results support a causal role for α-synuclein in the development of PD. Some studies also suggest that the cellular toxicity in dopamine neurons may be caused by the soluble cytoplasmic oligomeric α-synuclein protein, whereas the large insoluble protein aggregates may represent a cellular defense mechanism in which the cell eventually convert cytotoxic-soluble oligomeric proteins into insoluble inclusion bodies. The α-synuclein-containing fibrils in the degenerative dopamine neurons can disturb cell membrane, leading to increased membrane permeability and eventual cell death of affected neural cells [14, 15]. Some studies showed that genetic mutations in PD genes can affect protein trafficking and cellular degradation machinery and eventually lead to development of PD, but the precise role of these mutated genes in disease progression and interaction with need to be further explored. A recent study reported that accumulation of α-synuclein reduced lysosomal degradation capacity in human midbrain dopamine neurons. Continuous aggregation of α-synuclein in the neural cells disrupted the endoplasmic reticulum–Golgi localization of the key genes such as RAB1a for vesicular transport. Overexpression of RAB1a restored the protein trafficking in endoplasmic reticulum–Golgi pathway and reduced pathological accumulation of α-synuclein in neurons. This study proposes that enhancement of lysosomal trafficking probably play beneficial roles in synucleinopathies [16]. Another molecular mechanism of PD is lysosomal dysfunction and the accumulation of glucosylceramide induced by decreased activity of β-glucocerebrosidase (GBA). Glucosylceramide played roles in stabilizing toxic oligomeric forms of α-synuclein and blocking transport of newly synthesized β-glucocerebrosidase from the endoplasmic reticulum to endocytic compartments, increasing the pathological aggregation of α-synuclein in neuronal cells. A recent study revealed that mutation in GBA is a major risk factor for the development of PD and the molecular pathways of pathological accumulation of glucosylceramide, related lipids, and α-synuclein will need to be studied for the identification of new therapeutic drugs for PD [12, 17].

4. Current stem cell sources for cell-based therapy of PD

Stem cell sources for the treatment of PD have been studied in the past decades. These cells mainly include mesenchymal stem cells from bone marrow and placenta; neural stem cells

(NSCs) and dopamine neurons from fetal brain tissue; embryonic stem cells (ESCs) of the blastocysts from in vitro fertilization; and induced pluripotent stem cells (iPSCs) reprogrammed from autologous somatic cells by expressing transgenes of OCT4, SOX2, c-MYC, and KLF4.

4.1. Mesenchymal stem cells

Mesenchymal stem cells (MSCs) were first reported in 1966, and were described as plastic-adherent colony-forming-unit fibroblastic (CFU-F) cells. MSCs are multipotent with potential to differentiate into different cells of mesodermal lineage and transdifferentiate into epithelial, endothelial, and neuronal cells. MSCs can be isolated from various neonatal and adult tissues such as bone marrow, adipose tissue, umbilical cord, cord blood, amnion, placenta, peripheral blood, and dental pulp [18]. Bone marrow-derived MSCs (BM-MSCs) are a potentially promising source of cells for use in regenerative medicine because they are abundantly available, easy to isolate from the patient themselves, an autologous tissue, and there is no ethical dispute over their use. Several studies have shown that BM-MSCs have the potential to regenerate DA neurons for the treatment of PD. Human BM-MSCs also have a protective effect on the progressive loss of DA neurons induced by carbobenzoxy-L-leucyl-L-leucyl-L-leucinal (MG-132) in vitro and in PD rats [19]. After grafted into the striatum, BM-MSCs were shown to exert neuroprotective effects against nigrostriatal degeneration and to improve motor function in 6-OHDA lesioned rats [20]. BM-MSCs grown in neuronal differentiation medium have more pronounced effect and improve the motor defects in a 6-OHDA fully lesioned rat PD model. BM-MSCs were induced to have neural morphology and expressed markers of DA neurons, such as tyrosine hydroxylase (TH), and most of the cells survived in striatum, expressed TH and behavioral recovery was observed after the cells were transplanted to a 6-OHDA mouse model. A human MSCs-induced DA subpopulation combined with pharmacologically active microcarriers grafted in a rat PD model also led to protection and repair of the nigrostriatal pathway and behavioral recovery.

The role of genetically modified MSCs for the protection and repair of damaged DA neurons and their therapeutic effects have been studied after implanted into PD models. Park et al. investigated the potential of MSCs genetically engineered with glial derived neurotrophic factor (GDNF) by viral transduction to deliver this potent neurotrophic factor for DA neurons in the brain. They found that MPTP(1-Methyl-4-phenyl-1,2,3,6-tetrahydropyridine) mice that were intravenously injected with GDNF-modified BM-MSCs possessed more TH-IR neurons and fibers and showed more prominent behavioral recovery compared with control mice that were implanted naive BM-MSCs [21]. Barzilay et al. reprogrammed the BM-MSCs toward dopaminergic differentiation through delivery of LMX1a, which was reported to be a key transcriptional factor of dopaminergic differentiation in both embryonic stem cells and developmental animal models. They found that the LMX1a protein was concentrated in the cell nuclei, and the cells with forced expression of LMX1a expressed higher levels of tyrosine hydroxylase, secreted significantly higher level of dopamine comparison with nontransduced cells [22]. Wang et al. tested a cytotherapeutic strategy combining cell transplantation and NTN/Lmx1α gene therapy to ameliorate disease progression in hemiparkinsonian rhesus.

They found induced rh-BMSCs exhibited gene/protein expression phenotypes resembling nigral dopaminergic neurons, and these cells survived and retained dopaminergic function following stereotaxic injection into the MPTP-lesioned hemiparkinsonian rhesus [23].

4.2. Neural stem cells and dopamine neurons from fetal brain tissue

Neural stem cells (NSCs) were first described as granule cells with a high proliferative activity in the brain cortex and middle brains. These cells have self-renewal and neural differentiation potential and can differentiate into neurons, astrocytes, and oligodendrocytes. In the developing brain, the distribution of NSCs demonstrate regionalization. For instance, only NSCs isolated from the midbrain have been reported to differentiate into A9 mesencephalic DA neurons necessary for treatment of PD patients. Moreover, NSCs can also be isolated from the other regions of fetal brain or from the subventricular zone (SVZ) and hippocampus of the adult mammalian brain, the regions where neurogenesis continues throughout the mammalian's lifespan [24, 25]. Since initial discoveries of NSCs in 1965, research advances in the isolation, expansion, and differentiation of NSCs have been made [26]. After transplantation in the adult rat brain, undifferentiated NSCs show some promise in treatment of PD. Human NSCs transplanted into the rat brain migrate and differentiate to neurons in a site-specific manner. Moreover, in PD rats with depleted host DA levels, engrafted NSCs were sensitive to environmental factors, appearing to differentiate preferentially to DA neurons.

NSCs can also be modified to overexpress the neurotrophic factors, which can increase the survival of the transplanted cells. Cai et al. studied some homeodomain proteins selectively expressed in DA progenitor cells in the ventral midbrain, and found that Lmx1a and Msx1 function as key factors triggering generation of DA neurons. Overexpressing the transcription factor ASCL1 was reported to be able to regain neurogenesis from human neural progenitor cells and to produce larger neurons with more neurites [27]. Animal study showed that forcing expression of Nurr1 promoted the mouse NSCs to differentiate into DA neurons and survive in 6-OHDA-lesioned PD rats. After transplantation of rodent and human fetal brain dopamine neurons to the midbrain of the 6-OHDA-lesioned rats, the cells survived well in the host brains and the motor defects of the PD rats were improved [28, 29]. Based on the results of animal studies, Lindvall et al. started the first clinical trials by transplanting fetal dopaminergic neurons or tissue to PD patients. Since then the clinical assessment protocols have been modified and significant effects were found by detecting behavioral and histological improvement [30, 31]. Moreover, younger PD patients showed more significant improvements, implying that the treatment efficiency may be limited in certain subpopulations. Generally, long-term graft survival was poor and did not convincingly justify the use of three to five human embryos per procedure [32]. In general, variable functional outcome has been showed from the clinical trials, but solid improvements need to be determined by clinical and imaging evaluations in the future [33, 34]. Transplantation of NSCs in PD patients also showed some side-effects. Olanow et al. reported that 56% of patients transplanted with fetal midbrain tissue developed persistent dyskinesia after overnight withdrawal of dopaminergic medication [35], which was much more than Freed et al.'s result of 15% of patients showing dyskinesias [31]. Its exact prevalence may be argued, while the recurrence of dyskinesia following neural transplantation has been well-proved. Some evidence showed that grafts containing serotonin neurons were easier to have this detrimental effect, therefore dyskinesias symptom may be alleviated by ensuring a homogeneous cell population in transplanted tissue [36].

Long-term follow-up results were shown in three individual clinical studies. One study found transplanted fetal midbrain DA neurons survived up to 14 years without pathology [37], whereas others found that α-synuclein-positive Lewy bodies in eventual spread to the transplanted DA neurons in PD patients [38, 39]. These findings suggest that PD can be an ongoing process with pathological changes. The controversy may be the reason of the difference between environmentally and genetically caused PD—a case of PD caused by environmental factors might be cured by the infusion of healthy cells, whereas a case of PD, which has been caused by genetic mutations would be an ongoing process. In general, DA neuron engraftment cannot be stated as a universally permanent treatment for PD; follow-up implantations may be further required for optimal effectiveness. Like all other allogeneic treatments, there is also a risk of graft rejection which must be repressed in the study [40]. Overall, the clinical trials with NSCs of fetal brains showed the survival of the transplanted cells and some improvements of symptoms in PD patients, whereas some results are over in dispute because of the diversities or limited cases of the PD patients [34]. **Table 1** summarized some of the clinical trials with fetal brain-derived NSCs or dopamine neurons.

No. of patients transplanted with NSC	Observation time	Symptom improvement 0/0	Side effect of dyskinesia	References and publication year
1	12 months	1/1	No	[41]
6	10–72 months	4/6	No	[42]
5	18–24 months	2/5	No	[43]
20/40	3 years	17/20	No	[31]
23/34	24 months	6/23	Yes	[35]
2	8 years	2/2	Yes	[44]
5	9–14 years	Not available	Not available	[37]
1	14 years	1/1	Yes	[39]
2	11–16 years	Not available	Not available	[38]
33	2–4 years	45%	Not available	[45]
3	13–16 years	Yes	Not available	[46]
2	18 and 15 years	2/2	Not available	[47]

Note: 23/34 indicates that 23 of 34 cases are in the group transplanted with NSCs and the other cases are in the control group.

Table 1. The clinical trials in PD patients transplanted with fetal brain-derived neural stem cells.

To further address the clinical therapeutic effects of the transplanted NSCs, and to provide new guidelines for clinical trials of fetal brain-derived cell therapy for PD treatment, a new, multicenter and collaborative study of European Union (TRANSEURO) was formed in 2010. These need careful selection of patients: early in the course of their disease (disease duration 2–10 years); aged 30–68 at the time of inclusion, showing a good response to levodopa; systematically evaluation of cell preparation, and location of transplantation; immunosuppression after transplantation and follow-up time; numbers of patients and clinical assessment standards. The new clinical trial for more than 100 patients suffered with PD has completed in this study, and results are in the analysis [48, 49].

4.3. Human embryonic stem cells (hESCs)-derived neural stem cells and dopamine neurons

Embryonic stem cells (ESCs) are self-renewing, pluripotent, and isolated from the inner cell mass cells of the preimplantation blastocysts. ESC can be differentiated into any kind of tissue cells including neural stem cells (NSCs), neurons, and DA neurons under special microenvironment. The differentiated neural stem cells, or fully differentiated neurons and dopamine neurons from mouse embryonic stem cell have been proved to have effects for PD neuroprotection [50].

Originally, human embryonic stem cells (hESCs) were isolated through culturing inner cell mass cells using mouse embryonic fibroblasts (MEFs) as feeder cells [51]. Since then, many groups have developed methods to direct the hESC differentiation to the neural stem cells and neurons, in particular dopamine neurons for the treatment of PD. Cooper et al. employed sonic hedgehog (SHH) and FGF8a as patterning factors in DA neuron induction [52]. The differentiation of hESCs to mesencephalic dopamine neurons was promoted by the application of specific patterning molecules that regulate mesencephalon development [53] or by applying growth factors SHH and FGF8a in a specific sequence [54]. Early exposure of FGF8a and SHH instructs early precursors to adopt a region identity which promotes DA neuron differentiation from mesencephalic neuroepithelial cells. These hESC-derived dopamine neurons were able to improve the motor deficiency of PD rat models, suggesting that grafted hESC-derived dopamine neurons played a role in vivo. The efficiency of DA production from pluripotent stem cells was greatly improved by Chamber et al. using a developed protocol through inhibiting SMAD signaling using Noggin and SB431542, with enhancing survival of mesencephalic DA neurons from hESCs [55]. They found that addition of Noggin and SB431542 for inhibiting SMAD signaling is sufficient to induce complete neural conversion of more than 80% of hESCs under adherent culture conditions. Fasano et al. found complimentary results, showing that neurons in development did not form toward anterior regionalization, but may be shifted toward a midbrain-like identity after FGF8 or Wnt1 treatment [56]. The same group developed a floor-plate-based protocol for generating hESCs-derived DA neurons in differentiation medium containing activators of sonic hedgehog (SHH) and canonical WNT signaling in vitro, further improved complete conversion of hESCs to the dopamine neurons and decreased the teratoma formation in vivo. They found that these DA neurons efficiently grew for several months in vitro and restored the amphetamine-induced rotation behaviors and improvements in tests of akinesia and forelimb use after transplanted to Parkinsonian monkeys and 6-OHDA-lesioned rats [57]. Sanchez-Danes et al. reported that using lentiviral expression of LMX1A, the key DA neuron-regulating gene, in hESCs to obtain more than 60% ventral mesencephalic DA neurons of the A9 subtype of all neurons differentiated from LMX1A-modified hESC [58]. Grealish et al. studied the functional properties of hESC-derived DA neurons in vivo by implanting hESC-derived mesencephalic dopamine neurons and fetal brain DA neurons into the brains of PD rats. They found that grafted hESC-DA neurons survived, projected long neural branches and played functions to improve the locomotive deficits of PD rats as similar as fetal brain DA neurons by MRI and PET imaging analysis, which provided further preclinical basis of hESC-derived dopamine neurons for PD patients' treatment [59].

To dissolve the major concerns for clinical use with stromal cells as feeder cells for culturing hESCs, some groups developed the implementation of factors which substitute for feeder cells. For example, Schulz et al. used a serum-free suspension system for generating the neurons, which are clinically applicable use [60]. Vazin et al. succeeded in substituting growth factors SDF-1, PTN, IGF2, and EFNB1 for the PA6 stromal cells, resulting in the induction of differentiating hESCs directly to TH-positive DA neurons without requiring this initial induction step [61]. During differentiating hESCs to NSCs, Swistowski et al. reported that growth factors SHH and FGF8 substitute for PA6 stromal cells for generating DA cells after an initial induction step. They endeavored a culture protocol applicable to the clinic and following to the standards of good manufacturing protocol (GMP). In their culture process, serum is not involved, but they found cells could be stored at each of the intermediate stages in their four-step process (propagation of ESC→generation of neural stem cells (NSC)→induction of dopaminergic precursors→maturation of dopaminergic neurons) without loss of functional ability, which is an important discovery that allowing cells to be transplanted at an appropriate time point in neural development [62].

Though many studies demonstrated hESCs can be differentiated to DA neurons efficiently in vitro and showed solid functional results to restore the motor defects in PD animal models including mice, rats, and nonhuman primates, clinical trials have not been performed for treating the PD patients because of the immune-rejection and ethical issues.

4.4. Induced pluripotent stem cells (iPSCs)-derived neural stem cells or dopamine neurons

Previous studies showed an undifferentiated state of cells could be reprogrammed from differentiated somatic cells using the somatic cell nuclear transfer (SCNT). SCNT technology is available to make the cloned lambs and cows. However, no studies were described generating patient-specific cells using this SCNT technique [63, 64]. The successful induction of mouse iPSCs from mouse embryonic and adult fibroblasts were first demonstrated in Yamanaka lab in 2006 by introducing four transcription factors of Oct3/4, Sox2, c-Myc, and Klf4 [65]. Soon afterward, human iPSCs and patient-specific iPSCs with different diseases including PD were also generated from several labs by introducing the human orthologs of these four transcription factors (OCT4, SOX2, c-MYC, and KLF4) or OCT4, SOX2, NANOG, and LIN28 [66, 67]. The implication of Oct3/4 and Sox2 was shown to play an essential role in the propagation of undifferentiated ESCs in culture. The roles of Klf4 and c-Myc were equally undecided. Later studies described that the only genes indispensable in generating iPSCs were Oct3/4 and Sox2 but not Klf4 and c-Myc [68]. Similar to ESCs, iPSCs are self-renew indefinitely and pluripotent. However, iPSCs overcome the problems associated with BM-MSCs, fetal NSCs and hESCs, as they reprogram from the already-differentiated somatic cells of an organism back to their embryonic-like pluripotent state. iPSCs generated from patients will have wide applications for exploring the molecular mechanisms and cell-based therapy of neurodegenerative diseases such as PD [69, 70].

In clinical applications, one of the major advantages of iPSCs over BM-MSCs, fetal NSCs, and hESCs is that iPSCs can be generated from the cells of the individual being treated. As the cultured cells will be autologous, this key trait of iPSCs theoretically enhances their integration into the brain tissues of PD patients and minimizes the risk of rejection. Furthermore, the ethical problems of using aborted fetuses as a cell source are avoided. Once reprogrammed into iPSC state from the mature cells, the iPSCs can be systematically exposed to specific factors that promote their differentiation into a specific lineage (such as NSCs or DA neurons) [71]. Until now, a ton of work has been done to improve the generation, differentiation, and potential clinical applications of iPSCs, especially with great efforts made to bring these therapeutic cells to meet GMP (good manufacturing practice) standards, to translate them to the clinic for treatment of neurodegenerative diseases like PD. iPSCs have also been used in other fields such as diseases model to study the molecular mechanisms of the disease and as drug screening and discovery.

To determine the clinical potential of iPSCs-derived cells, the therapeutic effects of mouse iPSCs were analyzed after transplanting them into the rat brains. Wernig et al. reported that grafted iPSCs matured into midbrain-like dopamine neurons, resulting in behavioral improvements in rat PD models [72].

It was found that DA neurons from the iPSCs with LRRK2 mutation (G2019S) were sensitive to oxidative stress and had α-synuclein aggregation and more expression of key oxidative stress-response genes. The phenotypic neurodegeneration of the differentiated DA neurons could be rescued by correction of LRRK2 G2019S mutation in iPSCs, supporting LRRK2 mutation playing an important role in the pathogenesis of PD [73]. The virus-free PD-iPS cells-derived DA neurons were transplanted to the 6-OHDA-lesioned rats and it was found that these DA neurons survived and provided functional improvements in PD rats by alleviating motor defects induced by apomorphine [74]. Recently, our lab made efforts to generate of iPS cells by retrovirus-mediated expression of OCT4, SOX2, c-MYC, and KLF4 from skin fibroblasts of PD patients and control individuals, and studied the differentiation of iPSCs to NSCs and DA neurons, and then transplanted the iPSCs-derived NSCs into the striatums of the 6-OHDA-induced PD rats. iPSCs carrying the transgenes can also be differentiated to the NSCs and be fully differentiated to neurons and DA neurons in vitro and in vivo. The grafted iPS cells-derived NSCs significantly improved the rotational asymmetry of PD rats [4]. Further work are needed to improve the differentiation efficiency of neurons and DA neurons by incorporating growth factors and iPSCs together for transplantation, or elevating the dose of immune-suppressive agents to lower the immune-rejection against the human-derived cells, or renewing the cell culture protocols.

Much work has been done toward improving the efficiency of iPSCs generation in absence of c-Myc. Stadtfeld et al. reprogrammed mouse liver cells into iPSCs using nonintegrating, replication-incompetent adenoviruses carrying the classic four transcription factors [75]. Okita et al. developed an approach that repeated transfection of plasmids containing the appropriate genes (one containing the complementary DNAs of Oct3/4, SOx2, and Klf4; the other, c-Myc) into embryonic fibroblasts could generate iPSCs [76]. Yu et al. developed a further protocol to iPSC generation by using nonintegrating episomal vectors, which allows the derivation of iPSCs free of vector and transgene sequences completely [77]. The direct protein transduction system free of DNA vector was also proposed to generate iPSCs to remove potential risks in association with chromosomal integrations and mutations [78].

This claim is verified by the follow-up study through comparing the cellular properties of human iPSCs (hiPSC) generated by chromosome integrating with nonintegrating methods. They found consistent differences in cellular and differentiation properties between hiPSCs from nonintegrating and integrating reprogramming factors. According to their results, protein-based reprogramming of cells into hiPSCs resulted in cells showed no obvious exogenous reprogramming gene expression, therefore behaved most similar to hESCs [79].

Many efforts have been done to achieve clinical-grade DA neurons with a stable phenotype, the A9 subtype DA neurons. From both human ES/iPS cells, a strategy for efficient differentiation and sorting DA neurons has been developed by Isacson et al. From iPSC-differentiated neural cells, the NCAM (+)/CD29 (low)-enriched ventral mesencephalic DA neurons were sorted. The sorted neurons were positive for EN1/TH and FOXA2/TH and had elevated expression levels of GIRK2, FOXA2, PITX3, LMX1A, NURR1, TH, and EN1 which indicated that the sorted neural cells are DA neurons. These iPSC-derived DA neurons were able to restore behavior activity of PD rats after transplantation. The sorted cells transplanted to the PD rats were integrated into the brain tissue. Their results provided molecular basis for the safety and feasibility of iPSC-derived cell therapies [80].

The similarity and differences between iPSCs and ESC is another issue about iPSCs. Many studies succeeded in generating both human iPSCs and mouse iPSCs identical to ESCs developmentally and epigenetically by improving end points for the reprogramming process [81]. Other groups have also made modifications to reduce the mutagenic potential of the lentiviruses and retroviruses By using non-integrating methods or omitting the KLF4 or c-MYC. For instance, Muller et al. found that substituting Nanog and Lin28 for Klf4 and c-Myc [67] was one way to reduce this risk. The reactivation of the c-Myc retrovirus particularly promotes the risk of mutations, because of tumorigenicity [82]. However, the efficiency of iPSC formation was far lower after eliminations of c-Myc from the protocol. This suggests that the role of c-Myc is not being necessary in the establishing pluripotency itself but to accelerate proliferation or otherwise enhance the speed of events establishing pluripotency [83]. Although the generated iPSCs in morphology, growth properties, and differentiation into different germ layers were very similar to ESCs, differences between iPSCs and ESCs were detected, which may be the reason by using different iPSC lines [84]. Recently at the molecular levels, the similarity and difference between iPSCs and hESCs were studied. In one study, Koyanagi-Aoi et al found that only two hiPSC lines had different gene expression and DNA methylation through analyzing 49 hiPSC lines and 10 hESC lines. And they found that only seven hiPSC lines formed some undifferentiated cells by comparing neural differentiation in vitro between 40 hiPSC lines and 10 hESC lines. This study showed that hiPSCs are very similar to hESCs [85].

The important point is that such protocols need to meet a xeno-free, scalable system for the clinic. A suspension culture system was created for the neural differentiation of hESCs and hiPSCs [86]. Such systems allowed long-term cell culture while keeping appropriate marker expression, normal karyotype, and pluripotency. To decrease the effects of transgenes on iPSCs functions, several labs developed protocols to use two or three factors to generate iPSCs. Using single factor of OCT4 in combination of small molecules of VPA, TGF-β inhibitor (616452), CHIR 99021, iPSCs can be reprogrammed from mouse adult and embryonic fibroblasts [68]. Omitting the OCT4, the naive iPSCs derived from rhesus monkey fibroblasts can be obtained with only small molecules, which provided a valuable cell source for further use in disease modeling and preclinical study [87]. Though iPSCs bring great potentials to the cell-based PD therapy, much work is needed for the researchers to find other convenient method to obtain DA neurons as the complicated procedures for generation, characterization, and differentiation to the DA neurons. Directly reprograming the fibroblasts of PD patients to DA neurons is one of the other approaches. Using different combinations of transcription factors such as Nurr1 (Nr4a2), Mash1 (Ascl1), Sox2, Ngn2, Lmx1a, and Pitx3, DA neurons were directly reprogrammed from the fibroblasts [88, 89]. Since the lentiviral vectors were used to express the genes related in most direct reprogramming methods for development of DA neurons, this can cause the safety concerns for use of the directly reprogrammed DA neurons in PD patients. However, the research advance will overcome these issues and finally bring these cells to clinical trials for PD.

5. Future aspects and challenges for clinical application of iPSCs

The NSCs and DA neurons from fetal brain and hESCs are not suitable for wide clinical use because of their immune-rejections and ethical issues. The availability of iPSCs has great potential for autologous cell-based therapy of PD. The treatment of eye-disorders using iPSCs for clinical trial has been initiated in Japan. However, several aspects of iPSCs are further needed to be resolved for clinical use. These include genetic and epigenetic abnormalities, low yields of DA neurons, and the safety of iPSC-derived cells.

5.1. Low yield

Low yield of fully reprogrammed cells is by no means an inherent property of iPSC generation and there will continue to be yield improvements in the future. Low yield is a potential problem, addition of VPA and other chemicals increased the original yields of 0.05% [90]. iPSCs can theoretically be sourced from anywhere on the adult human, such as stomach cells, liver cells, and human hair cells, with varying yields across experiments [75]. In fact, Aasen et al. generated keratinocyte-derived iPSCs using cells from adult human hairs with a 100-fold increase in efficiency compared to human fibroblast reprogramming, and found these iPSCs were indistinguishable from ESCs [91]. In any case, with the goal of optimizing methods for maximum cell yield of iPS cells, avenues must include comparisons between method efficiencies in the future.

5.2. Genetic and epigenetic abnormalities

It is unclear whether iPSCs cells toward a cell fate related to their donor source or otherwise maintaining a reprogramming signature after differentiation [92]. For the generation of clinical applicable iPS cells, the lentivirus or retrovirus-mediated reprogramming methods should be replaced by nonintegrating vectors to express the reprogramming genes or combine with small molecules [93]. Some iPSCs from PD patients may also have gene mutations such as chromosomal structure variation, point mutation, gene deletions, and duplications [12, 94]. It is not suitable to use the cells derived from iPSCs with genetic mutations for direct transplantation as the functions of cells are affected by the genetic mutations. Many reports developed protocols to correct the mutation in PD patient-derived iPSCs. Reinhardt et al. showed that iPSCs with *LRRK2* G2019S mutation was corrected and the *LRRK2* correction produced phenotype rescue in differentiated neurons [73]. Soldner et al. reported that the iPSCs with *SNCA* mutation (A53T) was repaired using zinc-finger nuclease (ZFN)-mediated nuclease approach and genetic repair of the A53T mutation in the patient-derived iPSCs did not affect the differentiation ability to dopaminergic neurons. The correctly repaired patient-derived iPSC lines were confirmed through PCR genotyping and sequencing analysis [95].

5.3. Safety and purity

It is required that the residues of undifferentiated iPSCs should be less than 1% to avoid the teratoma formation after transplantation, in the aim to obtain iPSC-derived NSCs or DA neurons for transplantation. FACS or other noninvasive magnetic selections were used for developing the approaches to sort the iPSC-derived cells. Moreover, the cell culture in feeder-free conditions are needed to avoid the contamination of animal sources. Currently, murine-derived feeder cells are widely used to maintain hESCs and hiPSCs. In addition, these feeder cells are normally cultured in culture medium including fetal bovine serum (FBS). This would enhance the possibility to cause the allogenic cell contamination of the iPSC-derived cells. Nakagawa et al. developed a new feeder-free system to culture the hESCs and iPSCs in StemFit™ medium, which made a big step to make clinically applicable GMP-standard cells [96].

6. Conclusion: moving forward to the clinic

Cell-based therapy holds clinical potential for the treatment of many neurodegenerative disorders including PD. The use of BM-MSCs, fetal NSCs, and ESCs is facing with safety and ethical concerns. However, recently great advance is making in developing iPSC-derived cells for PD. Animal studies using injection iPSCs and their derivatives into animal models have shown promise in treatment of disorders such as PD. However in clinical trials for PD, iPSCs have not been used until their limitations are overcome. Therefore, a relevant therapeutic progenitor or mature cell type may be identified and grafted in such treatments; in the case of PD, the options are of course iPSC-derived DA neurons and iPSC-derived NSCs.

Acknowledgements

This work was supported by National Natural Science Foundation of China (NSFC 81571241) and Program of high-educated Foreign Scholars, Shandong Province, China (201309116SDWZ). The author also thanks Jing Duan and Qingfa Chen for their technical and editing the manuscript.

Author details

Fabin Han*

Address all correspondence to: fhan2013@126.com

The Institute for Tissue Engineering and Regenerative Medicine, Liaocheng University/The Liaocheng People's Hospital, Shandong, China

References

[1] Berg, D., R.B. Postuma, B. Bloem, P. Chan, B. Dubois, T. Gasser, C.G. Goetz, G.M. Halliday, J. Hardy, A.E. Lang, I. Litvan, K. Marek, J. Obeso, W. Oertel, C.W. Olanow, W. Poewe, M. Stern, and G. Deuschl. Time to redefine PD? Introductory statement of the MDS Task Force on the definition of Parkinson's disease. Mov Disord. 2014; 29(4): 454–62.

[2] Olanow, C.W., R.L. Watts, and W.C. Koller. An algorithm (decision tree) for the management of Parkinson's disease (2001): treatment guidelines. Neurology. 2001; 56(11 Suppl 5): S1–S88.

[3] Takahashi, K., K. Tanabe, M. Ohnuki, M. Narita, T. Ichisaka, K. Tomoda, and S. Yamanaka. Induction of pluripotent stem cells from adult human fibroblasts by defined factors. Cell. 2007; 131(5): 861–72.

[4] Han, F., W. Wang, B. Chen, C. Chen, S. Li, X. Lu, J. Duan, Y. Zhang, Y.A. Zhang, W. Guo, and G. Li. Human induced pluripotent stem cell–derived neurons improve motor asymmetry in a 6-hydroxydopamine–induced rat model of Parkinson's disease. Cytotherapy. 2015; 17(5): 665–79.

[5] Lesage, S. and A. Brice. Parkinson's disease: from monogenic forms to genetic susceptibility factors. Hum Mol Genet. 2009; 18(R1): R48–59.

[6] Chen, M.L., C.H. Lin, M.J. Lee, and R.M. Wu. BST1 rs11724635 interacts with environmental factors to increase the risk of Parkinson's disease in a Taiwanese population. Parkinsonism Relat Disord. 2014; 20(3): 280–3.

[7] Tanner, C.M., R. Ottman, S.M. Goldman, J. Ellenberg, P. Chan, R. Mayeux, and J.W. Langston. Parkinson disease in twins: an etiologic study. JAMA. 1999; 281(4): 341–6.

[8] Polymeropoulos, M.H., C. Lavedan, E. Leroy, S.E. Ide, A. Dehejia, A. Dutra, B. Pike, H. Root, J. Rubenstein, R. Boyer, E.S. Stenroos, S. Chandrasekharappa, A. Athanassiadou, T. Papapetropoulos, W.G. Johnson, A.M. Lazzarini, R.C. Duvoisin, G. Di Iorio, L.I. Golbe, and R.L. Nussbaum. Mutation in the alpha-synuclein gene identified in families with Parkinson's disease. Science. 1997; 276(5321): 2045–7.

[9] Grimes, D.A., L. Racacho, F. Han, M. Panisset, and D.E. Bulman. LRRK2 screening in a Canadian Parkinson's disease cohort. Can J Neurol Sci. 2007; 34(3): 336–8.

[10] Martin, I., J.W. Kim, V.L. Dawson, and T.M. Dawson. LRRK2 pathobiology in Parkinson's disease. J Neurochem. 2014; 131(5): 554–65.

[11] Grimes, D.A., F. Han, M. Panisset, L. Racacho, F. Xiao, R. Zou, K. Westaff, and D.E. Bulman. Translated mutation in the Nurr1 gene as a cause for Parkinson's disease. Mov Disord. 2006; 21(7): 906–9.

[12] Yu, Z., T. Wang, J. Xu, W. Wang, G. Wang, C. Chen, L. Zheng, L. Pan, D. Gong, X. Li, H. Qu, F. Li, B. Zhang, W. Le, and F. Han. Mutations in the glucocerebrosidase gene are responsible for Chinese patients with Parkinson's disease. J Hum Genet. 2015; 60(2): 85–90.

[13] Dawson, T.M., H.S. Ko, and V.L. Dawson. Genetic animal models of Parkinson's disease. Neuron. 2010; 66(5): 646–61.

[14] Gonzalez-Horta, A. The Interaction of Alpha-synuclein with Membranes and its Implication in Parkinson's Disease: a literature review. Nat Prod Commun. 2015; 10(10): 1775–8.

[15] Fares, M.B., N. Ait-Bouziad, I. Dikiy, M.K. Mbefo, A. Jovicic, A. Kiely, J.L. Holton, S.J. Lee, A.D. Gitler, D. Eliezer, and H.A. Lashuel. The novel Parkinson's disease linked mutation G51D attenuates in vitro aggregation and membrane binding of alpha-synuclein, and enhances its secretion and nuclear localization in cells. Hum Mol Genet. 2014; 23(17): 4491–509.

[16] Mazzulli, J.R., F. Zunke, O. Isacson, L. Studer, and D. Krainc. alpha-Synuclein-induced lysosomal dysfunction occurs through disruptions in protein trafficking in human midbrain synucleinopathy models. Proc Natl Acad Sci U S A. 2016; 113(7): 1931–6.

[17] Blanz, J. and P. Saftig. Parkinson's disease: acid-glucocerebrosidase activity and alpha-synuclein clearance. J Neurochem. 2016.

[18] Hass, R., C. Kasper, S. Bohm, and R. Jacobs. Different populations and sources of human mesenchymal stem cells (MSC): a comparison of adult and neonatal tissue-derived MSC. Cell Commun Signal. 2011; 9: 12.

[19] Park, H.J., P.H. Lee, O.Y. Bang, G. Lee, and Y.H. Ahn. Mesenchymal stem cells therapy exerts neuroprotection in a progressive animal model of Parkinson's disease. J Neurochem. 2008; 107(1): 141–51.

[20] Blandini, F., L. Cova, M.T. Armentero, E. Zennaro, G. Levandis, P. Bossolasco, C. Calzarossa, M. Mellone, B. Giuseppe, G.L. Deliliers, E. Polli, G. Nappi, and V. Silani. Transplantation of undifferentiated human mesenchymal stem cells protects against 6-hydroxydopamine neurotoxicity in the rat. Cell Transplant. 2010; 19(2): 203–17.

[21] Park, K.W., M.A. Eglitis, and M.M. Mouradian. Protection of nigral neurons by GDNF-engineered marrow cell transplantation. Neurosci Res. 2001; 40(4): 315–23.

[22] Barzilay, R., T. Ben-Zur, S. Bulvik, E. Melamed, and D. Offen. Lentiviral delivery of LMX1a enhances dopaminergic phenotype in differentiated human bone marrow mesenchymal stem cells. Stem Cells Dev. 2009; 18(4): 591–601.

[23] Wang, W.P., Z.L. He, S.Y. Lu, M. Yan, Y. Zhou, T.H. Xie, N. Yin, W.J. Wang, D.H. Tang, H.J. Li, and M.S. Sun. Dopaminergic neuron-like cells derived from bone marrow mesenchymal stem cells by Lmx1alpha and neurturin overexpression for autologous cytotherapy in hemiparkinsonian rhesus monkeys. Curr Stem Cell Res Ther. 2015; 10(2): 109–20.

[24] Eriksson, P.S., E. Perfilieva, T. Bjork-Eriksson, A.M. Alborn, C. Nordborg, D.A. Peterson, and F.H. Gage. Neurogenesis in the adult human hippocampus. Nat Med. 1998; 4(11): 1313–7.

[25] Taupin, P. and F.H. Gage. Adult neurogenesis and neural stem cells of the central nervous system in mammals. J Neurosci Res. 2002; 69(6): 745–9.

[26] Kallur, T., V. Darsalia, O. Lindvall, and Z. Kokaia. Human fetal cortical and striatal neural stem cells generate region-specific neurons in vitro and differentiate extensively to neurons after intrastriatal transplantation in neonatal rats. J Neurosci Res. 2006; 84(8): 1630–44.

[27] Kim, H.J., E. McMillan, F. Han, and C.N. Svendsen. Regionally specified human neural progenitor cells derived from the mesencephalon and forebrain undergo increased neurogenesis following overexpression of ASCL1. Stem cells. 2009; 27(2): 390–8.

[28] Studer, L., V. Tabar, and R.D. McKay. Transplantation of expanded mesencephalic precursors leads to recovery in parkinsonian rats. Nat Neurosci. 1998; 1(4): 290–5.

[29] Monni, E., C. Cusulin, M. Cavallaro, O. Lindvall, and Z. Kokaia. Human fetal striatum-derived neural stem (NS) cells differentiate to mature neurons in vitro and in vivo. Curr Stem Cell Res Ther. 2014; 9(4): 338–46.

[30] Lindvall, O., G. Sawle, H. Widner, J.C. Rothwell, A. Bjorklund, D. Brooks, P. Brundin, R. Frackowiak, C.D. Marsden, P. Odin, et al. Evidence for long-term survival and function of dopaminergic grafts in progressive Parkinson's disease. Ann Neurol. 1994; 35(2): 172–80.

[31] Freed, C.R., P.E. Greene, R.E. Breeze, W.Y. Tsai, W. DuMouchel, R. Kao, S. Dillon, H. Winfield, S. Culver, J.Q. Trojanowski, D. Eidelberg, and S. Fahn. Transplantation of embryonic dopamine neurons for severe Parkinson's disease. N Engl J Med. 2001; 344(10): 710–9.

[32] Hagell, P. and P. Brundin. Cell survival and clinical outcome following intrastriatal transplantation in Parkinson disease. J Neuropathol Exp Neurol. 2001; 60(8): 741–52.

[33] Lindvall, O. and A. Bjorklund. Cell therapy in Parkinson's disease. NeuroRx. 2004; 1(4): 382–93.

[34] Barker, R.A., J. Barrett, S.L. Mason, and A. Bjorklund. Fetal dopaminergic transplantation trials and the future of neural grafting in Parkinson's disease. Lancet Neurol. 2013; 12(1): 84–91.

[35] Olanow, C.W., C.G. Goetz, J.H. Kordower, A.J. Stoessl, V. Sossi, M.F. Brin, K.M. Shannon, G.M. Nauert, D.P. Perl, J. Godbold, and T.B. Freeman. A double-blind controlled trial of bilateral fetal nigral transplantation in Parkinson's disease. Ann Neurol. 2003; 54(3): 403–14.

[36] Politis, M., K. Wu, C. Loane, N.P. Quinn, D.J. Brooks, S. Rehncrona, A. Bjorklund, O. Lindvall, and P. Piccini. Serotonergic neurons mediate dyskinesia side effects in Parkinson's patients with neural transplants. Sci Transl Med. 2010; 2(38): 38ra46.

[37] Mendez, I., A. Viñuela, A. Astradsson, K. Mukhida, P. Hallett, H. Robertson, T. Tierney, R. Holness, A. Dagher, and J.Q. Trojanowski. Dopamine neurons implanted into people with Parkinson's disease survive without pathology for 14 years. Nat Med. 2008; 14(5): 507.

[38] Li, J.Y., E. Englund, J.L. Holton, D. Soulet, P. Hagell, A.J. Lees, T. Lashley, N.P. Quinn, S. Rehncrona, A. Bjorklund, H. Widner, T. Revesz, O. Lindvall, and P. Brundin. Lewy bodies in grafted neurons in subjects with Parkinson's disease suggest host-to-graft disease propagation. Nat Med. 2008; 14(5): 501–3.

[39] Kordower, J.H., Y. Chu, R.A. Hauser, T.B. Freeman, and C.W. Olanow. Lewy body-like pathology in long-term embryonic nigral transplants in Parkinson's disease. Nat Med. 2008; 14(5): 504–6.

[40] Michel-Monigadon, D., V. Nerriere-Daguin, X. Leveque, M. Plat, E. Venturi, P. Brachet, P. Naveilhan, and I. Neveu. Minocycline promotes long-term survival of neuronal

transplant in the brain by inhibiting late microglial activation and T-cell recruitment. Transplantation. 2010; 89(7): 816–23.

[41] Lindvall, O., P. Brundin, H. Widner, S. Rehncrona, B. Gustavii, R. Frackowiak, K.L. Leenders, G. Sawle, J.C. Rothwell, C.D. Marsden, and et al. Grafts of fetal dopamine neurons survive and improve motor function in Parkinson's disease. Science. 1990; 247(4942): 574–7.

[42] Wenning, G.K., P. Odin, P. Morrish, S. Rehncrona, H. Widner, P. Brundin, J.C. Rothwell, R. Brown, B. Gustavii, P. Hagell, M. Jahanshahi, G. Sawle, A. Bjorklund, D.J. Brooks, C.D. Marsden, N.P. Quinn, and O. Lindvall. Short- and long-term survival and function of unilateral intrastriatal dopaminergic grafts in Parkinson's disease. Ann Neurol. 1997; 42(1): 95–107.

[43] Hagell, P., A. Schrag, P. Piccini, M. Jahanshahi, R. Brown, S. Rehncrona, H. Widner, P. Brundin, J.C. Rothwell, P. Odin, G.K. Wenning, P. Morrish, B. Gustavii, A. Bjorklund, D.J. Brooks, C.D. Marsden, N.P. Quinn, and O. Lindvall. Sequential bilateral transplantation in Parkinson's disease: effects of the second graft. Brain. 1999; 122 (Pt 6): 1121–32.

[44] Pogarell, O., W. Koch, F.J. Gildehaus, A. Kupsch, O. Lindvall, W.H. Oertel, and K. Tatsch. Long-term assessment of striatal dopamine transporters in Parkinsonian patients with intrastriatal embryonic mesencephalic grafts. Eur J Nucl Med Mol Imaging. 2006; 33(4): 407–11.

[45] Ma, Y., C. Tang, T. Chaly, P. Greene, R. Breeze, S. Fahn, C. Freed, V. Dhawan, and D. Eidelberg. Dopamine cell implantation in Parkinson's disease: long-term clinical and (18)F-FDOPA PET outcomes. J Nucl Med. 2010; 51(1): 7–15.

[46] Politis, M., K. Wu, C. Loane, N.P. Quinn, D.J. Brooks, W.H. Oertel, A. Bjorklund, O. Lindvall, and P. Piccini. Serotonin neuron loss and nonmotor symptoms continue in Parkinson's patients treated with dopamine grafts. Sci Transl Med. 2012; 4(128): 128ra41.

[47] Kefalopoulou, Z., M. Politis, P. Piccini, N. Mencacci, K. Bhatia, M. Jahanshahi, H. Widner, S. Rehncrona, P. Brundin, A. Bjorklund, O. Lindvall, P. Limousin, N. Quinn, and T. Foltynie. Long-term clinical outcome of fetal cell transplantation for Parkinson disease: two case reports. JAMA Neurol. 2014; 71(1): 83–7.

[48] Moore, S.F., N.V. Guzman, S.L. Mason, C.H. Williams-Gray, and R.A. Barker. Which patients with Parkinson's disease participate in clinical trials? One centre's experiences with a new cell based therapy trial (TRANSEURO). J Parkinsons Dis. 2014; 4(4): 671–6.

[49] Evans, J.R., S.L. Mason, and R.A. Barker. Current status of clinical trials of neural transplantation in Parkinson's disease. Prog Brain Res. 2012; 200: 169–98.

[50] Liu, T.W., Z.G. Ma, Y. Zhou, and J.X. Xie. Transplantation of mouse CGR8 embryonic stem cells producing GDNF and TH protects against 6-hydroxydopamine neurotoxicity in the rat. Int J Biochem Cell Biol. 2013; 45(7): 1265–73.

[51] Thomson, J.A., J. Itskovitz-Eldor, S.S. Shapiro, M.A. Waknitz, J.J. Swiergiel, V.S. Marshall, and J.M. Jones. Embryonic stem cell lines derived from human blastocysts. Science. 1998; 282(5391): 1145–1147.

[52] Cooper, O., G. Hargus, M. Deleidi, A. Blak, T. Osborn, E. Marlow, K. Lee, A. Levy, E. Perez-Torres, A. Yow, and O. Isacson. Differentiation of human ES and Parkinson's disease iPS cells into ventral midbrain dopaminergic neurons requires a high activity form of SHH, FGF8a and specific regionalization by retinoic acid. Mol Cell Neurosci. 2010; 45(3): 258–66.

[53] Zeng, X., J. Cai, J. Chen, Y. Luo, Z.B. You, E. Fotter, Y. Wang, B. Harvey, T. Miura, C. Backman, G.J. Chen, M.S. Rao, and W.J. Freed. Dopaminergic differentiation of human embryonic stem cells. Stem Cells. 2004; 22(6): 925–40.

[54] Yan, Y., D. Yang, E.D. Zarnowska, Z. Du, B. Werbel, C. Valliere, R.A. Pearce, J.A. Thomson, and S.C. Zhang. Directed differentiation of dopaminergic neuronal subtypes from human embryonic stem cells. Stem Cells. 2005; 23(6): 781–90.

[55] Chambers, S.M., C.A. Fasano, E.P. Papapetrou, M. Tomishima, M. Sadelain, and L. Studer. Highly efficient neural conversion of human ES and iPS cells by dual inhibition of SMAD signaling. Nat. Biotechnol. 2009; 27(3): 275–80.

[56] Fasano, C.A., S.M. Chambers, G. Lee, M.J. Tomishima, and L. Studer. Efficient derivation of functional floor plate tissue from human embryonic stem cells. Cell Stem Cell. 2010; 6(4): 336–47.

[57] Kriks, S., J.W. Shim, J. Piao, Y.M. Ganat, D.R. Wakeman, Z. Xie, L. Carrillo-Reid, G. Auyeung, C. Antonacci, A. Buch, L. Yang, M.F. Beal, D.J. Surmeier, J.H. Kordower, V. Tabar, and L. Studer. Dopamine neurons derived from human ES cells efficiently engraft in animal models of Parkinson's disease. Nature. 2011; 480(7378): 547–51.

[58] Sanchez-Danes, A., A. Consiglio, Y. Richaud, I. Rodriguez-Piza, B. Dehay, M. Edel, J. Bove, M. Memo, M. Vila, A. Raya, and J.C. Izpisua Belmonte. Efficient generation of A9 midbrain dopaminergic neurons by lentiviral delivery of LMX1A in human embryonic stem cells and induced pluripotent stem cells. Hum Gene Ther. 2012; 23(1): 56–69.

[59] Grealish, S., E. Diguet, A. Kirkeby, B. Mattsson, A. Heuer, Y. Bramoulle, N. Van Camp, A.L. Perrier, P. Hantraye, A. Bjorklund, and M. Parmar. Human ESC-derived dopamine neurons show similar preclinical efficacy and potency to fetal neurons when grafted in a rat model of Parkinson's disease. Cell Stem Cell. 2014; 15(5): 653–65.

[60] Schulz, T.C., S.A. Noggle, G.M. Palmarini, D.A. Weiler, I.G. Lyons, K.A. Pensa, A.C. Meedeniya, B.P. Davidson, N.A. Lambert, and B.G. Condie. Differentiation of human

embryonic stem cells to dopaminergic neurons in serum-free suspension culture. Stem Cells. 2004; 22(7): 1218–38.

[61] Vazin, T., K.G. Becker, J. Chen, C.E. Spivak, C.R. Lupica, Y. Zhang, L. Worden, and W.J. Freed. A novel combination of factors, termed SPIE, which promotes dopaminergic neuron differentiation from human embryonic stem cells. PLoS One. 2009; 4(8): e6606.

[62] Swistowski, A., J. Peng, Y. Han, A.M. Swistowska, M.S. Rao, and X. Zeng. Xeno-free defined conditions for culture of human embryonic stem cells, neural stem cells and dopaminergic neurons derived from them. PLoS One. 2009; 4(7): e6233.

[63] Wilmut, I., A.E. Schnieke, J. McWhir, A.J. Kind, and K.H. Campbell. Viable offspring derived from fetal and adult mammalian cells. Nature. 1997; 385(6619): 810–3.

[64] Jullien, J., V. Pasque, R.P. Halley-Stott, K. Miyamoto, and J.B. Gurdon. Mechanisms of nuclear reprogramming by eggs and oocytes: a deterministic process? Nat Rev Mol Cell Biol. 2011; 12(7): 453–9.

[65] Takahashi, K. and S. Yamanaka. Induction of pluripotent stem cells from mouse embryonic and adult fibroblast cultures by defined factors. Cell. 2006; 126(4): 663–76.

[66] Park, I.H., R. Zhao, J.A. West, A. Yabuuchi, H. Huo, T.A. Ince, P.H. Lerou, M.W. Lensch, and G.Q. Daley. Reprogramming of human somatic cells to pluripotency with defined factors. Nature. 2008; 451(7175): 141–6.

[67] Yu, J., M.A. Vodyanik, K. Smuga-Otto, J. Antosiewicz-Bourget, J.L. Frane, S. Tian, J. Nie, G.A. Jonsdottir, V. Ruotti, R. Stewart, Slukvin, II, and J.A. Thomson. Induced pluripotent stem cell lines derived from human somatic cells. Science. 2007; 318(5858): 1917–20.

[68] Li, Y., Q. Zhang, X. Yin, W. Yang, Y. Du, P. Hou, J. Ge, C. Liu, W. Zhang, X. Zhang, Y. Wu, H. Li, K. Liu, C. Wu, Z. Song, Y. Zhao, Y. Shi, and H. Deng. Generation of iPSCs from mouse fibroblasts with a single gene, Oct4, and small molecules. Cell Res. 2011; 21(1): 196–204.

[69] Isobe, K., Z. Cheng, N. Nishio, T. Suganya, Y. Tanaka, and S. Ito. Reprint of "iPSCs, aging and age-related diseases". N Biotechnol. 2015; 32(1): 169–79.

[70] Han, F. The Applications of the Induced Pluripotent Stem Cells in Studying the Neurodegenerative Diseases. Chin J Cell Biol. 2012; 34(5): 13.

[71] Kiskinis, E. and K. Eggan. Progress toward the clinical application of patient-specific pluripotent stem cells. J Clin Invest. 2010; 120(1): 51–9.

[72] Wernig, M., J.-P. Zhao, J. Pruszak, E. Hedlund, D. Fu, F. Soldner, V. Broccoli, M. Constantine-Paton, O. Isacson, and R. Jaenisch. Neurons derived from reprogrammed fibroblasts functionally integrate into the fetal brain and improve symptoms of rats with Parkinson's disease. Proc Natl Acad Sci. 2008; 105(15): 5856–61.

[73] Reinhardt, P., B. Schmid, L.F. Burbulla, D.C. Schondorf, L. Wagner, M. Glatza, S. Hoing, G. Hargus, S.A. Heck, A. Dhingra, G. Wu, S. Muller, K. Brockmann, T. Kluba, M. Maisel,

R. Kruger, D. Berg, Y. Tsytsyura, C.S. Thiel, O.E. Psathaki, J. Klingauf, T. Kuhlmann, M. Klewin, H. Muller, T. Gasser, H.R. Scholer, and J. Sterneckert. Genetic correction of a LRRK2 mutation in human iPSCs links parkinsonian neurodegeneration to ERK-dependent changes in gene expression. Cell Stem Cell. 2013; 12(3): 354–67.

[74] Hargus, G., O. Cooper, M. Deleidi, A. Levy, K. Lee, E. Marlow, A. Yow, F. Soldner, D. Hockemeyer, P.J. Hallett, T. Osborn, R. Jaenisch, and O. Isacson. Differentiated Parkinson patient-derived induced pluripotent stem cells grow in the adult rodent brain and reduce motor asymmetry in Parkinsonian rats. Proc Natl Acad Sci U S A. 2010; 107(36): 15921–6.

[75] Stadtfeld, M., M. Nagaya, J. Utikal, G. Weir, and K. Hochedlinger. Induced pluripotent stem cells generated without viral integration. Science. 2008; 322(5903): 945–9.

[76] Okita, K., M. Nakagawa, H. Hyenjong, T. Ichisaka, and S. Yamanaka. Generation of mouse induced pluripotent stem cells without viral vectors. Science. 2008; 322(5903): 949–53.

[77] Yu, J., K. Hu, K. Smuga-Otto, S. Tian, R. Stewart, Slukvin, II, and J.A. Thomson. Human induced pluripotent stem cells free of vector and transgene sequences. Science. 2009; 324(5928): 797–801.

[78] Kim, D., C.H. Kim, J.I. Moon, Y.G. Chung, M.Y. Chang, B.S. Han, S. Ko, E. Yang, K.Y. Cha, R. Lanza, and K.S. Kim. Generation of human induced pluripotent stem cells by direct delivery of reprogramming proteins. Cell Stem Cell. 2009; 4(6): 472–6.

[79] Rhee, Y.H., J.Y. Ko, M.Y. Chang, S.H. Yi, D. Kim, C.H. Kim, J.W. Shim, A.Y. Jo, B.W. Kim, H. Lee, S.H. Lee, W. Suh, C.H. Park, H.C. Koh, Y.S. Lee, R. Lanza, and K.S. Kim. Protein-based human iPS cells efficiently generate functional dopamine neurons and can treat a rat model of Parkinson disease. J Clin Invest. 2011; 121(6): 2326–35.

[80] Sundberg, M., H. Bogetofte, T. Lawson, J. Jansson, G. Smith, A. Astradsson, M. Moore, T. Osborn, O. Cooper, and R. Spealman. Improved cell therapy protocols for Parkinson's disease based on differentiation efficiency and safety of hESCcy ion -, and non-human primate iPSC-derived dopaminergic neurons. Stem Cells. 2013; 31(8): 1548–62.

[81] Maherali, N., R. Sridharan, W. Xie, J. Utikal, S. Eminli, K. Arnold, M. Stadtfeld, R. Yachechko, J. Tchieu, R. Jaenisch, K. Plath, and K. Hochedlinger. Directly reprogrammed fibroblasts show global epigenetic remodeling and widespread tissue contribution. Cell Stem Cell. 2007; 1(1): 55–70.

[82] Okita, K., T. Ichisaka, and S. Yamanaka. Generation of germline-competent induced pluripotent stem cells. Nature. 2007; 448(7151): 313–7.

[83] Muller, L.U., G.Q. Daley, and D.A. Williams. Upping the ante: recent advances in direct reprogramming. Mol Ther. 2009; 17(6): 947–53.

[84] Hu, B.Y., J.P. Weick, J. Yu, L.X. Ma, X.Q. Zhang, J.A. Thomson, and S.C. Zhang. Neural differentiation of human induced pluripotent stem cells follows developmental principles but with variable potency. Proc Natl Acad Sci U S A. 2010; 107(9): 4335–40.

[85] Koyanagi-Aoi, M., M. Ohnuki, K. Takahashi, K. Okita, H. Noma, Y. Sawamura, I. Teramoto, M. Narita, Y. Sato, T. Ichisaka, N. Amano, A. Watanabe, A. Morizane, Y. Yamada, T. Sato, J. Takahashi, and S. Yamanaka. Differentiation-defective phenotypes revealed by large-scale analyses of human pluripotent stem cells. Proc Natl Acad Sci U S A. 2013; 110(51): 20569–74.

[86] O'Brien, C. and A.L. Laslett. Suspended in culture--human pluripotent cells for scalable technologies. Stem Cell Res. 2012; 9(2): 167–70.

[87] Fang, R., K. Liu, Y. Zhao, H. Li, D. Zhu, Y. Du, C. Xiang, X. Li, H. Liu, Z. Miao, X. Zhang, Y. Shi, W. Yang, J. Xu, and H. Deng. Generation of naive induced pluripotent stem cells from rhesus monkey fibroblasts. Cell Stem Cell. 2014; 15(4): 488–96.

[88] Caiazzo, M., M.T. Dell'Anno, E. Dvoretskova, D. Lazarevic, S. Taverna, D. Leo, T.D. Sotnikova, A. Menegon, P. Roncaglia, G. Colciago, G. Russo, P. Carninci, G. Pezzoli, R.R. Gainetdinov, S. Gustincich, A. Dityatev, and V. Broccoli. Direct generation of functional dopaminergic neurons from mouse and human fibroblasts. Nature. 2011; 476(7359): 224–7.

[89] Kim, H.S., J. Kim, Y. Jo, D. Jeon, and Y.S. Cho. Direct lineage reprogramming of mouse fibroblasts to functional midbrain dopaminergic neuronal progenitors. Stem Cell Res. 2014; 12(1): 60–8.

[90] Wang, Q., X. Xu, J. Li, J. Liu, H. Gu, R. Zhang, J. Chen, Y. Kuang, J. Fei, C. Jiang, P. Wang, D. Pei, S. Ding, and X. Xie. Lithium, an anti-psychotic drug, greatly enhances the generation of induced pluripotent stem cells. Cell Res. 2011; 21(10): 1424–35.

[91] Aasen, T., A. Raya, M.J. Barrero, E. Garreta, A. Consiglio, F. Gonzalez, R. Vassena, J. Bilic, V. Pekarik, G. Tiscornia, M. Edel, S. Boue, and J.C. Izpisua Belmonte. Efficient and rapid generation of induced pluripotent stem cells from human keratinocytes. Nat Biotechnol. 2008; 26(11): 1276–84.

[92] Lister, R., M. Pelizzola, Y.S. Kida, R.D. Hawkins, J.R. Nery, G. Hon, J. Antosiewicz-Bourget, R. O'Malley, R. Castanon, S. Klugman, M. Downes, R. Yu, R. Stewart, B. Ren, J.A. Thomson, R.M. Evans, and J.R. Ecker. Hotspots of aberrant epigenomic reprogramming in human induced pluripotent stem cells. Nature. 2011; 471(7336): 68–73.

[93] Hou, P., Y. Li, X. Zhang, C. Liu, J. Guan, H. Li, T. Zhao, J. Ye, W. Yang, K. Liu, J. Ge, J. Xu, Q. Zhang, Y. Zhao, and H. Deng. Pluripotent stem cells induced from mouse somatic cells by small-molecule compounds. Science. 2013; 341(6146): 651–4.

[94] Laurent, L.C., I. Ulitsky, I. Slavin, H. Tran, A. Schork, R. Morey, C. Lynch, J.V. Harness, S. Lee, M.J. Barrero, S. Ku, M. Martynova, R. Semechkin, V. Galat, J. Gottesfeld, J.C. Izpisua Belmonte, C. Murry, H.S. Keirstead, H.S. Park, U. Schmidt, A.L. Laslett, F.J. Muller, C.M. Nievergelt, R. Shamir, and J.F. Loring. Dynamic changes in the copy

http://dx.doi.org/10.5772/63340

number of pluripotency and cell proliferation genes in human ESCs and iPSCs during reprogramming and time in culture. Cell Stem Cell. 2011; 8(1): 106–18.

[95] Soldner, F., J. Laganiere, A.W. Cheng, D. Hockemeyer, Q. Gao, R. Alagappan, V. Khurana, L.I. Golbe, R.H. Myers, S. Lindquist, L. Zhang, D. Guschin, L.K. Fong, B.J. Vu, X. Meng, F.D. Urnov, E.J. Rebar, P.D. Gregory, H.S. Zhang, and R. Jaenisch. Generation of isogenic pluripotent stem cells differing exclusively at two early onset Parkinson point mutations. Cell. 2011; 146(2): 318–31.

[96] Nakagawa, M., Y. Taniguchi, S. Senda, N. Takizawa, T. Ichisaka, K. Asano, A. Morizane, D. Doi, J. Takahashi, M. Nishizawa, Y. Yoshida, T. Toyoda, K. Osafune, K. Sekiguchi, and S. Yamanaka. A novel efficient feeder-free culture system for the derivation of human induced pluripotent stem cells. Sci Rep. 2014; 4: 3594.

Chapter 16

Surgical Therapy of Parkinson's Disease

Massimo Piacentino, Giacomo Beggio and
Lorenzo Volpin

Additional information is available at the end of the chapter

http://dx.doi.org/10.5772/62884

Abstract

The history of surgical treatment of Parkinson's disease (PD) covers more than 100 years. It started from lesional approach and evolved to the final deep brain stimulation (DBS) only in the 1990s. The aim of this treatment was to reduce clinical manifestation of PD and drug intake by acting directly on the altered motor pathways. The typical targets are represented by ventralis intermedius thalamic nucleus (VIM), internal globus pallidus nucleus (GPi), and subthalamic nucleus (STN) with more recent extension on other anatomical structures as pedunculopontine nucleus (PPN). Patients are selected according to CAPSIT protocol and undergo DBS when medical treatment has failed to effectively control the symptoms. Clinical benefits are represented by the reduction of "off" time and "on" time with dyskinesia. However, even DBS treatment is characterized by complications and side effects, as intracerebral hemorrhages, infections, ischemia, and seizures. The recent introduction of neuronavigation systems and the amelioration in neuroradiological imaging quality simplified preoperative DBS planning and consequently reduced surgical-related problems

Keywords: Deep brain stimulation, Parkinson surgical treatment, DBS target, surgical outcome, DBS complications

1. Introduction

The first experiences concerning surgical treatment of Parkinson's disease (PD) were made between the end of the nineteenth century and the beginning of twentieth century by Sir V. Horsely with surgery performed on cortical motor area. In the same period, Leriche et al. [1] attempted to improve rigidity and tremor by focusing on pyramidal tracts, in particular trying to interrupt abnormal motor signals by removing motor cortex, lesioning cervical spinal cord, or cerebral peduncle. Just before the World War II, the focus of surgical interest shifted to the basal ganglia with the work of Meyers on pallidofugal fibers and Russell, which completed a transventricular approach to remove the anterior two thirds of the caudate nucleus. However, the modern era can be traced by Spiegel [2] with the first stereotactic technique approaching globus pallidus (GPi). This author introduced the idea of a three-dimensional spatial target identification based on pneumoencephalography, ventriculography, and spatial relationship of targets in relation to a reference line connecting the foramen of Monro to the posterior commissure. In 1952, stereotactic thalamotomies were made in Freiburg, and between 1950 and 1960, surgical treatment of Parkinson was conducted in a quite homogeneous way by pallidotomy and thalamotomy with remarkable improvement of both tremor and rigidity. During the 1960s, the discovery of levodopa effect on PD symptoms induced a loss of interest on surgical treatment for almost three decades [3].

In the 1990s, the amelioration of diagnostic systems, with the introduction of computed tomography (CT), and the awareness of the inevitability of levodopa side effects gave a renewed strength to surgical approach to PD. However, Benabid and colleagues with chronic deep brain stimulation (DBS) introduced the real change of PD surgical therapy [4]. The first DBS target to be identified was ventral intermediate nucleus (Vim), followed later by subthalamic nucleus (STN) and internal segment of globus pallidus (GPi). In the following years, after the approval of US FDA to STN and GPi DBS (2002), this technique rapidly obtained the title of recognized therapy for advanced PD.

Recently, the introduction of magnetic resonance imaging (MRI)—Angio CT neuronavigation, intraoperative neurophysiologic evaluation and frameless systems gave rise to further improvements opening the doors to possible alternatives to the utilization of the classic stereotactic frames.

2. Stereotactic systems

In almost all neurosurgical centers, stereotactic surgery is conducted by the utilization of classic stereotactic frames in combination with either MRI or MRI and CT scan. This system is based on the determination of spatial relationship between an identified target into the brain contest and the frame rods visible on the MRI or CT images. Therefore, it is possible to determine the exact location of the target in relation to the Cartesian axes as well as the trajectories angles and the entry point. The computation of the coordinates and angles is performed by dedicated computer systems and more frequently by the neuronavigation devices available on the market. Finally, obtained coordinates and angle values are reported on specific millimetric scales of the stereotactic frame in order to have a chosen position of the electrodes on the entry point and along the planned trajectory to the target. During surgery, it is possible to perform X-ray control to confirm the exact position of the electrode in relation to the chosen target (**Figure 1**).

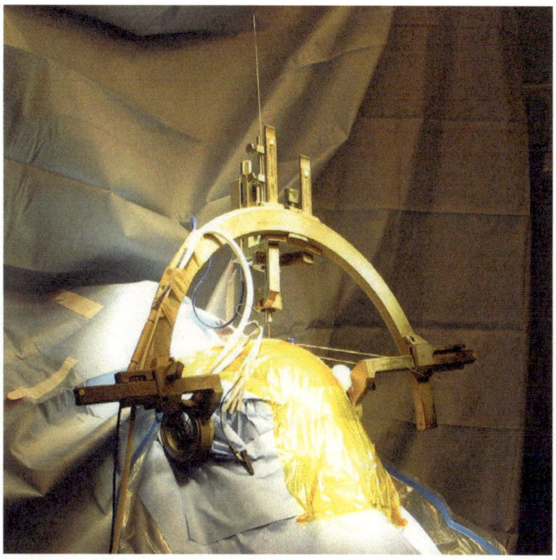

Figure 1. Stereotactic frame.

More recently, different companies have launched new frameless systems. This tools are based on the utilization of external fiducials (usually 6) fixed to the skull and consequently recorded on radiological studies (MRI and CT) acquired on the navigation system in order to reconstruct the entire head volume and report chosen targets, entry points, and trajectories. This new approach leaves the patient free from obliged and fixed position with less discomfort and fatigue. Moreover, these new systems do not differ in accuracy from classic stereotactic frame (**Figures 2** and **3**).

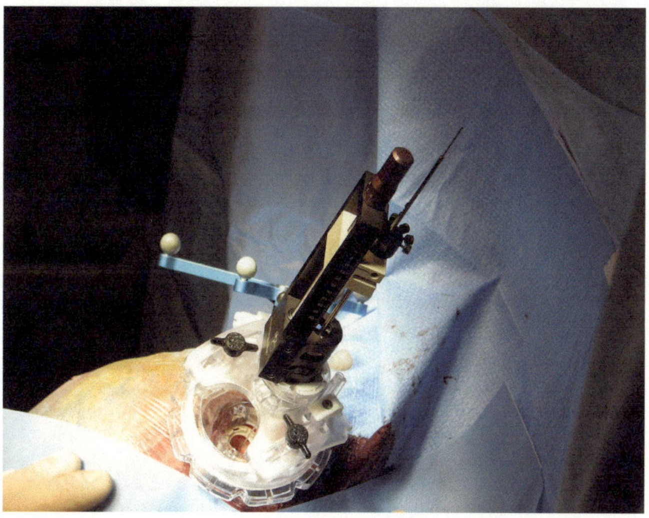

Figure 2. Frameless system.

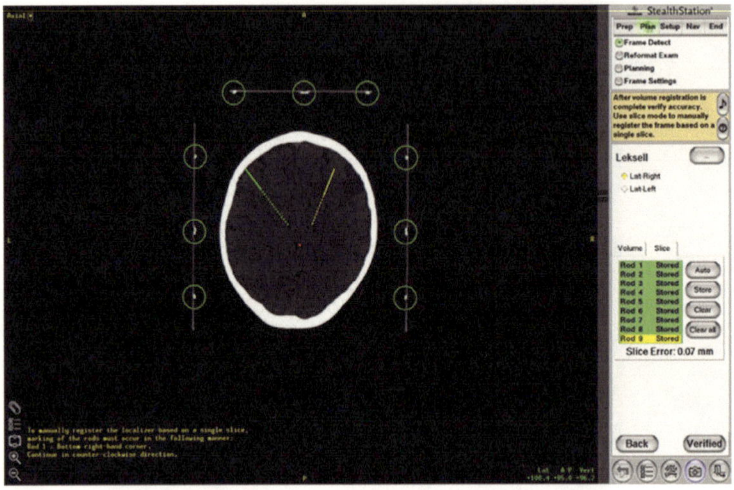

Figure 3. Fiducials image on neuronavigation system.

3. Target identification

Although in recent years, we assisted to a progressive improvement of technology, there are still strongholds that come from the past. In fact, neurosurgeons still consider the classical

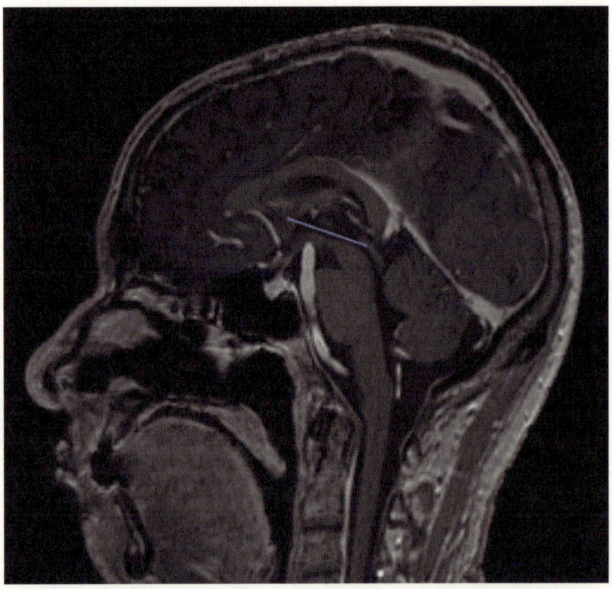

Figure 4. Intercommissural line marked in blue on Gadolinium T1-weighted sagittal MRI.

Intercommissural Line (anterior commissure AC—posterior commissure PC line, AC-PC line, IC line) as a reference to determine stereotactic coordinates, which are consequently used as starting points to find specific anatomical targets (indirect targeting methodology) (**Figure 4**).

However, recent amelioration of MRI quality allowed a direct visualization of most of anatomical structures and a consequent easier direct surgical targeting (direct targeting methodology). Although this technical progress, it is always recommended to use both methods to adjust indirect final position to anatomical structures visible on MRI (**Figure 5**).

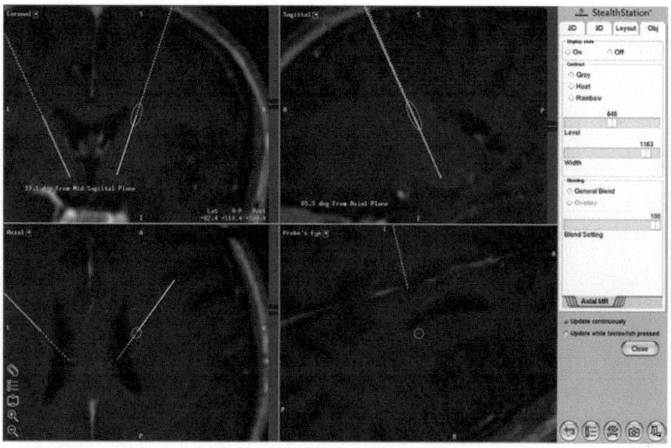

Figure 5. Trajectory planning on neuronavigation system.

The introduction of neuronavigation systems brought amelioration in pre-surgical determination of entry point and trajectory. Angio CT merged to Gadolinium T1-weighted MRI can better visualize vessels, bundles, and nuclei. Even if some authors do not consider strictly necessary to have both T1-weighted MRI and Angio CT for trajectories planning, sometimes the resolution of a single exam could not allow a complete and satisfactory vision in particular for small deep vessels (**Figure 6**).

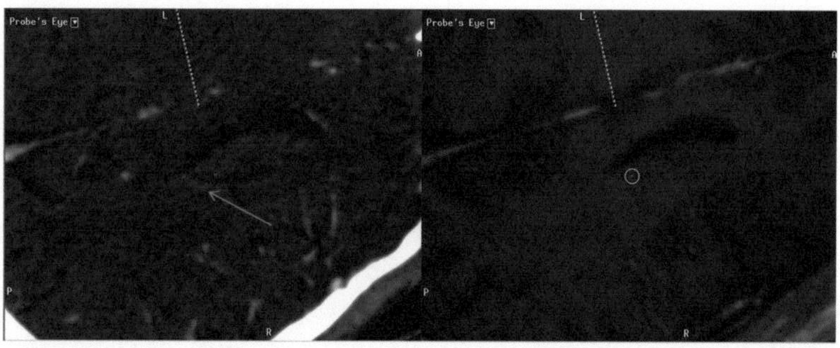

Figure 6. Confrontation between Angio CT and Gadolinium T1-weighted axial MRI; the arrow shows a vessel posterior to the trajectory only visible on Angio CT.

Finally, it is important to remark the role of T2-weighted or inversion recovery sequences for the location of some anatomical structures, as STN or GPi, respectively, and proton density studies for direct determination of PPN.

Generally, implantation procedure is made with an awoken patient because of the necessity to stimulate the chosen target and avoid postoperative side effects. However, some authors reported experience of DBS in Parkinson's patients under general anesthesia considering secondary the neurophysiological aspect, and others just performed stimulation with macro electrode.

Once the electrodes have been positioned in the proper targets, the stimulation device (internal pulse generator, IPG) is hosted in a subclavicular subcutaneous pouch, and connections among IPG, extension, and intracerebral electrodes are performed under general anesthesia. An important consideration must be made about the number of electrode utilized during intraoperative recording that could vary from 1 to 5. An important concern, in relation to this aspect, is in fact particularly linked to the necessity to find the best compromise between an efficient neurophysiologic test and the risk of hemorrhages.

Intraoperative electrical activity recording may give rise to a typical electrical pattern depending on the anatomical structure found along the electrode trajectory. Stimulation could also produce improvement of Parkinson's symptoms or induce different side effects giving important information about the exact targeting and possible correction to be made in relation to the obtained results.

4. Surgical aspects

In present times, deep brain stimulation (DBS) surgery can be performed with different systems that share however two common starting points. These are represented by the selection of PD patients and the choice of anatomical target.

4.1. Patient selection

The first attempt to standardize patient selection was developed in 1992 with the publication of CAPIT (core assessment program for intracerebral transplantation) that had the purpose of evaluate the outcome of patients selected for intracerebral transplantation of fetal dopamine neurons [5]. The evolution of this protocol, which included also patients treated by ablative and neurostimulation procedures, is represented by core assessment program for surgical interventional therapies (CAPSIT), which have been published in 1999 [6]. This protocol gained a growing importance during the last years and now represents the base for a correct selection of PD patients. In fact, it is mandatory to choose patients in which the clinical benefits of DBS overcome surgical risks connected to the procedure. Patients not only should be characterized by PD but also should be prepared in term of cognition, emotion, and social relations to the DBS procedure in order to maximize the treatment effect.

CAPSIT–PD inclusion criteria are as follows: idiopathic Parkinson's disease; duration of illness >5 years; age between 35 and 70 years; improving UPDRS motor part of at least 40% at the L-Dopa test; persistence of severe disability at certain times of the day despite all the adopted therapeutic strategies; antiparkinsonian therapy stabilized during the month before the implant; absence of dementia (MMSE >24); absence of severe depression with suicidal ideations; absence of psychosis; MRI within normal limits without evidence of marked atrophy, or multiple abnormalities of vascular origin, or diseases interfering with the surgical procedure (e.g., tumors); no history of drug addiction; absence of disease or medication interfering with the coagulation.

These criteria describe three major groups of PD patients that could effectively benefit from DBS surgery. The first group is represented by patients affected by idiopathic PD with normal cognitive capacities that show motor fluctuations and dyskinesia despite optimal levodopa therapy. Patients with controlled PD with persistent medication-resistant tremor compose the second group. Patients who do not tolerate medical treatment with consequently poor symptoms control represent the third category of DBS candidates.

4.2. DBS target identification

Since Vim chronic stimulation has proven its efficacy only for tremor control, this nucleus is not considered as a useful target for PD patient [7]. For this reason, possible stimulation sites are chosen between internal globus pallidus (GPi) and subthalamic nucleus (STN) associated in certain cases to pedunculopontine nucleus (PPN) [8]. The difference between STN and GPi stimulation consists in a greater effect in controlling tremor by STN stimulation with a consistent reduction of therapy intake and a consequent better control of psychiatric side effects due to L-Dopa. Conversely, targeting of GPi leads to a major anti-dyskinetic effect but leaves pharmacological dosage unchanged with all possible consequences on the psychiatric condition. Nevertheless, even STN stimulation could produce psychiatric side effects concerning mood and behavioral troubles. Some authors consider the possibility to stimulate PPN in order to obtain an improvement in axial manifestations such as postural instability or gait dysfunction [9, 10].

4.2.1. Targeting of internal globus pallidus (GPi)

Internal globus pallidus nucleus could be identified using a direct or an indirect method. According to the scheme reported by Laitinen, indirect targeting of the GPi is obtained, 2–3 mm in front of the mid-AC-PC-point, 3–6 mm caudal to intercommissural (IC) plane, and 20–21 mm lateral to the AC-PC line.

The planning requires the utilization of T2-weighted or inversion recovery (IR) MRI to locate the intercommissural line and draw the coordinate projection. T1-contrast images are also used to identify sulci gyri and vessels for the identification of safe trajectories avoiding vessels. GPi can be found in the medial part of the globus pallidus, medial to the lamina medullaris interna and lateral to the genu/posterior limb of internal capsule on the axial plane. Coronal plane can be used to obtain a better definition of GPi's relationship with optic radiations. Once the target is reached, intraoperative recording shows a specific electrical pattern consisting in a high frequency activity with 40 spikes/s of tonic firing [11]. Visual spots are conversely evocated when the electrode trespasses on the optic radiations. This sign is important to determine the lower boundary of the GPI and to avoid visual impairments once the device is completely implanted and programmed (**Figures 7** and **8**).

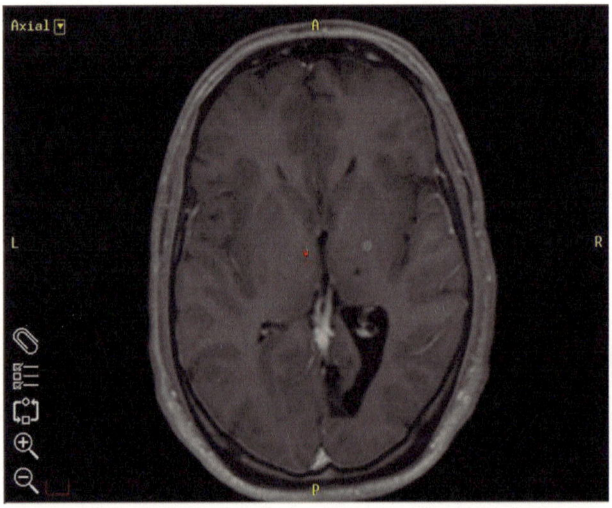

Figure 7. Electrode final position in GPI.

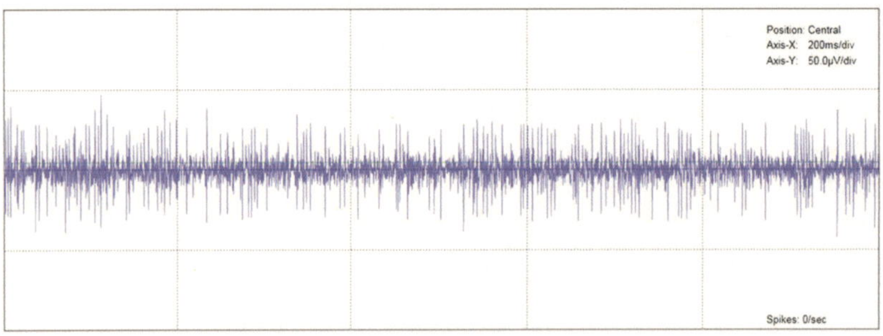

Figure 8. Intraoperative GPI recording.

4.2.2. Targeting of subthalamic nucleus (STN)

Indirect coordinates of the STN are reported as 3–4 mm posterior to mid-AC-PC-point, 3–5 mm below the AC-PC line, 11–12 mm lateral to AC-PC line. MRI images and in particular T2-weighted acquisitions may give a clear vision of the subthalamic nucleus as well as its anatomical relationship with other structures such as red nucleus, Forel's fields, and zona incerta (**Figure 9**).

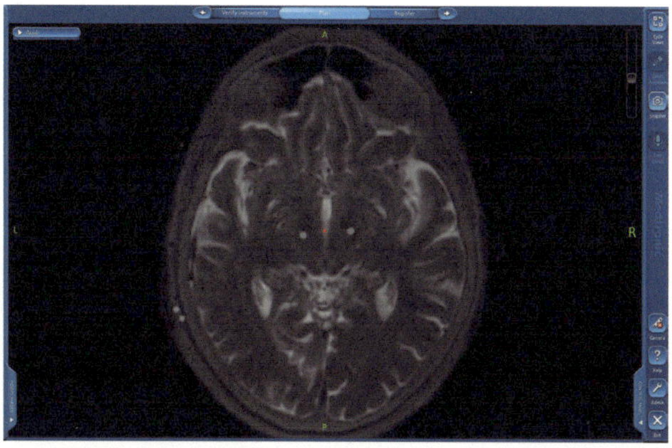

Figure 9. Final electrode position showed on CT merged to T2-axial MRI.

Neurophysiological intraoperative monitoring could give important information not only evidencing the typical electrical pattern of STN (STN neurons are characterized by a mean firing rate of 42.30 ± 22.00 spikes/sec (mean ± SD); the STN cells exhibited irregular or bursty discharge pattern) but also inducing improvement of Parkinson's symptoms or even side effects as paresthesias, muscular spasticity, diplopia, speech difficulties, and neurovegetative alterations [11, 12]. Therefore, neurophysiological intraoperative tests play an important role for the determination of the final electrode position, in order to maximize the benefit and avoid side effects lied to a possible brain shift secondary to CSF leakage and air penetration. During target planning, an important step is to avoid the anterior part of the STN, which is involved not only in extrapyramidal pathways but also in limbic circuits. Effectively, a stimulus that involves the anterior part of STN may cause behavioral changes, depression, maniac episodes,

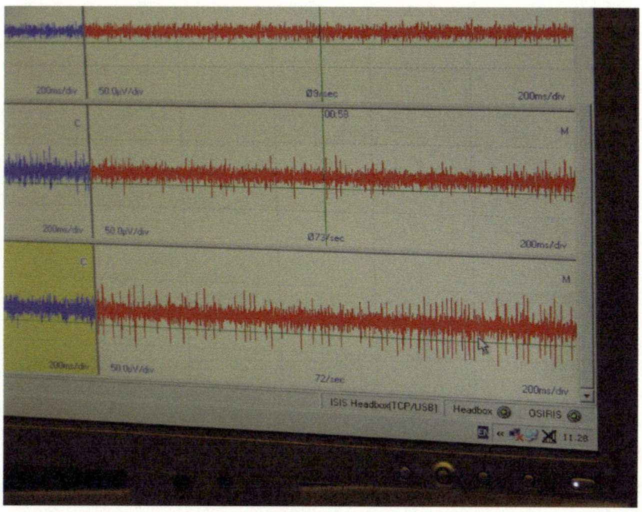

Figure 10. Intraoperative recording of STN electrical activity.

and other psychiatric complications. The diffusion of the stimulus to the substantia nigra may also give rise to psychiatric problems such as major depression and hypomania [13] (**Figure 10**).

4.2.3. Targeting ventralis intermedius thalamic nucleus (VIM)

VIM stimulation is used in patients affected by tremor (parkinsonian or essential), and its indirect target is 25–50% of AC-PC length from PC at IC plane, ½ (third ventricular width) +11.5 mm. These coordinates are actually reported on MRI images, where the nucleus is not normally visible on 3 Tesla MRI. Recorded electrical pattern has no specific features and does not differ from other sites within the thalamus. Conversely, the stimulation test can be very useful not only in reducing or abolishing tremor immediately but also in defining the boundaries of the VIM by evocating paresthesia or other sensitive symptoms secondary to the stimulation of the VPL nucleus [14] (**Figures 11** and **12**).

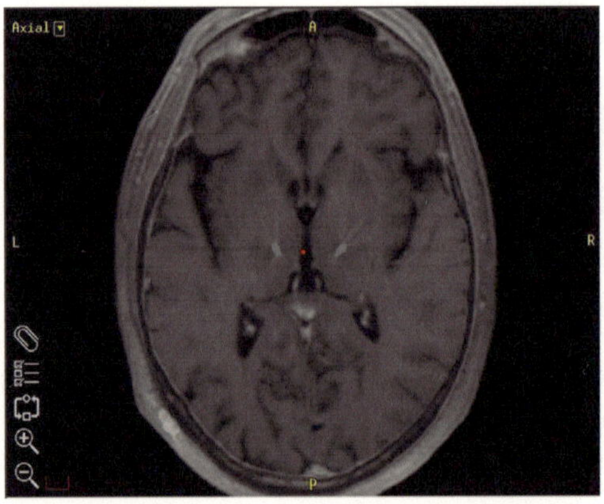

Figure 11. Final electrodes position in VIM showed on neuronavigation system.

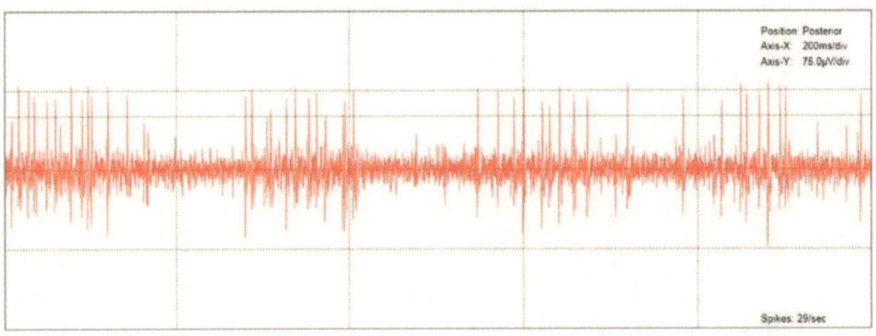

Figure 12. Intraoperative VIM recording showing typical low-frequency spikes synchronized with tremor.

4.2.4. Targeting of pedunculopontine nucleus (PPN)

The stimulation of this nucleus is utilized to reduce or abolish gait disturbances and freezing. The indirect localization may be obtained considering a line passing anterior to the floor of the fourth ventricle on a line running along the pontomesencephalic longitudinal axis (**Figure 13**).

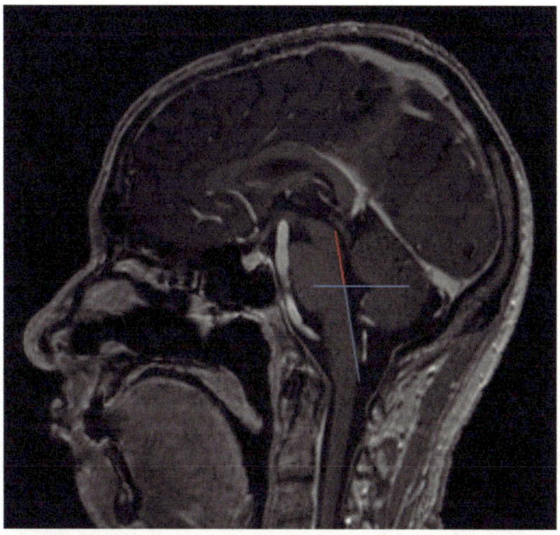

Figure 13. Gadolinium T1-sagittal MRI showing indirect localization of PPN; the red tract above the fastigial line indicates the location of PPN.

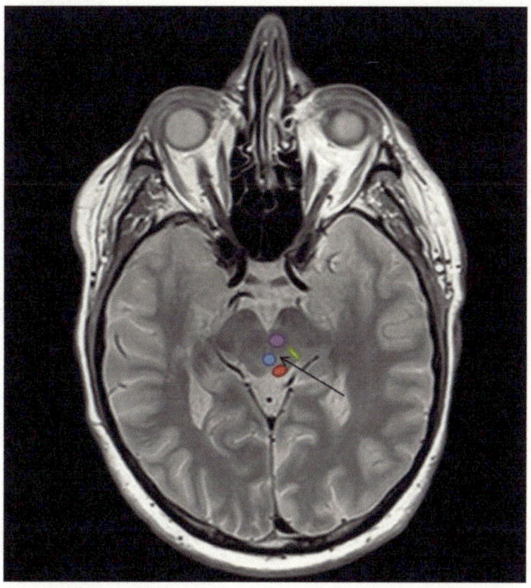

Figure 14. Proton density axial MRI; the arrow shows the PPN location; the blue area indicates the periaqueductal grey matter, the violet circle indicates the red nucleus/decussation of anterior cerebellar peduncle, the green oval indicates lateral lemniscus and the red area indicates the medial lemniscus/spinothalamic tract; on the left side of the image, the anatomical structures are visible in the real grey scale.

This line is crossed by an orthogonal line traced through the fastigium in order to identify a superior and inferior component of the previous identified line. Using this reference system, the PPN is identified 6 mm lateral and 4 mm anterior to the pontomesencephalic/fastigial lines,

16 mm above the crossing point between the base point fastigial line. The direct localization may be obtained by MRI identification using proton density images. The target is identified on an axial slice passing through the inferior colliculus in an area localized among the decussation of anterior cerebellar peduncle anteriorly, medial lemniscus anterolaterally, lateral lemniscus and spinothalamic tracts posterolaterally, periaqueductal gray matter and middle longitudinal fasciculus medially (**Figure 14**).

Recording of this area does not give specific information, while stimulation may be helpful in determining the exact position of the electrode contacts in relation to the absence of evoked side effects. The diffusion of the stimulus to the close structures could cause sensitive disturbances in case of stimulation of the lemniscal/spinothalamic bundles, hearing and vertigo stimulating medial lemniscus, diplopia secondary to the activation of third cranial nerve subnuclei, neurovegetative imbalance for the stimulation of central tegmental neurons [15].

5. IPG programming

IPG programming takes place after a first period of postoperative rest in order to focalize better the real effect of DBS without the bias related to the surgical damage secondary to leads introduction. The optimization of IPG stimulation pattern could necessitate several months, usually from 4 to 6. Each electrode can range from four to eight contacts that could be spaced 0.5 or 1.5 mm, and the stimulation could be made in a monopolar or bipolar way. The chosen configuration should be characterized by the best clinical effect with the smallest amount of side effects, which could derive from the extension of electrical stimulation to neighboring anatomical structures.

Once IPG setting is completed, the attention is focalized on stimulation amplitude, which is usually increased gradually in order to obtain a reduction in antiparkinsonian drug intake while preserving clinical wellness [16].

Finally, it is important to pay attention to frequency stimulation. Since the beginning of DBS treatment, high-frequency stimulation (above 130 Hz) has been considered the base of clinical improvement. However, more recently several authors showed the great potential of intermediate frequencies (60–80 Hz) in particular on freezing and gait even if the clinical benefit could be only temporary [17, 18].

6. Outcomes

Recent randomized controlled clinical trials on GPi and STN DBS showed that these treatments are superior to PD medical management alone [19].

As reported in a review by Duker et al. [16] PD DBS patients could obtain almost 4.4–4.6 h per day of "on" time without dyskinesia and a reduction of 1–2.6 h per day of "on" time with dyskinesia and 2.4–4.2 h per day of "off" time.

Since it has been proved that STN and GPi DBS are characterized by the absence of difference in motor function, the selection of the anatomical target should rely on patient peculiarities and surgeon preference [10].

7. Timing of DBS in Parkinson patients

In the last years, several authors focused their attention on DBS timing, reporting the hypothesis of a larger and more lasting amelioration of PD symptoms with early surgical treatment. As reported by Schuepbach et al. [20] in 2013, an earlier DBS could in fact improve patient quality of life better than medication alone even only after 2 years of PD. Conversely till nowadays, DBS solution was reserved usually for patients that had a minimum history of 5 years of disease and motor symptoms that did not improved with optimized medical therapy [6]. More studies are, however, necessary in order to further verify this hypothesis and to clarify long-term efficacy of this early surgical approach [16].

8. Complications and side effects

Although DBS is a relatively safe and effective procedure, complications and side effects represent a rare but unavoidable constant in this surgical treatment. As reported by recent literature reviews, adverse effects can be divided into 3 time-related categories: intraoperative, perioperative (<2 weeks), and long-term postoperative complications (>2 weeks). Intraoperative adverse events are represented by intracerebral (ICH) and intraventricular (IVH) hemorrhage, acute perilesional edema, cortical/subcortical ischemic infarction, vasovagal response and hypotension, confusion, anxiety, seizure, arrhythmia, and aborted procedure. Perioperative complications, which arise during the first 2-week postop, are headache, hemiparesis, confusion, agitation, respiratory distress, seizure, hallucinations, somnolence, and falls. Conversely, long-term postoperative complications are represented by wound complications (infection, skin erosion, wound dehiscence), hardware complications (lead fracture/malposition/migration/malfunction, flipped IPG, malpositioned/uncomfortable/malfunctioning internal pulse generator (IPG), lead extension malfunction/fracture), and satisfaction-related complications (loss of system efficacy over time, decreased efficacy over time) [21].

The recent improvement in pre-surgical target planning, with the introduction of neuronavigation systems, and the quality improvement of neuroradiological imaging are decreasing the rate of intracranial hematomas connected to electrodes placement. However, this complication remains possible with all consequent damages ranging from minor asymptomatic bleedings to huge hemorrhages with fatal consequences. Medical treatment is based on administration of mannitol or steroids, depending on the clinical and radiological characteristics of the hematoma, and could be associated to surgical cloth evacuation.

Infections represent another important DBS complication. Infection sites are frequently located at the level of the pouch created for the device, more rarely along the extension cables (usually due to a propagation from the infected device pouch) or on the intracranial extension of the electrodes, with consequent meningitis, subdural empyema, or intracerebral abscess. Antibiogram, specific antibiotic treatment, and removal of the infected components are mandatory except in case of superficial skin infection with no propagation of the components of the implanted system.

Wound dehiscence is usually caused by cutaneous decubitus of stimulation device. This complication is often related to a subsequent infection frequently caused by saprophytes cutaneous germs. It requires wound reopening, tissue debridement, and change or increase of the pouch volume.

Dislocation may be possible due to the relative tenderness of the electrode tip that could deviate from the chosen target. In order to reduce this possibility, it is advisable to use long cannulas to guide the electrode to the target.

Sometimes the electrode may move upward or downward from the target. This problem is often related to a blockage failure and requires the removal of the electrode and a new surgical positioning.

The brain is normally contained in a liquid environment formed by cerebrospinal fluid (CSF). During surgery, a certain volume of CSF leaks trough the surgical opening giving rise to a change in spatial relationship between the brain and the skull. In order to minimize, this problem many authors planned different solutions but a minimal amount of brain shift is still unavoidable. Obviously, a careful and minimal opening of the skull and meninges and the neurophysiological intraoperative recording may minimize this effect without affecting the surgical outcome (**Figure 15**).

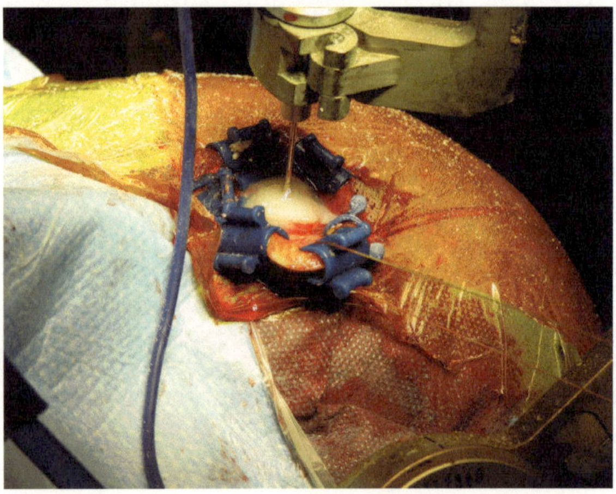

Figure 15. Fibrin glue and hemostatic sponge used as a plug to minimize CSF leakage.

A careful planning and intraoperative neurophysiological evaluation is usually sufficient to avoid side effects. However, complications as brain shift, electrode dislocation, or difficulty to evidence the evoked symptoms due to poor cooperation and reliability of the patient could cause postoperative problems. Propagation of the stimulus outside the planned target could induce pyramidal symptoms occurring by to the internal capsule, eye movement imbalance, appraisal, or worsening of dysarthria, psychiatric alteration, paresthesia, or skin numbness (this last complication normally disappears rapidly thanks to neuronal adaptation). Moreover, attention must be paid during trajectory planning to avoid caudate nucleus, in order to prevent cognitive deterioration.

Author details

Massimo Piacentino*, Giacomo Beggio and Lorenzo Volpin

*Address all correspondence to: massimo.piacentino@ulssvicenza.it

Department of Neurosurgery, San Bortolo Hospital, Vicenza, Italy

References

[1] Leriche R. Ueber Chirurgischen Eingriff bei Parkinson's scher Krankheit. Neurol Zeitblaetter. 1912;13:1093–1096.

[2] Spiegel EA, Wycis HT, Marks M, Lee AJ. Stereotaxic apparatus for operations on the human brain. Science. 1947;106(2754):349–350.

[3] Cotzias GC, Van Woert MH, Schiffer LM. Aromatic amino acids and modification of parkinsonism. N Engl J Med. 1967;276(7):374–379.

[4] Benabid AL, Pollak P, Louveau A, Henry S, De Rougemont J. Combined (thalamotomy and stimulation) stereotactic surgery of the VIM thalamic nucleus for bilateral Parkinson disease. Appl Neurophysiol. 1987;50ca(1–6):344–346.

[5] Langston JW, Widner H, Goetz CG, Brooks D, Fahn S, Freeman T, et al. Core assessment program for intracerebral transplantations (CAPIT). Mov Disord. 1992;7(1):2–13.

[6] Defer GL, Widner H, Marie RM, Remy P, Levivier M. Core assessment program for surgical interventional therapies in Parkinson's disease (CAPSIT-PD). Mov Disord. 1999;14:572–584.

[7] Rehncrona S, Johnels B, Widner H, Törnqvist A-L, Hariz M, Sydow O. Long-term efficacy of thalamic deep brain stimulation for tremor: double-blind assessments. Mov Disord. 2003;18(2):163–170.

[8] Odekerken VJ, Boel JA, Schmand BA, de Haan RJ, Figee M, van den Munckhof P, et al. GPi vs STN deep brain stimulation for Parkinson disease: three-year follow-up. Neurology. 2016; 86(8):755–61. doi:10.1212/WNL.0000000000002401

[9] Yousif N, Bhatt H, Bain PG, Nandi D, Seemungal BM. The effect of pedunculopontine nucleus deep brain stimulation on postural sway and vestibular perception. Eur J Neurol. 2016; 23(3):668-70. doi:10.1111/ene.12947

[10] Follett KA, Torres-Russotto D. Deep brain stimulation of globus pallidus interna, subthalamic nucleus, and pedunculopontine nucleus for Parkinson's disease: which target? Parkinsonism Relat Disord. 2012;18(Suppl 1):S165–7. doi:10.1016/S1353-8020(11)70051-7

[11] Bour LI, Contarino MF, Foncke EM, de Bie RM, van den Munckhof P, Speelman JD, et al. Long-term experience with intraoperative microrecording during DBS neurosurgery in STN and GPi. Acta Neurochir (Wien). 2010;152(12):2069–77. doi:10.1007/s00701-010-0835-y.

[12] Benazzouz A, Breit S, Koudsie A, Pollak P, Krack P, Benabid AL. Intraoperative microrecordings of the subthalamic nucleus in Parkinson's disease. Mov Disord. 2002;17(Suppl 3):S145–9.

[13] Ulla M, Thobois S, Llorca PM, Derost P, Lemaire JJ, Chereau-Boudet I, et al. Contact dependent reproducible hypomania induced by deep brain stimulation in Parkinson's disease: clinical, anatomical and functional imaging study. J Neurol Neurosurg Psychiatry. 2011;82(6):607–14. doi:10.1136/jnnp.2009.199323.

[14] Huss DS, Dallapiazza RF, Shah BB, Harrison MB, Diamond J, Elias WJ. Functional assessment and quality of life in essential tremor with bilateral or unilateral DBS and focused ultrasound thalamotomy. Mov Disord. 2015;30(14):1937–43. doi:10.1002/mds.26455.

[15] Golestanirad L, Elahi B, Graham SJ, Das S, Wald LL. Efficacy and safety of pedunculopontine nuclei (PPN) deep brain stimulation in the treatment of gait disorders: a meta-analysis of clinical studies. Can J Neurol Sci. 2016;43(1):120–6. doi:10.1017/cjn.2015.318

[16] Duker AP, Espay AJ. Surgical treatment of Parkinson disease: past, present, and future. Neurol Clin. 2013;31(3):799–808. doi:10.1016/j.ncl.2013.03.007.

[17] Moreau C, Defebvre L, Destée A, Bleuse S, Clement F, Blatt JL, et al. STN-DBS frequency effects on freezing of gait in advanced Parkinson disease. Neurology. 2008;71(2):80–84.

[18] Ricchi V, Zibetti M, Angrisano S, Merola A, Arduino N, Artusi CA, et al. Transient effects of 80 Hz stimulation on gait in STN DBS treated PD patients: a 15 months follow-up study. Brain Stimul. 2012;5(3):388–392.

[19] Williams A, Gill S, Varma T, Jenkinson C, Quinn N, Mitchell R, et al. Deep brain stimulation plus best medical therapy versus best medical therapy alone for advanced Parkinson's disease (PD SURG trial): a randomised, open-label trial. Lancet Neurol. 2010;9(6):581–591.

[20] Schuepbach WMM, Rau J, Knudsen K, Volkmann J, Krack P, Timmermann L, et al. Neurostimulation for Parkinson's disease with early motor complications. N Engl J Med. 2013;368(7):610–622.

[21] Fenoy AJ, Simpson RK Jr. Risks of common complications in deep brain stimulation surgery: management and avoidance. J Neurosurg. 2014;120(1):132–9. doi: 10.3171/2013.10.JNS131225.

Chapter 17

Neuro-Ophthalmologic Evaluation as a Biomarker for Diagnosis and Progression in Parkinson Disease

María Satue, Vicente Polo, Sofía Otin,
Jose M. Larrosa, Javier Obis and Elena Garcia-Martin

Additional information is available at the end of the chapter

http://dx.doi.org/10.5772/62877

Abstract

Objectives: The purpose of current neuro-ophthalmologic research is to evaluate visual dysfunction and its correlation with structural changes in the retina of patients with Parkinson's disease and to examine whether there is an association between retinal thinning and disease progression.

Methods: Patients with Parkinson's disease and controls were included in a series of observational cross-sectional studies and underwent visual function evaluation. Structural measurements of different layers of the retina were obtained using spectral domain optical coherence tomography (SD-OCT). Disease severity was assessed using the Schwab–England Activities of Daily Living scale, the Unified Parkinson Disease Rating Scale, and the Hoehn and Yahr (HY) scale. Comparison of obtained data and correlation analysis between functional and structural results and disease severity was performed. The diagnostic ability of SD-OCT for the detection of Parkinson disease was also tested by the development of two linear discriminant functions (LDFs).

Results: Patients with Parkinson's disease had altered visual function and presented retinal thinning in different sectors. Disease progression correlated with retinal parameters and measurements of retinal thickness was differentiated between healthy subjects and those with advanced Parkinson's disease.

Keywords: Parkinson's disease, optical coherence tomography, retinal nerve fiber layer, retinal ganglion cells, macular thickness

1. Introduction

Parkinson's disease (PD) is well known for its motor symptoms, such as bradykinesia, rigidity, resting tremor, and postural instability. However, the loss of dopaminergic neurons also leads to non-motor alterations, such as depression, dementia, and autonomic dysfunction [1].

Vision is one of the non-motor systems altered in PD. Patients suffering from Parkinson´s are reported to have decreased visual acuity (VA), contrast sensitivity, and color vision [2–8]. Recent research demonstrated that retinal thinning in PD patients and axonal damage can be detected and quantified using ocular imaging technologies, such as optical coherence tomography (OCT). The retina is part of the central nervous system and is easily accessible to clinical examination. The retinal nerve fiber layer (RNFL) comprises mainly non-myelinated axons of retinal ganglion cells (RGCs), so RNFL thickness measurements provide a relatively direct assessment of the axons and axonal damage.

OCT provides cross-sectional images of the retina and optic disc based on interference patterns produced by low coherence light reflected from retinal tissues. This technology includes the development of parameters to provide quantitative, objective, and reproducible measurements of the different retinal layers. Recent research on segmentation and analysis of different retinal layers has shown that measures of specific layers, such as the RGC layer provide more accurate information about axonal loss in neurodegenerative diseases [9].

Dopamine in the human retina is released by a set of amacrine cells. These dopaminergic cells are located in the proximal inner nuclear layer of the retina and send long processes to other retinal layers. Dopamine in the mammalian retina modulates color vision and contrast sensitivity through dopaminergic receptors (D1 and D2), which are differentially located in the retinal layers. A complete lack of D1 and D2 receptor activation leads to signal dispersion and alterations in color vision and contrast sensitivity.

The diagnosis of idiopathic PD is based on medical history and neurologic examination, and it sometimes takes several years to obtain a definitive diagnosis. Thus, new technologies and accurate tests are needed to improve and accelerate the diagnostic procedure in early stages of PD.

Recent research using OCT technology has demonstrated that parameters provided by OCT are accurate to detect various inner retinal or optic nerve pathologies, such as multiple sclerosis, PD, or Alzheimer disease [10–15]. At present, no clear guidelines are available on whether one, several, or all of the retinal parameters provided by OCT can be used in the diagnosis of PD.

Current research in the field of neuro-ophthalmology focuses on the evaluation of visual dysfunction in PD and its correlation with retinal alterations in these patients. Recent studies in PD have evaluated the association between macular, ganglion cell layer, and RNFL defects and PD severity, as well as the possible diagnostic ability of OCT technology [9, 15, 16].

The main objective of this study was to provide a better understanding of the role of retinal layers in PD and a diagnostic tool for the early detection of this neurodegenerative pathology.

2. Neuro-ophthalmologic evaluation of PD patients

2.1. Visual dysfunction in PD

Vision comprises many simultaneous functions that are important for daily life activities, such as mobility, reading, driving, and facial recognition [17–20]. Thus, it is important to assess the functional capability of the visual pathways by measuring VA, color vision, visual fixation, objects visual tracking, and contrast sensitivity and to evaluate the impact of vision loss on a person's ability to perform everyday visual tasks.

PD patients are reported to have decreased contrast sensitivity and color vision [2–8]. Previous studies have indicated that PD patients lose foveal contrast sensitivity to patterns to which normal observers are most sensitive (that is, requiring the least contrast for detection of letters, shapes, and figures) [3, 4]. In the retina, ganglion cells adapt to visual contrast and pool the visual information of their receptive fields through a network of parallel bipolar cells with smaller receptive fields [21]. Additionally, contrast sensitivity and color vision are modulated through dopaminergic receptors, which are located in the inner retinal layers. A complete lack of activation of these receptors leads to signal dispersion and alterations in color vision and contrast sensitivity [22].

In our hospital, we evaluated a cohort of 37 patients with PD and analyzed possible alterations in their visual function. We assessed VA, contrast sensitivity vision (CSV), and color vision in these patients and compared the results with healthy controls.

The diagnosis of PD was based on standard clinical and neuroimaging criteria [23]. Patients with significant refractive errors (>5 diopters of spherical equivalent refraction or 3 diopters of astigmatism), intraocular pressure ≥21 mm Hg, media opacifications, concomitant ocular diseases including history of glaucoma or retinal pathology, and systemic conditions that could affect the visual system were excluded from the study. The healthy controls had no history and no evidence of ocular or neurologic disease of any nature, and their best-corrected visual acuity (BCVA) was >20/30 based on the Snellen scale, to ensure all of them could complete the visual function evaluation tests. All subjects underwent a complete neuro-ophthalmic evaluation that included pupillary, anterior segment, and funduscopic examination. All procedures adhered to the tenets of the Declaration of Helsinki, and all participants provided informed consent to participate in the study.

Visual function was assessed by evaluating different functional parameters: BCVA using an ETDRS chart; CSV using the CVS-1000E test and Pelli–Robson chart; and color vision using the Farnsworth D15 and L'Anthony D15 tests.

VA is a measure of the spatial resolution of the visual processing system and is dependent on optical and neural factors, that is, the sharpness of the retinal focus within the eye, the health and functioning of the retina, and the sensitivity of the interpretative faculty of the brain. Thus, the VA in a patient with PD and a healthy eye will depend solely on their neurologic condition. VA can be evaluated using different optotypes (with letters or numbers). For clinical research, the ETDRS chart is considered the gold standard and consists of a set of 10 letters from the Roman alphabet, each of them equally visible (**Figure 1**).

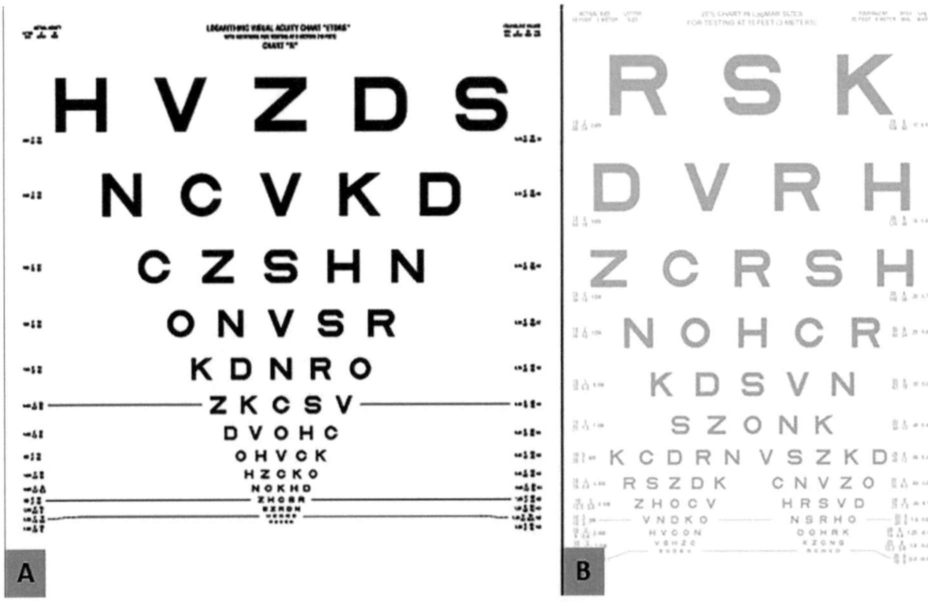

Figure 1. ETDRS charts for evaluation of high and low contrast visual acuity. (A): 100% contrast ETDRS chart. (B:) 2.50% contrast ETDRS chart.

The letters are arranged in 14 rows, with 5 letters each, and decrease in size progressively. Results can be expressed as 6/6, 10/10, decimal value or logarithmic scale (LogMar). In the expression 6/6, at 6 m, a human eye with a VA of 6/6 is able to separate contours that are approximately 1.75 mm apart; 6/12 means that a person with 6/6 vision would discern the same optotype from 12 m away (i.e., at twice the distance). The equivalent to 6/6 in decimal digits would be 1.0 and 0.0 in logarithmic scale (LogMar). In our patients, LogMAR VA was evaluated at three different contrast levels: 100, 2.50, and 1.25% (using Low-Contrast Sloan Letter Charts), the percentage indicating the level of contrast, that is, 100% representing black letters over white background and 1.25% light grey letters over white background (**Figure 1**).

CSV provides more complete information about visual function than VA tests. CSV was evaluated in our patients using the Pelli–Robson chart and the CSV-1000E test. The Pelli–Robson is a commonly used test for the evaluation of contrast sensitivity, assessing CSV at one spatial frequency (1 cycle/degree [cpd]). This chart comprises horizontal lines of capital letters organized into groups of three (triplets) with two triplets per line. Within each triplet, all letters have the same contrast. The contrast decreases from one triplet to the next, even within each line. All patients were evaluated at a distance of 1 m from the chart and under controlled fotopic conditions (85 cd/m^2). The score corresponding to the last triplet of letters seen by the patient was recorded. The CSV-1000E instrument is used worldwide for standardized CSV and glare testing and evaluates CSV at 4 different spatial frequencies (3, 6, 12, and 18 cpd). The chart comprises four rows with 17 circular patches each. The patches present a grating that decreases in contrast moving from left to right across the row (**Figure 2**). Each contrast value for each spatial frequency was transformed into a logarithmic scale according to standardized values.

http://dx.doi.org/10.5772/62877

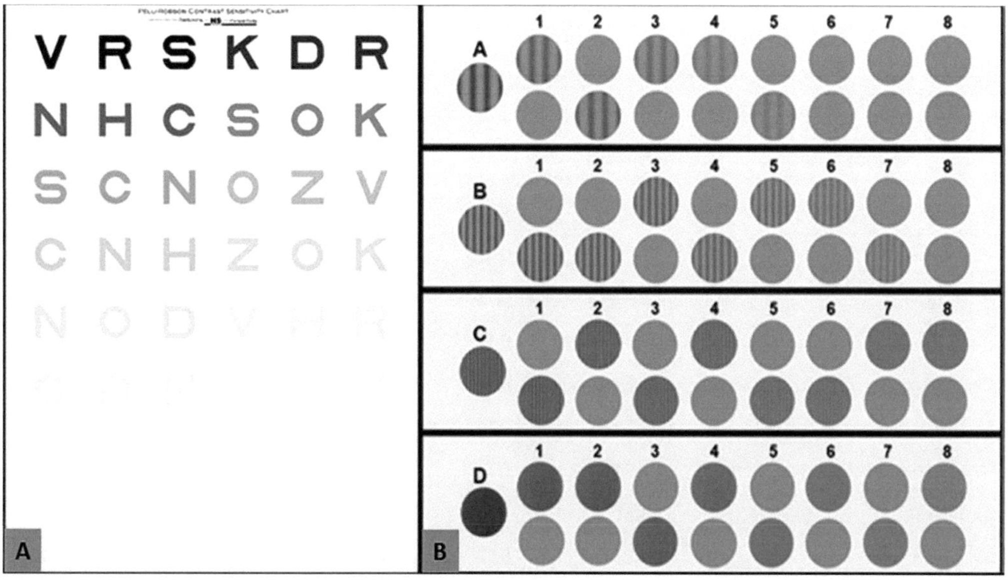

Figure 2. Contrast sensitivity vision tests. (A) Pelli–Robson chart explores contrast sensitivity in one spatial frequency (1 cycle per degree). (B) CSV 1000E test evaluates contrast sensitivity at four different spatial frequencies (3, 6, 12, and 18 cycles per degree).

Color vision was evaluated using the Color Vision Recorder (CVR) program. CVR software is designed for the Windows operating system and analyzes chromatic discrimination by classification of colors (color arrangement using colored caps). CVR includes several classic color tests. All patients in the study were evaluated using the Farnsworth D15 and L´Anthony D15 tests. These tests are often used to differentiate between subjects with severe loss of color vision and those with milder color defects or normal color vision. Different output parameters, such as the age-corrected color confusion index (AC CCI, which represents the ratio between the radius or distance between caps), the Confusion angle (Conf angle, which represents the axis of color deficiency), and the Scatter index (S-index, which represents the parallelism of confusion vectors to the personal confusion angle) were recorded [24, 25]. All these parameters evaluate the severity of dyschromatopsia. For example, an AC CCI score higher than 1, indicates altered color vision perception; the higher the score in the AC CCI and the S-index, the worse the color deficiency.

We found that our patients with PD had a lower BCVA at all three contrast levels of the ETDRS chart compared to the controls (0.18 ± 0.26 in patients vs. −0.065 ± 0.9 in controls at 100%, p = 0.001; 0.59 ± 0.21 vs. 0.44 ± 0.13 at 2.50%, p = 0.01; and 0.61 ± 0.23 vs. 0.58 ± 0.16 at 1.25%, p = 0.009). The Pelli– Robson results revealed a significant reduction in CSV in PD patients (p = 0.02). CSV was also affected in patients at all four spatial frequencies of the CSV 1000E chart (3, 6, 12, and 18 cpd; p = 0.001, <0.001, <0.001, and 0.004 respectively). Color vision was also affected in PD: In our patients, only the L´Anthony test results were significantly altered. L´Anthony test is less saturated than the Farnsworth color test; thus, it is designed to detect very subtle color deficiencies. Our patients performed worse than controls in both tests (higher C-index and S-index, reaching ranges similar to protanomalies), although only the differences in L′Anthony S-index were statistically significant, indicating that our patients had a (subtle) protanomaly (**Table 1**).

	Healthy controls		Parkinson's disease		P
	Mean	SD	Mean	SD	
VA ETDRS 100	−0.06	0.096	0.18	0.26	**0.001**
VA ETDRS 2.5	0.44	0.13	0.59	0.22	**0.010**
VA ETDRS 1.25	0.58	0.16	0.62	0.23	**0.009**
Pelli–Robson	1.89	0.11	1.71	0.17	**0.002**
CSV 1000 3 cpd	1.72	0.16	1.49	0.35	**0.001**
CSV 1000 6 cpd	1.94	0.13	1.62	0.34	**0.000**
CSV 1000 12 cpd	1.62	0.17	1.26	0.41	**0.000**
CSV 1000 18 cpd	1.11	0.22	0.73	0.34	**0.004**
Farnsworth AC CCI	1.11	0.22	0.73	0.34	0.851
Farnsworth Conf Angle	63.90	11.15	65.84	7.49	0.392
Farnsworth S-index	1.56	0.22	1.64	0.39	0.278
Farnsworth time	78.67	28.96	82.91	33.10	0.616
L′Anthony AC CCI	1.05	0.19	1.02	0.18	0.489
L′ Anthony Conf Angle	62.31	14.74	71.91	9.25	**0.002**
L′ Anthony S-index	1.69	0.43	1.95	0.48	**0.020**
L′ Anthony time	77.14	25.99	84.09	39.31	0.431

Results in bold letters indicate statistical significance ($p < 0.05$).
AC CCI, age-corrected color confusion index; Conf Angle, confusion angle; cpd, cycles per degree; ETDRS, early treatment diabetic retinopathy study; PD, Parkinson disease; S-index, scatter index; VA, visual acuity.

Table 1. Mean and standard deviation (SD) of visual functional parameters in healthy controls and subjects with Parkinson's disease. Results in bold letters indicate statistical significance ($p < 0.05$).

Ganglion cells in the retina show adaptation to visual contrast. The parvo- and magnocellular ganglion cells are located in the RGC layer and take two different pathways for the identification of color and contrast at different frequencies [26]. RGC loss was recently identified as the cause of visual impairment in patients suffering from another neurodegenerative process (multiple sclerosis) [27]. Thus, a similar process could be the cause of the contrast and color deficiencies in PD.

The results found in this study highlight the importance of visual function tests in the evaluation of PD patients and may have important implications for clinical diagnosis of functional deficits in these patients.

http://dx.doi.org/10.5772/62877

2.2. Retinal changes in PD

Parkinson´s disease has been associated with alterations in foveal vision. This visual alteration seems to be caused by a dysfunction of the intraretinal dopaminergic circuitry and final retinal output to the brain [2].

Thanks to the new digital imaging technologies applied in the field of ophthalmology, an objective assessment of the retinal layers is now possible. OCT provides a rapid, objective, non-invasive, and reproducible method for the assessment of eye structures thicknesses and volumes.

OCT is an established medical imaging technique that uses light to capture micrometer-resolution, three-dimensional images from within optical scattering media. OCT is based on low-coherence interferometry, usually employing near-infrared light. The use of relatively long wavelength light allows it to penetrate into the scattering medium. The interference of light (caused by the different tissues) occurs at a distance of micrometers. Light with broad bandwidths can be generated using superluminescent diodes or lasers with extremely short pulses.

The OCT device combines the reflected light from two arms (one arm containing the object of study, and a second arm containing usually a mirror) to rise an interference pattern. A reflectivity profile of the sample is obtained by scanning the mirror in the reference arm [28]. Parts of the sample that reflect a lot of light will create greater interference than areas that do not. These higher interference areas will be seen as bright patterns and will correlate with fibrosis or dense retinal layers, whereas low interference areas will be seen as dark patterns and will correlate with fluid. Any light that is outside the short coherence length will not interfere.

There are many studies on neurodegenerative diseases using OCT to detect changes in the RNFL thickness and macular morphology. Regarding PD and the alteration of macular thickness, recent studies have shown a significant thinning in the retinal inner layers of the macular area in patients with PD. Alterations of the retinal layers in PD patients were first demonstrated in 2004 [29]. Since then, various studies have reported different results [29–33].

For the past 5 years, the neuro-ophthalmology research team of Miguel Servet University Hospital has studied retinal structural alterations in PD patients using different OCT devices. Various software applications were used in the evaluation of these patients.

A first cohort of 153 subjects with PD underwent OCT examinations using the Cirrus high-definition (HD) OCT device and the Spectralis OCT device. Two different applications were used for Spectralis OCT, for the analysis of the optic nerve: the *Glaucoma* application (which scans the optic nerve head starting and finishing in the temporal quadrant), and the *Axonal Analytics* application for neurodegenerative diseases (which scans the optic nerve from and to the temporal quadrant) (**Figure 3.**).

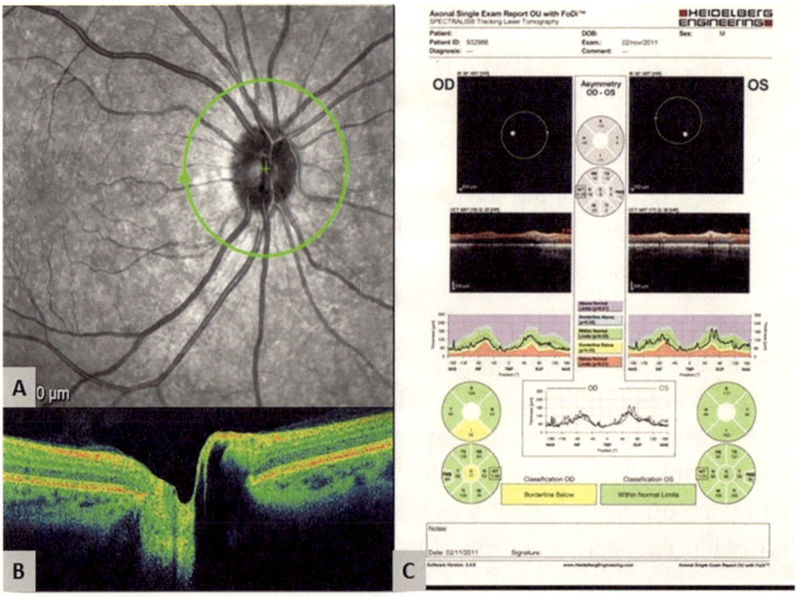

Figure 3 Evaluation of the retinal nerve fiber layer using Axonal Analytics application for Spectralis OCT. (A) Arrow marks the direction of the scan in the optic nerve head. (B) Cross-sectional image of the peripapillary retinal thickness. The retinal layers can be observed in different colors, depending on their interference pattern. (C) OCT report with measurements of the retinal nerve fiber layer in μm.

The difference between both applications resides in the sector with the most accurate measurements: With Glaucoma application, the most accurate sector is nasal, and with Axonal Analytics application is the temporal sector, which is precisely the sector with earlier affectation in neurodegenerative diseases. Macular and peripapillary RNFL thicknesses were evaluated and compared with thicknesses of a group of 242 healthy individuals [9].

The Spectralis OCT measurements revealed significant differences in most of the RNFL sectors using the traditional *Glaucoma* application, and in the mean thickness, the inferior quadrant, the inferonasal, and the inferotemporal RNFL sectors using the *Axonal* Analytics application. The Cirrus OCT measurements revealed significant RNFL differences in mean thickness, and thickness of superior, inferior, and temporal quadrants. Macular thickness was also reduced in patients with PD for all measurements of the inner and outer macular sectors using the Spectralis OCT device; and for the central sector (fovea thickness) and the nasal outer and inferior outer sectors with the Cirrus OCT. Results from this study were published in the *British journal of Ophthalmology* in 2014.

A different cohort of patients underwent retinal evaluation with a new prototype technique for retinal segmentation using the Spectralis OCT [16]. This new software is designed to identify each retinal layer and to measure its thickness. Segmentation of the retinal layers in single horizontal foveal scans was performed automatically by the segmentation application into 10 different layers [16] (**Figure 4.**).

http://dx.doi.org/10.5772/62877

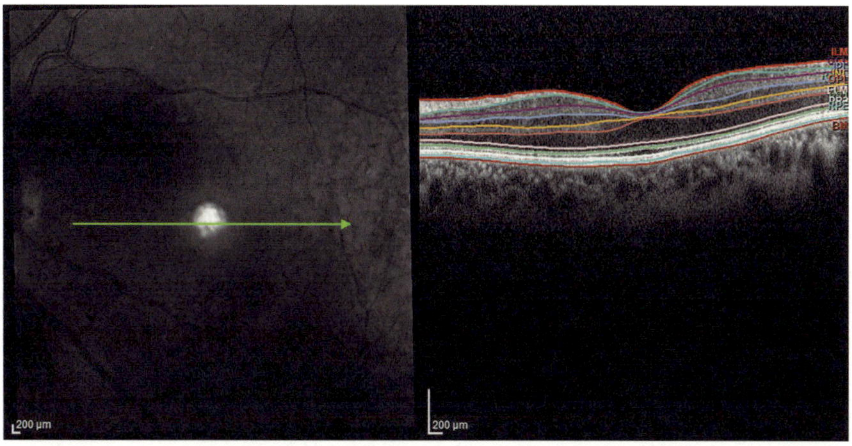

Figure 4 Macular cross-sectional image of a patient with Parkinson's disease, as provided by the segmentation application of Spectralis OCT. The different retinal layers can be observed marked in different colored lines.

All measurements of the macular and peripapillary thickness of the 10 layers were registered in a database for all eyes, and mean thickness of each retinal layer was calculated. A total of 129 eyes from 129 PD patients and 129 eyes of 129 healthy subjects were included in the study.

The segmentation application revealed a significant reduction of the RNFL, ganglion cell layer, the inner plexiform, and outer plexiform layer thickness in PD patients compared with controls. Surprisingly, the inner nuclear layer was significantly thicker in PD patients compared with healthy subjects (**Table 2**). These results were published in 2013 in the *American Journal of Ophthalmology*.

LAYER	Parkinson's disease (n = 129)	Healthy subjects (n = 129)	P*
Inner glial limiting membrane	5.69 ± 2.01	5.68 ± 1.72	0.563
Retinal nerve fiber layer	6.06 ± 1.90	6.26 ± 1.80	**0.036**
Ganglion cell layer	6.30 ± 1.89	6.49 ± 1.86	**0.011**
Inner plexiform layer	6.64 ± 1.95	6.77 ± 1.92	**0.016**
Inner nuclear layer	7.39 ± 1.94	7.14 ± 1.90	**0.033**
Outer plexiform layer	7.17 ± 1.93	7.31 ± 1.91	**0.028**
Outer nuclear layer	7.89 ± 1.91	7.95 ± 1.92	0.085
Outer glial limiting membrane	8.20 ± 1.90	8.25 ± 1.96	0.220
Photoreceptors	8.26 ± 1.98	8.29 ± 1.95	0.139
Retinal pigment epithelium	8.58 ± 1.88	8.63 ± 1.89	0.397

Table 2. Mean and standard deviation of retinal thickness in the 10 different retinal layers automatically provided by the segmentation application of the Spectralis optical coherence tomography and comparison between patients with Parkinson's disease and healthy subjects.

The correlation between retinal changes and visual dysfunction in patients suffering from PD was also investigated. A small cohort of 37 patients with PD (37 eyes) underwent visual function tests (see previous section *Visual dysfunction in Parkinson´s disease*) and structural analysis of macular thickness, ganglion cell layer (GCL) and RNFL thickness, and linear correlations between functional and structural results were calculated using Pearson's correlation coefficient.

Results demonstrated that CSV was the functional parameter most frequently associated with structural measurements in PD. The Pelli– Robson CSV results correlated with GCL thickness in all sectors, although the association was not strong ($r < 0.5$, $p < 0.05$). The Pelli– Robson measurements also correlated with the thicknesses in different sectors of the peripapillary RNFL (average, superior, and inferior sectors). The CSV-1000E measurements at different spatial frequencies correlated significantly with most GCL measurements: The spatial frequency of 6 cpd correlated with the superonasal thickness ($r = 0.40$, $p = 0.013$), with the superotemporal thickness ($r = 0.44$, $p = 0.006$), with the average GCL + IPL thickness ($r = 0.40$, $p = 0.012$), and with the minimum GCL + IPL ($r = 0.40$, $p = 0.011$). The spatial frequency of 18 cpd correlated with the superotemporal thickness ($r = 0.41$, $p = 0.01$) and the minimum GCL + IPL thickness ($r = 0.43$, $p = 0.006$), showing here the strongest correlations with GCL thickness. Spatial frequencies of 6 and 18 cpd were strongly correlated with average macular thickness ($r = 0.79$, $p = 0.012$; $r = 0.77$, $p = 0.016$, respectively) and macular volume ($r = 0.78$, $p = 0.013$; $r = 0.78$, $p = 0.014$, respectively). Color vision was also associated with the structural parameters, but only those measurements (the C-index and CCI) assessed by the L´Anthony test were significantly correlated with all outer macular parameters and most of the GCL measurements. A significant association between color vision and the RNFL parameters was only found in isolated sectors.

The VA ETDRS results (high and low contrast) correlated strongly with average macular thickness and macular volume (**Table 3**). This was particularly interesting, since this is the first time such a strong correlation between macular thickness, macular volume, and functional parameters (VA and CSV) is reported ($r > 0.70$).

	Macular thickness (correlation coefficient)	P value	Macular volume (correlation coefficient)	P value
VA ETDRS 100	−0.765	**0.006**	−0.761	**0.007**
VA ETDRS 1.25	−0.718	**0.013**	−0.715	**0.013**
VA ETDRS 2.50	−0.738	**0.010**	−0.729	**0.011**

Correlation data in bold type are statistically significant (p value < 0.05).
ETDRS, early treatment diabetic retinopathy study; VA, visual acuity.

http://dx.doi.org/10.5772/62877

Table 3. Correlation between visual acuity measured with ETDRS chart at different levels of contrast (in %) and macular structural measurements (thickness and volume) in patients with Parkinson disease. Results in bold letters indicate statistical significance ($p < 0.05$).

The study on the association between structural and functional parameters is currently pending acceptance for its publication in a peer- reviewed journal.

2.3. Correlation between structural changes and disease severity

The stage and severity of PD were determined in all our patients based on three different rating scales: the Hoehn and Yahr (HY), the Schwab–England activities of daily living (ADL), and the Unified Parkinson's disease rating score (UPDRS). Patients were tested by a trained neurologist who was blind to the ophthalmology results. Disease duration was also recorded, setting the appearance of the first symptoms as the onset time of the disease.

A correlation analysis between disease severity and structural changes as measured by OCT was performed in the first cohort of patients (153 patients with PD). Correlations between structural data (measured with Cirrus OCT and Spectralis OCT) and the different rating scales were examined by Pearson's test. The results of this study were published in the *British Journal of Ophthalmology*, in 2014 [9].

The correlation analysis revealed an inverse correlation between most macular thickness measurements assessed by Spectralis OCT and the scores on the HY scale. This means that increased neurological effects and severity of PD progression are linked to thinning of macular tissue. There was a significant correlation between the Schwab–England ADL scores and the outer temporal macular thickness measured with the Cirrus OCT device ($r = 0.284$, $p = 0.010$); and between the Schwab–England ADL scores and the inner inferior macular thickness measured with the Spectralis OCT device ($r = 0.217$, $p = 0.039$). The UPDRS scores were significantly correlated with the inner inferior macular thickness and measured using the Cirrus OCT device ($r = -0.331$, $p = 0.032$). Disease duration was correlated with RNFL thickness measured by the Spectralis OCT device (nasal quadrant using glaucoma application, $p = 0.036$; nasal quadrant and mean thickness using axonal application, $p = 0.016$ and $p = 0.038$, respectively). No correlation between disease duration and Cirrus OCT values was found.

In the second cohort (129 patients and 129 healthy controls), PD patients were divided into two groups depending on disease duration: <10 years (67% of the patients) or at least 10 years (33%). The thickness of the different retinal layers was compared between both patient's groups using Student's t-test. Linear agreement between the mean thickness of each retinal layer and three neurologic parameters (duration of disease, HY, and UPDRS scores) was obtained using the Pearson correlation coefficient. A logistical regression analysis was performed to identify which retinal layer thicknesses predicted axonal damage in PD patients.

When analyzing the results, the inner retinal layer thicknesses (RNFL, ganglion cell, and inner plexiform layers) were more affected in PD patients with disease duration of at least 10 years (**Table 4**). GCL thickness correlated inversely with PD duration ($r = -0.221$, $p = 0.046$) and the HY scale ($r = -0.311$, $p = 0.041$), but not the UPDRS scale.

Layer	Parkinson's disease patients with disease duration < 10 years (n:86)	Parkinson's disease patients with disease duration ≥ 10 years (n:43)	P*
Inner glial limiting membrane	5.70 ± 1.95	5.68 ± 1.96	0.211
Retinal nerve fiber layer	6.06 ± 1.87	5.89 ± 1.91	**0.028**
Ganglion cell layer	6.40 ± 1.92	5.96 ± 1.85	**0.031**
Inner plexiform layer	6.47 ± 1.91	6.11 ± 1.89	**0.009**
Inner nuclear layer	7.37 ± 1.91	7.41 ± 1.75	0.111
Outer plexiform layer	7.19 ± 1.91	7.08 ± 1.99	0.136
Outer nuclear layer	7.89 ± 1.98	7.82 ± 1.93	0.356
Outer glial limiting membrane	8.21 ± 1.79	8.20 ± 1.95	0.457
Photoreceptors	8.27 ± 1.90	8.24 ± 1.89	0.665
Retinal pigment epithelium	8.60 ± 1.85	8.57 ± 1.93	0.763

Table 4. Mean and standard deviation of thicknesses in the 10 retinal layers automatically provided by the new segmentation application of the Spectralis optical coherence tomography and comparison between Parkinson disease patients with disease duration of <10 years or at least 10 years.

The regression analysis showed that only the GCL thickness could predict axonal atrophy in PD. Based on the OCT measurements, PD patients with thinner GCL thickness showed a greater decrease in average RNFL thickness. However, thickness of the other retinal layers was not predictive of axonal damage. These results were published in the *American Journal of Ophthalmology*, in 2013 [16].

Our data clearly revealed that disease duration has an impact on the thickness of the RNFL, the GCL, and the inner plexiform layer. The negative correlation between macular thickness, the thickness of the RNFL, and the Hoehn and Yahr score indicates that patients with greater axonal damage tend to have more severe PD symptoms. Our results also indicated that GCL thickness could predict axonal damage in PD patients. GCL atrophy is thought to be a component of RNFL loss, which is suggested to produce consecutive degeneration of the RGC layer and its axons as disease progresses [34, 35].

2.4. The role of OCT in the diagnosis of Parkinson´s disease

Because of the difficulty in diagnosing PD, medical organizations have created diagnostic criteria to standardize and simplify the diagnostic process. Diffusion magnetic resonance imaging is a specific technique that may help discriminate between typical and atypical parkinsonism, but its exact diagnostic value is still under investigation.

A definitive diagnosis for PD may take years. Thus, new technologies and accurate tests are needed to improve and accelerate the diagnostic procedure in early stages of the disease. Currently, there are no clear guidelines available on which retinal or RNFL parameters provided by OCT can be used in the diagnosis of PD. Previous research demonstrated that

http://dx.doi.org/10.5772/62877

overall RNFL mean thickness provided by OCT is a good parameter to detect various inner retinal or optic nerve pathologies, such as glaucoma [11], and neurodegenerative disease [10]. Optimal neurodegenerative disease detection, however, is liable to depend on a combination of several parameters. In 2013, our research team published a study in the journal *Retina* that evaluated whether a selective combination of RNFL and retinal OCT parameters could further optimize PD diagnosis. The purpose of this study was to evaluate the diagnostic ability of a linear discriminant function (LDF) for PD, based exclusively on ophthalmologic parameters.

Two independent samples of 100 consecutive healthy subjects and 60 idiopathic patients with PD were recruited from two clinics in the hospital area. The diagnosis of PD was based on the United Kingdom's BrainBank criteria and the United States National Institute of Neurological Disorders and Stroke criteria [36].

All subjects underwent OCT evaluation to obtain measurements of the peripapillary RNFL and retinal thickness using the Spectralis OCT device. Regression analysis was used, when the dependent variable (to have PD) was dichotomous (yes/no) and the independent variables (all OCT measurements) were of any kind. For logistic regression analysis, the probability that a subject has PD was set as the predicted-dependent variable. The relative importance of each independent variable was evaluated using the forward Wald method, which tests the unique contribution of each predictor in the context of the other predictors. The LDF was calculated by taking the weighted sum of the predictor variables. The significant OCT parameters were combined to generate a new variable (LDF) in such a way that the measurable differences between healthy eyes and eyes with PD were maximized. One hundred and eleven eyes from 60 patients with PD were evaluated. All RNFL scans and retinal measurements provided by the Spectralis OCT were analyzed to calculate three LDFs: the Retinal LDF using the 9 retinal measurements (macular area), the RNFL LDF with 768 RNFL measurements, and the definitive LDF (which combined all OCT measurements). The statistical analysis showed that the Retinal LDF was the best formula. Retinal LDF was defined as follows: 31.173 + temporal outer thickness × 0.026 − superior outer thickness × 0.267 + nasal outer thickness × 0.159 − inferior outer thickness × 0.197 − superior inner thickness × 0.060 + foveal thickness × 0.049 [36].

For the Retinal LDF, the area under the ROC curves was 0.900 (**Table 5**).

OCT parameters	AUC	95% CI	AUC P-value	Cut-off point	Sens (%)	Spec (%)
Retinal LDF	0.900	0.862–0.933	**<0.001**	>–58.4	89.5	80.5
Foveal thickness	0.467	0.409–0.525	0.345	>305	22.4	96.5
Temporal inner thickness	0.737	0.684–0.787	**<0.001**	≤327	66.3	75.5
Temporal outer thickness	0.680	0.624–0.733	**<0.001**	≤277	47.2	83.5
RNFL LDF	0.824	0.777–0.865	**<0.001**	>–0.84	85.6	63.5
RNFL average thickness	0.535	0.478–0.592	0.185	<86	17.1	96.5
RNFL temporal thickness	0.574	0.517–0.630	0.083	>77	32.4	86.5

OCT parameters	AUC	95% CI	AUC P-value	Cut-off point	Sens (%)	Spec (%)
RNFL PMB sector	0.567	0.510–0.623	**0.037**	>52	65.7	50.0
RNFL N/T index	0.586	0.529–0.641	**0.016**	≤1.16	65.7	52.5

AUC, area under the receiver operating characteristic curve; CI, confidence interval; LDF, linear discriminant function; OCT, optical coherence tomography; RNFL, retinal nerve fiber layer; Sens, Sensitivity; Spec, Specificity.

Table 5. In the validating set, areas under the receiver operating characteristic curves, best sensitivity-specificity balance, and likelihood ratios of retinal nerve fiber layer parameters of the Nsite Axonal Analytics software of Spectralis optical coherence tomography (OCT) to discriminate between normal subjects and patients with Parkinson's disease.

The largest areas under the ROC curves were those for the Temporal Inner and Outer retinal thickness [36].

3. Discussion

Parkinson's disease patients present decreased high and low contrast VA and CSV, and mild anomalies in color perception. Visual dysfunction in PD is frequently underdiagnosed, since tests designed to detect abnormalities in visual function are not routinely performed in eye examination, and symptoms often go unnoticed by patients.

Neurodegeneration caused by PD can be detected using OCT. Our studies, along with previous research, revealed a reduction in retinal thickness (specifically in the macular area), RNFL and RGC thicknesses in patients suffering from PD. The loss of RGCs has been linked to visual dysfunction and may also be responsible for visual function anomalies in PD patients.

The loss of RGCs leads to a corresponding decrease in retinal and RNFL thicknesses that can be detected using OCT [37, 38]. In PD patients, this loss could be due to primary neurodegeneration of the RGCs and their axons or to retrograde degeneration of the RGC layer plus its axons produced by PD lesions of the posterior visual pathways [39]. Retrograde RGC degeneration produced by retrogeniculate lesions was previously reported in patients with homonymous hemianopia [40], which suggests that OCT measurements reveal combined anterior and posterior visual pathway disease [40, 41].

Our results revealed macular thinning of all areas in patients with PD compared with controls, an inverse correlation with HY and UPDRS severity, and a positive correlation with the Schwab–England ADL scale. Therefore, increased neurologic alterations and severity of PD progression are linked to thinning of macular tissue. The degree of correlation, although significant, was low moderate. These results, however, are consistent with findings in other neurodegenerative diseases [42].

Our segmentation analysis revealed that the GCL thickness was inversely correlated with disease duration and PD severity and was predictive of axonal damage in PD patients. We believe that further research with segmentation application is needed to establish the extent to which each retinal layer can predict PD in particular circumstances (e.g., recognizing PD when in an early stage), or to evaluate the effectiveness of different treatments.

The retinal measurements provided by Fourier domain OCT technology are tools that can be used in combination with other parameters and clinical explorations. LDF calculated upon OCT parameters may be more sensitive and specific than the methods currently used for diagnosis. Our Retinal LDF yielded higher sensitivity (at a high specificity) than any single parameter determined using OCT. The high sensibility and specificity demonstrated by OCT may be better than some of the accepted neuroimaging criteria in the current PD diagnosis procedure.

The LDFs presented in our study, however, demonstrate better accuracy for PD diagnosis in patients with advanced disease. Clinical application of our findings may help diagnosis in patients who suffer from movement alterations, and PD is suspected. Our results indicate that retinal thinning may be useful for detecting patients with PD. However, larger studies using OCT technology are needed to evaluate the sensitivity, specificity, and the ability of retinal thickness measurements to detect PD. Longitudinal prospective studies should be carried out in the future, to assess disease progression and treatment effectiveness.

Author details

María Satue*, Vicente Polo, Sofía Otin, Jose M. Larrosa, Javier Obis and Elena Garcia-Martin

*Address all correspondence to: mariasatue@gmail.com

IIS Aragon, Ophthalmology Department, Institute for Health Sciencies of Aragon (IACS), Miguel Servet University Hospital, Zaragoza, Spain

References

[1] Park A, Stacy M. Non-motor symptoms in Parkinson's disease. J Neurol 2009; 256(Suppl 3): 293–298.

[2] Bodis-Wollner I. Retinopathy in Parkinson disease. J Neural Transm 2009;116:1493–501.

[3] Bodis-Wollner I. Visual acuity and contrast sensitivity in patients with cerebral lesions. Science 1972;178:769–71.

[4] Bodis-Wollner I, Diamond S. The measurement of spatial contrast sensitivity in cases of blurred vision associated with cerebral lesions. Brain 1976;99:695–710.

[5] Price MJ, Feldman RG, Adelberg D, Kayne H. Abnormalities in color vision and contrast sensitivity in Parkinson's disease. Neurology 1992;42:887–90.

[6] Oh YS, Kim JS, Chung SW, Song IU, Kim YD, Kim YI, Lee KS. Color vision in Parkinson's disease and essential tremor. Eur J Neurol 2011;18: 577–83.

[7] Hipp G, Diedericha NJ, Pieria V, Vaillant M. Primary vision and facial emotion recognition in early Parkinson's disease. J Neurol Sci 2014;338: 178–82.

[8] Archibald NK, Clarke MP, Mosimann UP, Burn DJ. Retinal thickness in Parkinson's disease. Parkinsonism Relat Disord 2011; 17(6):431–6.

[9] Satue M, Seral M, Otin S, Alarcia R, Herrero R, Bambo MP, Fuertes MI, Pablo LE, Garcia-Martin E. Retinal thinning and correlation with functional disability in patients with Parkinson's disease. Br J Ophthalmol 2014;98(3):350–5.

[10] Garcia-Martin E, Pueyo V, Ara JR, Almarcegui C, Martin J, Pablo L, Dolz I, Sancho E, Fernandez FJ. Effect of optic neuritis on progressive axonal damage in multiple sclerosis patients. Mult Scler 2011;17:830–837.

[11] Burgansky-Eliash Z, Wollstein G, Chu T, Glymour C, Noecker RJ, Ishikawa H, Schuman JS. Optical coherence tomography machine learning classifiers for glaucoma detection: a preliminary study. Investig Ophthalmol Vis Sci 2005;46:4147–4152.

[12] Garcia-Martin E, Pueyo V, Martin J, Almarcegui C, Ara JR, Dolz I, Honrubia FM, Fernandez FJ. Progressive changes in the retinal nerve fiber layer in patients with multiple sclerosis. Eur J Ophthalmol 2010;20:167–173.

[13] Garcia-Martin E, Pablo LE, Herrero R, Satue M, Polo V, Larrosa JM, Martin J, Fernandez J. Diagnostic ability of a linear discriminant function for Spectral domain optical coherence tomography in multiple sclerosis patients. Ophthalmology 2012;119(8): 1705–11.

[14] Larrosa JM, Garcia-Martin E, Bambo MP, Pinilla J, Polo V, Otin S, Satue M, Herrero R, Pablo LE. Potential new diagnostic tool for Alzheimer's disease using a linear discriminant function for Fourier domain optical coherence tomography. Investig Ophthalmol Vis Sci 2014;55(5):3043–51.

[15] Garcia-Martin E, Satue M, Otin S, Fuertes I, Alarcia R, Larrosa JM, Polo V, Pablo LE. Retina measurements for diagnosis of Parkinson disease. Retina 2014;34(5):971–80.

[16] Garcia-Martin E, Larrosa JM, Polo V, Satue M, Marques ML, Alarcia R, Seral M, Fuertes I, Otin S, Pablo LE. Distribution of retinal layer atrophy in patients with Parkinson disease and association with disease severity and duration. Am J Ophthalmol 2014;157(2):470–478.

[17] Turano KA, Broman AT, Bandeen-Roche K, Munoz B, Rubin GS, West SK. Association of visual field loss and mobility performance in older adults: salisbury eye evaluation study. Optom Visi Sci 2004;81(5):298–307.

[18] Leat SJ, Woo GC. The validity of current clinical tests of contrast sensitivity and their ability to predict reading speed in low vision. Eye 1997;11(6):893–9.

[19] Wood JM. Age and visual impairment decrease driving performance as measured on a closed-road circuit. Hum Factors 2002;44(3):482–94.

[20] West SK, Rubin GS, Broman AT, Muñoz B, Bandeen-Roche K, Turano K. How does visual impairment affect performance on tasks of everyday life? The SEE project. Arch Ophthalmol 2002;120(6):774–80.

[21] Kim, KJ, Rieke, F. Temporal contrast adaptation in the input and output signals of salamander retinal ganglion cells. J. Neurosci 2001;21:287–99.

[22] Hajee ME, March WF, Lazzaro DR, Wolintz AH, Shrier EM, Glazman S, Bodis-Wollner IG. Inner retinal layer thinning in Parkinson's disease. Arch Ophthalmol 2009;127:737–41.

[23] Gelb DJ, Oliver E, Gilman S. Diagnostic criteria for Parkinson disease. Arch Neurol 1999;56:33–9.

[24] Vingrys AJ, King-Smith PE. A quantitative scoring technique for panel tests of color vision. Investig Ophthalmol Vis Sci 1988;29(1):50–63.

[25] Bowman AJ. A method for quantitive scoring of the Farnsworth panel D15. Acta Ophthalmol 1982;60:907–16.

[26] Laycock R, Crewther SG, Crewther DP. A role for the 'magnocellular advantage' in visual impairments in neurodevelopmental and psychiatric disorders. Neurosci Biobehav Rev 2007;31:363–76.

[27] Lampert EJ, Andorra M, Torres-Torres R, Ortiz-Pérez S, Llufriu S, Sepúlveda M, Sola N, Saiz A, Sánchez-Dalmau B, Villoslada P, Martínez-Lapiscina EH. Color vision impairment in multiple sclerosis points to retinal ganglion cell damage. J Neurol 2015;262(11):2491–7.

[28] Besharse J, Dana J, editors. Corneal Imaging: Clinical. Encyclopedia of the Eye, 1st ed. Academic Press Inc; Elsevier 2010. 9780123741981.

[29] Inzelberg R, Ramirez JA, Nisipeanu P, Ophir A. Retinal nerve fiber layer thinning in Parkinson's disease. Vis Res 2004;44:2793–7.

[30] Cubo E, Tedejo RP, Rodriguez Mendez V. Retina thickness in Parkinson's disease and essential tremor. Mov Disord 2010;25:2461–77.

[31] Satue M, Garcia-Martin E, Fuertes I, Otin S, Alarcia R, Herrero R, Bambo MP, Pablo LE, Fernandez FJ. Use of Fourier-domain OCT to detect retinal nerve fiber layer degeneration in Parkinson's disease patients. Eye (Lond) 2013;27:507–14.

[32] Garcia-Martin E, Satue M, Fuertes, Otin S, Alarcia R, Herrero R, Bambo MP, Fernandez J, Pablo LE. Ability and reproducibility of Fourier domain optical coherence tomography to detect retinal nerve fiber layer atrophy in Parkinson's disease. Ophthalmology 2012;119:2161–7.

[33] Altintaş O, Işeri P, Ozkan B, Cağlar Y. Correlation between retinal morphological and functional findings and clinical severity in Parkinson's disease. Doc Ophthalmol 2008;116:137–46.

[34] Almarcegui C, Dolz I, Pueyo V, Garcia E, Fernandez FJ, Martin J, Ara JR, Honrubia F. Correlation between functional and structural assessments of the optic nerve and retina in multiple sclerosis patients. Neurophysiol Clin 2010;40(3):129–135.

[35] Davies EC, Galetta KM, Sackel DJ, Talman LS, Frohman EM, Calabresi PA, Galetta SL, Balcer LJ. Retinal ganglion cell layer volumetric assessment by spectral-domain optical coherence tomography in multiple sclerosis: Application of a high precision manual estimation technique. J Neuroophthalmol 2011;31(3):260–264.

[36] Garcia-Martin E, Satue M, Otin S, Fuertes I, Alarcia R, Larrosa JM, Polo V, Pablo LE. Retina measurements for diagnosis of Parkinson disease. Retina 2014;34(5):971–80.

[37] Maresca A, la Morgia C, Caporali L, Valentino ML, Carelli V. The optic nerve: a "mito-window" on mitochondrial neurodegeneration. Mol Cell Neurosci 2013;55:62–76.

[38] La Morgia C, Barboni P, Rizzo G, Carbonelli M, Savini G, Scaglione C, Capellari S, Bonazza S, Giannoccaro MP, Calandra-Buonaura G, Liguori R, Cortelli P, Martinelli P, Baruzzi A, Carelli V. Loss of temporal retinal nerve fibers in Parkinson disease: a mitochondrial pattern? Eur J Neurol 2013;20:198–201.

[39] Albrecht P, Ringelstein M, Müller AK, Keser N, Dietlein T, Lappas A, Foerster A, Hartung HP, Aktas O, Methner A. Degeneration of retinal layers in multiple sclerosis subtypes quantified by optical coherence tomography. Mult Scler 2012;18(10):1422–1429.

[40] Jindahra P, Petrie A, Plant GT. Retrograde trans-synaptic retinal ganglion cell loss identified by optical coherence tomography. Brain 2009;132(Pt3):628–634.

[41] Reich DS, Smith SA, Gordon-Lipkin EM, Ozturk A, Caffo BS, Balcer LJ, Calabresi PA. Damage to the optic radiation in multiple sclerosis is associated with retinal injury and visual disability. Arch Neurol 2009;66(8):998–1006.

[42] Garcia-Martin E, Rodriguez-Mena D, Herrero R, Almarcegui C, Dolz I, Martin J, Ara JR, Larrosa JM, Polo V, Fernández J, Pablo LE. Neuro-ophthalmologic evaluation, quality of life and functional disability in MS patients. Neurology 2013;81:1–8.

Chapter 18

Possible Treatments of Atypical Parkinsonism

Moretti Davide Vito

Additional information is available at the end of the chapter

http://dx.doi.org/10.5772/63948

Abstract

Success in treating patients with atypical parkinsonism remains exceedingly low. It is particularly important for both neurologists and general practitioners to have a guideline in the actual possible cure options. This study reviews the limited available literature reporting treatment trials about treatment in parkinsonism. Various therapeutical approaches have been tried with rasagiline, immunoglobulin, autologous mesenchymal stem cells, davunetide, lithium, and tideglusib. Recently, transdermal rotigotine (RTG) has been proposed for the treatment of atypical parkinsonism, as well as deep brain stimulation (DBS) of the pedunculopontine nucleus (PPN) alone or combined with globus pallidus internus (Gpi) stimulation. The outcomes reviewed here highlight the need for the development of randomized, placebo-controlled trials to validate outcomes about rotigotine, DBS, and all other new therapies directed at altering the underlying biological mechanisms involved in the disease process.

Keywords: atypical parkinsonism, treatment options, pharmacological intervention, deep brain stimulation, diagnosis

1. Introduction

Progressive supranuclear palsy (PSP), corticobasal degeneration (CBD), multiple system atrophy (MSA), Parkinson's disease with dementia (PDD), and dementia with Lewy bodies (DLB) are usually indicated as atypical parkinsonian syndromes (APS). Anyway, each of that syndrome is characterized by peculiar anatomo-pathological picture [1–5]. Up to date, the amount of pathophysiological data available regarding APS has progressively grown in the past two decades. Nonetheless, the etiology of APS is still under investigation and effective treatments are lacking [6,7]. Various therapeutical approaches have been tried with rasagiline, immunoglobulin, autologous mesenchymal stem cells, davunetide, lithium, and tideglusib [8]. Recently, the transdermal rotigotine (RTG) has been proposed for the treatment of atypical parkinsonism [9–11], as well as deep brain stimulation of the pedunculopontine nucleus (PPN) alone or combined with globus pallidus internus (Gpi) stimulation [12]. This study reviews the limited available literature reporting treatment trials. The outcomes reviewed here highlight the need for the development of novel therapies directed at altering the underlying biological mechanisms involved in the disease process.

2. Materials and methods

This study reviews all the limited available literature reporting treatment trials about treatment in atypical parkinsonism.

3. Clinical features

Diagnosis of AP has been performed in accordance with the primary diffuse tips and medical criteria [13–20]. PSP is characterized by vertical gaze abnormalities, early falls, postural instability, and presenile cognitive impairment. PSP has two principal clinical forms: classical PSP (or Richardson's syndrome) and PSP-parkinsonism (PSP-P). Respect to the classical form, PSP-P is characterized by the presence of tremor and an inconstant clinical response to levodopa. The classical CBD phenotype includes apraxia, cortical sensory loss, alien limb, as well as dystonia and myoclonus. MSA patients usually show a mix of cerebellar and pyramidal signs, parkinsonism, and autonomic dysfunction. The predominant phenotype at onset of MSA allows the classification into MSA-parkinsonism or MSA-cerebellar form. The diagnosis of PD was made following previously published criteria [21]. Only subjects with idiopathic PD were enclosed within the present study in order to get a homogeneous sample study population [22]. So, patients had unilateral onset and development of parkinsonian signs, two of the three cardinal signs among akinesia, rigidity, and postural abnormalities and resting tremor. A superb response to a dopaminoagonist treatment was a strong criterion. In the Parkison-dementia group, patients with idiopathic PD, who developed cognitive decline after a year of the onset of parkinsonism, were included. On the contrary, in Lewy Body Dementia (LBD) group, patients with cognitive impairment appeared within 1 year after the onset of movement disorders were included Moreover, in this group patients with Rapid Eye Movements (REM) sleep behavior disorders, vivid dreams, hallucinations and postural instability have been enclosed [22].

4. Results

4.1. Current pharmacological chances in APS

Table 1 summarizes the most important clinical trials aiming to find a drug therapy for APS.

Authors	Disease	Treatment	Duration	Outcomes
Poewe et al. [23]	MSA	Rasagiline	48 weeks	No improvement
Novak et al. [24]	MSA	Intravenous immunoglobulin	6 months	Improvement
Lee et al. [25]	MSA-cerebellar type	Autologous mesenchymal stem cells	12 months	Improvement
Hoglinger et al. [35]	PSP	Tideglusib	12 months	Improvement
www.allontherapeutics.com, 2012	PSP	Davunetide	52 weeks	No improvement
Stamelou et al. [40]	PSP	CoQ10	6 weeks	Improvement
Moretti et al. [9–11]	MSA-PSP-CBD-LBD	Transdermal rotigotine	24 months	Improvement
Servello et al. [12]	PSP	DBS of PPN	12 months	Improvement

Table 1. Synopsis of the main clinical trials for the treatment of atypical parkinsonism.

The monoamine oxidase-B inhibitor rasagiline with the dosage of 1 mg/day has been assessed in a randomized, placebo-controlled clinical trial for 48 weeks in 174 patients with possible or probable MSA-parkinsonism type. The total Unified Multiple System Atrophy Rating Scale (UMSARS) score did not found significant improvements in the treated when compared to placebo groups [23].

A monthly infusions of 0.4 g/kg intravenous immunoglobulin for 6 months in seven patients with MSA found significantly improved UMSARS part I (activities of daily living) and II (motor functions) score. A verification study has been programmed [24] to validate the anti-inflammatory approach.

Injections of autologous mesenchymal stem cells (MSCs) in 33 patients with probable MSA-cerebellar compared with placebo demonstrated a smaller increase in total and part II UMSARS scores in the MSC group. Anyway, a careful evaluation of the exact efficacy of the staminal cells is under investigation [25].

Due to the dangers of postural instability in MSA from orthostatic hypotension, considerable attention has been directed toward blood pressure control. A synthetic norepinephrine precursor was tested in 10 patients with MSA in a randomized, double-blind, placebo-controlled study, resulting in an increase in supine and upright blood pressure [26,27]. Moreover, the droxidopa has been evaluated in a phase III clinical trial in order to assess the efficacy in orthostatic hypotension, and recently FDA approved its clinical use (http://www.medscape.com/viewarticle/820786). As about other autonomic symptoms, oxybutynin or tolterodine can be helpful for neurogenic bladder and desmopressin can be helpful for nocturnal polyuria, whereas sildenafil may be efficacious in erectile dysfunction, but can dramatically worsen postural hypotension (Stamelou and Bathia). Recent large controlled studies with rasagiline and rifampicin have shown no neuroprotective effect [23,28].

In regard to PSP and CBD, in clinical practice, treatment options are limited to a levodopa trial (up to 1 g/d) and amantadine for parkinsonism and gait disturbance as well as valproate or levetiracetam for myoclonus [29]. Although not sufficiently studied, botulinum toxin injections can be helpful to relieve dystonic spasms of the hand or to treat levator inhibition [30]. Early clinical trials in PSP employed drug treatment to correct alterations in the dopaminergic, cholinergic, and gamma-amino butyric acid (GABA)ergic pathways and produced limited evidence of benefit. Trials with both physostigmine and donepezil were employed with a poor response in memory as well as motor function [31,32]. As about GABAergic agonists, trials with zolpidem [33] and gabapentin [34] found, respectively, transient improvement in eye movements and inhibitory frontal function. Anyway, these trials were limited by small sample size and little evidence of a long-term benefit of the treatment.

Progressive Supranuclear Palsy Rating Scale (PSPRS) and the Schwab and England Activities of Daily Living (SEADL) did not show significant outcomes in a multinational randomized, double-blind, placebo-controlled trial in which 313 patient with PSP received davunetide 30 mg twice daily or placebo (press release December 18, 2012 by Allon Therapeutics, www.allontherapeutics.com).

The inhibitors of glycogen synthase kinase-3 (GSK-3) such as lithium or tideglusib have been administered in PSP or CBD patients in two distinct trials. The lithium trial (ClinicalTrials.gov; identifier NCT00703677) a patient with PSP ended before the natural time because the drug was not tolerated. The tideglusib trial did not show significant improvement between the high-dose, low-dose, and placebo groups in the final clinical evaluation [35].

Methylene blue derivatives are inhibitors of tau protein aggregation. These agents could be a rational treatment for PSP and CBD. Anyway, the most advanced strategies for reducing tau protein are immunologic approaches targeting different tau epitopes [36]. Moreover, passive immunization approaches, which act through anti-tau monoclonal antibody directed against various tau epitopes, were shown to block seeding activity and improve cognitive deficits in transgenic mice [37].

Microtubule-stabilizing agents are also explored as potential therapies compensating the loss of tau protein function in PSP and CBD. In particular, taxanes, a class of cancer drugs and a related class of compounds called epothilones, are now being investigated as tau-related neurodegeneration. The epothilone D was found to improve axonal microtubule density and improved spatial learning in treated mice [38,39]. It has been suggested that mitochondrial dysfunction may contribute to pathogenesis of atypical parkinsonisms. This evidence has led to an interest in replacing the coenzyme Q10 (CoQ10), a component of the complex I of the mitochondrial chain. A small, double-blind, placebo-controlled, randomized trial involving 21 PSP patients treated with CoQ10 for 6 weeks has shown improvement in PSPRS scores, frontal assessment battery scores, and occipital energy when compared with placebo [40]. Currently, a large phase III trial with CoQ10 in PSP patients for 12 months is underway.

As about the LBD, the cholinergic deficit that affects in an important way these patients could benefit from the cholinesterase inhibitors; hallucinations, neuropsychiatric symptoms, and psychosis are all reduced in LBD [41].

In a large, randomized, double-blind controlled trial with 120 LBD patients over 20 weeks, rivastigmine treatment resulted in reduction of apathy, delusions, anxiety, and hallucinations, as well as improvements in cognitive assessment [42]. Furthermore, a 3-week post-treatment follow-up has also shown better Neuropsychiatric Inventory (NPI) scores [43]. A recent multicenter trial in Japan has administered donepezil to 140 patients with LBD showing clinical, cognitive, and behavioral improvement when compared to placebo [44].

Recently, the effect of memantine, an NMDA-receptor antagonist, has been evaluated in two clinical trials [45,46] in patients with both LBD and PDD. Although some clinical benefits have been reached, the effect of memantine remains inconclusive.

Atypical antipsychotic agents such as quetiapine are recommended because of the risk of extrapyramidal side effects in patients with LBD. Clonazepam at low dosage could be used in REM sleep behavior disorder. As about parkinsonian disorders, levodopa should be administered instead of dopaminergic agents with a particular care to the aggravation of psychotic symptoms.

4.2. Transdermal RTG as treatment option for atypical parkinsonian syndrome

Transdermal RTG seems to be effective and well tolerated in patients with APS. Recent studies [9–11] show significant improvement in UDPRS-III scores, maintained along the course of the 248 months follow-up. Only seven patients were dropped out, and 15 patients were affected by adverse events. In this study, behavioral or psychiatric adverse events and ICDs were not found. Moreover, results also show a reduction in NPI scores that became significant at the last follow-up evaluation (T18). Finally, during the study the patients did not suffer from congestive heart failure. These results confirm previous evidences obtained in patients with idiopathic Parkinson's disease showing positive effect on motor control and behavioral disturbances [47–55] as well as a good safety of RTG [56]. On the whole, these outcomes highlight that transdermal RTG should be considered as a therapeutic option for the treatment of atypical parkinsonism.

4.3. Deep brain stimulation in PSP

In a recent study [12], three patients with PSP were submitted to the deep brain stimulation of the pedunculopontine nucleus (PPN). A reduction of falls and an amelioration of postural balance were observed. The patients required less assistance for daily living activities. The clinical improvement was, however, not fully reflected in the evaluating scales. The mean PSPRS percentage decrease was of 26.3% (SD = 8.3) at the 12-month follow-up visit for the three patients. The diversity between the reported improvement and the PSPRS might be due to the phenomenological diversity of PSP, not fully captured by the PSPRS, and repeated scheduled postoperative evaluations are necessary to capture objectively the overall clinical improvement. That the greatest PSPRS percentage decrease (35.7%) was seen in the double-implanted GPi-PPN patient is possibly due to the improvement of the concomitant amelioration of his or her dystonic state. It remains of course speculative in light of a single case if this better clinical outcome seen in the GPi-PPN patient is reflection of an increased synergic effect of PPN and GPi secondary to stimulation, bearing in mind the strong connectivity between the basal ganglia and the PPN. An interesting observation was related to the stimulation parameters; we started with low-frequency stimulation, which was increased progressively to 130 Hz without noticing a significant change in clinical presentation.

4.4. Supportive therapies

The palliative therapies are highly recommended in APS patients. An assortment of physical, occupational, and language therapies should be considered, paying attention to the most invalidating symptom, that is, apraxia. If the risk of falls and postural instability become prevailing symptoms, a wheelchair has to be suggested and should be advised to patient and family. This acknowledgment can be shockingly testing and troublesome. Numerous families see the utilization of a wheelchair as a marker of the last loss of the capacity to ambulate and stay free. They should be persuaded that in addition to the fact that this is vital for the well-being of the patient, the wheelchair can give a more prominent level of flexibility than the constrained portability given by the patient's attempts to try to deambulate. At long last, it is vital to screen and support the prosperity of the caregivers. The especially troublesome mix of serious motor inability with cognitive and behavioral aggravations increases the risk of an overwhelming burnout.

4.5. Future treatment options

Different approaches such as "regenerative" or "restorative" (e.g., stem cells and trophic factors) are desirable to provide advance in the field of disease-modifying therapy. Trials of "neuroprotective" therapies are actively being planned or have been implemented (e.g., a trial of riluzole for PSP and multiple system atrophy has been initiated in Europe). Further discussion and evaluation of the best endpoints for clinical trials in these disorders are an important priority. One of the major obstacles to the design of the necessary clinical trials is the accuracy of clinical diagnosis. This finding emphasizes the need for developing biological markers for these neurodegenerative disorders. The similarities in the underlying neuropathology and molecular biology of these disorders suggest that critical advances in this field will equally impact on the treatment outcomes [1].

5. Conclusions

Up to date, the possibilities of the APS care are without no doubt very low. Two main goals are to achieve: the better understanding of the pathogenic mechanisms and the improvement of both symptomatic and disease-modifying treatments through controlled clinical trials. In the near future, every effort should be made to give hope to patients and caregivers whose number will not decrease.

http://dx.doi.org/10.5772/63948

Acknowledgements

Author contributions: Moretti DV was responsible for the conception and design of the study, acquisition, analysis, and interpretation of data, as well as for the drafting and revising of the article.

Author details

Moretti Davide Vito

Address all correspondence to: davide.moretti@afar.it

IRCCS S. Giovanni di Dio Fatebenefratelli, Brescia, Italy

References

[1] Litvan I, Bhatia KP, Burn DJ, et al. Movement Disorders Society Scientific Issues Committee report: SIC Task Force appraisal of clinical diagnostic criteria for Parkinsonian disorders. Mov Disord 2003;18:467–486.

[2] Williams DR, de Silva R, Paviour DC, et al. Characteristics of two distinct clinical phenotypes in pathologically proven progressive supranuclear palsy: Richardson's syndrome and PSP-parkinsonism. Brain 2005;128(Pt 6):1247–1258.

[3] Gilman S, Wenning GK, Low PA, et al. Second consensus statement on the diagnosis of multiple system atrophy. Neurology 2008;71:670–676.

[4] Stamelou M, Quinn N, Bhatia K. 'Atypical' parkinsonism: new genetic disorders presenting with features of PSP, MSA or CBD. Mov Disord 2013 (Epub ahead of print).

[5] Wenning GK, Geser F, Krismer F, et al. The natural history of multiple system atrophy: a prospective European cohort study. Lancet Neurol 2013;12:264–274.

[6] Antonini A, Cilia R. Behavioural adverse effects of dopaminergic treatments in Parkinson's disease: incidence, neurobiological basis, management and prevention. Drug Saf 2009;32(6):475–488.

[7] Vilas D, Pont-Sunyer C, Tolosa E. Impulse control disorders in Parkinson's disease. Parkinsonism Relat Disord 2012;18 Suppl 1:S80–S84.

[8] Lang AE. Treatment of progressive supranuclear palsy and corticobasal degeneration. Mov Disord 2005;20(Suppl 12):S83–S91.

[9] Moretti DV, Binetti G, Zanetti O, Frisoni GB. Rotigotine is safe and efficacious in Atypical Parkinsonism Syndromes induced by both α-synucleinopathy and tauopathy. Neuropsychiatr Dis Treat 2014;10:1003–1009. doi: 10.2147/NDT.S64015 (eCollection 2014a).

[10] Moretti DV, Binetti G, Zanetti O, Frisoni GB. Behavioral and neurophysiological effects of transdermal rotigotine in atypical parkinsonism. Front Neurol 2014;5:85. doi: 10.3389/fneur.2014.00085 (eCollection 2014b).

[11] Moretti DV, Binetti G, Zanetti O, Frisoni GB. Non-ergot dopamine agonist rotigotine as a promising therapeutic tool in atypical parkinsonism syndromes: a 24 months pilot observational open-label study. Neuropharmacology 2014;85:284–289. doi: 10.1016/j.neuropharm.2014.05.028 (Epub 2014 Jun 7).

[12] Servello D, Zekaj E, Saleh C, Menghetti C, Porta M. Long-term follow-up of deep brain stimulation of pedunculopontine nucleus in progressive supranuclear palsy: report of three cases. Surg Neurol Int 2014;5(Suppl 8):S416–S420. doi: 10.4103/2152-7806.140208 (eCollection 2014).

[13] Litvan I, Mangone CA, McKee A, et al. Natural history of progressive supranuclear palsy (Steele–Richardson–Olszewski syndrome) and clinical predictors of survival: a clinicopathological study. J Neurol Neurosurg Psychiatry 1996;60:615–620.

[14] Litvan I, Agid Y, Calne D, et al. Clinical research criteria for the diagnosis of progressive supranuclear palsy (Steele–Richardson–Olszewski syndrome): report of the NINDS-SPSP international workshop. Neurology 1996;47:1–9.

[15] Wenning GK, Ben-Shlomo Y, Magalhaes M, Daniel SE, Quinn NP. Clinicopathological study of 35 cases of multiple system atrophy. J Neurol Neurosurg Psychiatry 1995;58:160–166.

[16] Wenning GK, Tison F, Ben Shlomo Y, Daniel SE, Quinn NP. Multiple system atrophy: a review of 203 pathologically proven cases. Mov Disord 1997;12:133–147.

[17] Wenning GK, Scherfler C, Granata R, et al. Time course of symptomatic orthostatic hypotension and urinary incontinence in patients with postmortem confirmed parkinsonian syndromes: a clinicopathological study. J Neurol Neurosurg Psychiatry 1999;67:620–623.

[18] Wenning GK, Stefanova N, Jellinger KA, Poewe W, Schlossmacher MG. Multiple system atrophy: a primary oligodendrogliopathy. Ann Neurol 2008;64:239–246.

[19] Williams DR, Lees AJ. Progressive supranuclear palsy: clinicopathological concepts and diagnostic challenges. Lancet Neurol 2009;8:270–279.

[20] Ling H, O'Sullivan SS, Holton JL, et al. Does corticobasal degeneration exist? A clinicopathological re-evaluation. Brain 2010;133(Pt 7):2045–2057.

[21] Berardelli A, Wenning GK, Antonini A, Berg D, Bloem BR, Bonifati V, Brooks D, Burn DJ, Colosimo C, Fanciulli A, Ferreira J, Gasser T, Grandas F, Kanovsky P, Kostic V,

Kulisevsky J, Oertel W, Poewe W, Reese JP, Relja M, Ruzicka E, Schrag A, Seppi K, Taba P, Vidailhet M. EFNS/MDS-ES/ENS [corrected] recommendations for the diagnosis of Parkinson's disease. Eur J Neurol. 2013;20(1):16–34. doi: 10.1111/ene.12022. Review. Erratum in: Eur J Neurol 2013;20(2):406.

[22] McKeith I, Dickson D, Lowe J, et al. Diagnosis and management of dementia with Lewy bodies: third report of the DLB Consortium. Neurology 2005;65:1863–1872.

[23] Poewe W, Barone P, Gliadi N, et al. A randomized, placebo-controlled clinical trial to assess the effects of rasagiline in patients with multiple system atrophy of the parkinsonian subtype. Mov Disord 2012; 27(Suppl 1):1182.

[24] Novak P, Williams A, Ravin P, et al. Treatment of multiple system atrophy using intravenous immunoglobulin. BMC Neurol 2012; 12:131.

[25] Lee PH, Lee JE, Kim HS, et al. A randomized trial of mesenchymal stem cells in multiple system atrophy. Ann Neurol 2012; 72:32–40.

[26] Freeman R, Landsberg L, Young J. The treatment of neurogenic orthostatic hypotension with 3,4-dl-threo-dihydroxyphenylserine: a randomized, placebo-controlled, crossover trial. Neurology 1999;53(9):2151–2157.

[27] Tsai RM, Boxer AL. Clinical trials: past, current, and future for atypical parkinsonian syndromes. Semin Neurol 2014;34(2):225–234. doi: 10.1055/s-0034-1381739.

[28] Low PA, Robertson D, Gilman S, et al. Efficacy and safety of rifampicin for multiple system atrophy: a randomised, double-blind, placebo-controlled trial. Lancet Neurol 2014;13:268–275.

[29] Stamelou M, Hoeglinger GU. Atypical parkinsonism: an update. Curr Opin Neurol 2013;26:401–405.

[30] Stamelou M, Alonso-Canovas A, Bhatia KP. Dystonia in corticobasal degeneration: a review of the literature on 404 pathologically proven cases. Mov Disord 2012;27:696–702.

[31] Fabbrini G, Barbanti P, Bonifati V, Colosimo C, Gasparini M, Vanacore N, Meco G. Donepezil in the treatment of progressive supranuclear palsy. Acta Neurol Scand 2001;103(2):123–125.

[32] Litvan I, Phipps M, Pharr VL, Hallett M, Grafman J, Salazar A. Randomized placebo-controlled trial of donepezil in patients with progressive supranuclear palsy. Neurology 2001;57(3):467–473

[33] Daniele A, Moro E, Bentivoglio AR. Zolpidem in progressive supranuclear palsy. N Engl J Med 1999;341(7):543–544. No abstract available. Erratum in: N Engl J Med 1999;341(21):1632.

[34] Poujois A, Vidailhet M, Trocello JM, Bourdain F, Gaymard B, Rivaud-Péchoux S. Effect of gabapentin on oculomotor control and parkinsonism in patients with progressive supranuclear palsy. Eur J Neurol 2007;14(9):1060–1062.

[35] Hoeglinger GU, Huppertz HJ, Wagenpfeil FS, et al. Tideglusib reduces progression of brain atrophy in progressive supranuclear palsy in a randomized trial. In: Alzheimer's Association International Conference, Vancouver, British Columbia, Canada, 2012, proposal number: 34102.

[36] Yanamandra K, Kfoury N, Jiang H, Mahan TE, Ma S, Maloney SE, Wozniak DF, Diamond MI, Holtzman DM. Anti-tau antibodies that block tau aggregate seeding in vitro markedly decrease pathology and improve cognition in vivo. Neuron 2013;80(2): 402–414. doi: 10.1016/j.neuron.2013.07.046.

[37] Brunden KR, Ballatore C, Lee VM, Smith AB 3rd, Trojanowski JQ. Brain-penetrant microtubule-stabilizing compounds as potential therapeutic agents for tauopathies. Biochem Soc Trans 2012;40(4):661–666. doi: 10.1042/BST20120010 (review).

[38] Barten DM, Fanara P, Andorfer C, Hoque N, Wong PY, Husted KH, Cadelina GW, Decarr LB, Yang L, Liu V, Fessler C, Protassio J, Riff T, Turner H, Janus CG, Sankaranarayanan S, Polson C, Meredith JE, Gray G, Hanna A, Olson RE, Kim SH, Vite GD, Lee FY, Albright CF. Hyperdynamic microtubules, cognitive deficits, and pathology are improved in tau transgenic mice with low doses of the microtubule-stabilizing agent BMS-241027. J Neurosci 2012;32(21):7137–7145.

[39] Stamelou M, Pilatus U, Reuss A, Magerkurth J, Eggert KM, Knake S, Ruberg M, Schade-Brittinger C, Oertel WH, Höglinger GU. In vivo evidence for cerebral depletion in high-energy phosphates in progressive supranuclear palsy. J Cereb Blood Flow Metab 2009;29(4):861–870. doi: 10.1038/jcbfm.2009.

[40] Stamelou M, Reuss A, Pilatus U, Magerkurth J, Niklowitz P, Eggert KM, Krisp A, Menke T, Schade-Brittinger C, Oertel WH, Höglinger GU. Short-term effects of coenzyme Q10 in progressive supranuclear palsy: a randomized, placebo-controlled trial. Mov Disord 2008;23(7):942–949. doi: 10.1002/mds.22023.

[41] McKeith I, Del Ser T, Spano P, Emre M, Wesnes K, Anand R, Cicin-Sain A, Ferrara R, Spiegel R. Efficacy of rivastigmine in dementia with Lewy bodies: a randomised, double-blind, placebo-controlled international study. Lancet 2000;356(9247):2031–2036

[42] Wesnes KA, McKeith IG, Ferrara R, Emre M, Del Ser T, Spano PF, Cicin-Sain A, Anand R, Spiegel R. Effects of rivastigmine on cognitive function in dementia with Lewy bodies: a randomised placebo-controlled international study using the cognitive drug research computerised assessment system. Dement Geriatr Cogn Disord 2002;13(3): 183–192

[43] Mori E, Ikeda M, Kosaka K, Donepezil-DLB Study Investigators. Donepezil for dementia with Lewy bodies: a randomized, placebo-controlled trial. Ann Neurol 2012;72(1):41–52. doi: 10.1002/ana.23557.

[44] Aarsland D, Ballard C, Walker Z, Bostrom F, Alves G, Kossakowski K, Leroi I, Pozo-Rodriguez F, Minthon L, Londos E. Memantine in patients with Parkinson's disease dementia or dementia with Lewy bodies: a double-blind, placebo-controlled, multicentre trial. Lancet Neurol 2009;8(7):613–618. doi: 10.1016/S1474-4422(09)70146-2.

[45] Fernandez HH, Wu CK, Ott BR. Pharmacotherapy of dementia with Lewy bodies. Expert Opin Pharmacother 2003;4(11):2027–2037.

[46] Emre M, Tsolaki M, Bonuccelli U, Destée A, Tolosa E, Kutzelnigg A, Ceballos-Baumann A, Zdravkovic S, Bladström A, Jones R, 11018 Study Investigators. Memantine for patients with Parkinson's disease dementia or dementia with Lewy bodies: a randomised, double-blind, placebo-controlled trial. Lancet Neurol 2010;9(10):969–977. doi: 10.1016/S1474-4422(10)70194-0.

[47] LeWitt PA, Boroojerdi B, Surmann E, Poewe W, SP716 Study Group, SP715 Study Group. Rotigotine transdermal system for long-term treatment of patients with advanced Parkinson's disease: results of two open-label extension studies, CLEOPATRA-PD and PREFER. J Neural Transm 2013;120(7):1069–1081. doi: 10.1007/s00702-012-0925-5 (Epub 2012 Dec 4).

[48] LeWitt PA, Lyons KE, Pahwa R, SP 650 Study Group Advanced Parkinson disease treated with rotigotine transdermal system: PREFER study. Neurology 2007;68:1262–1267.

[49] Poewe WH, Rascol O, Quinn N, Tolosa E, Oertel WH, Martignoni E, Rupp M, Boroojerdi B, SP 515 Investigators. Efficacy of pramipexole and transdermal rotigotine in advanced Parkinson's disease: a double-blind, double-dummy, randomised controlled trial. Lancet Neurol 2007;6:513–520.

[50] Scheller D, Ullmer C, Berkels R, Gwarek M, Lübbert H. The in vitro receptor profile of rotigotine: a new agent for the treatment of Parkinson's disease. Naunyn Schmiedebergs Arch Pharmacol 2009;379(1):73–86.

[51] Scheller D, Stichel-Gunkel C, Lübbert H, Porras G, Ravenscroft P, Hill M, Bezard E. Neuroprotective effects of rotigotine in the acute MPTP-lesioned mouse model of Parkinson's disease. Neurosci Lett 2008;432(1):30–34 (Epub 2007 Dec 8).

[52] Georgiev D, Danieli A, Ocepek L, Novak D, Zupancic-Kriznar N, Trost M, Pirtosek Z. Othello syndrome in patients with Parkinson's disease. Psychiatr Danub 2010;22(1):94–98.

[53] Sanford M, Scott LJ. Rotigotine transdermal patch: a review of its use in the treatment of Parkinson's disease. CNS Drugs 2011;25(8):699–719.

[54] Ray Chaudhuri K, Martinez-Martin P, Antonini A, Brown RG, Friedman JH, Onofrj M, Surmann E, Ghys L, Trenkwalder C. Rotigotine and specific non-motor symptoms of Parkinson's disease: post hoc analysis of RECOVER. Parkinsonism Relat Disord 2013;19(7):660–665. doi: 10.1016/j.parkreldis.2013.02.018 (Epub 2013 Apr 1).

[55] Zhou CQ, Li SS, Chen ZM, Li FQ, Lei P, Peng GG. Rotigotine transdermal patch in Parkinson's disease: a systematic review and meta-analysis. PLoS One 2013;8(7):e69738. doi: 10.1371/journal.pone.0069738; 1–9.

Chapter 19

The Role of Nurses in Parkinson's Disease

Michelle Hyczy de Siqueira Tosin and
Beatriz Guitton Renaud Baptista de Oliveira

Additional information is available at the end of the chapter

http://dx.doi.org/10.5772/63162

Abstract

Background: The complexity of motor and nonmotor symptoms in patients with Parkinson's disease (PD) requires multidisciplinary health actions.

Objective: To describe the role of nurses as members of multidisciplinary teams tasked with treatment of motor and nonmotor symptoms and provide nursing protocols for the care of patients with Parkinson's disease.

Methods: Analysis of the main diagnoses, outcomes, and ICNP® interventions identified by cross-mapping empirical evidence described in 2123 nursing documents and data from medical records of patients with Parkinson's disease in the specialized rehabilitation program at the Sarah Network of Rehabilitation Hospitals in Brazil. The protocols were based on scientific evidence and international recommendations.

Results: Clinical nursing protocols were developed based on a standardized nursing language of diagnoses, outcomes, and interventions focused on motor and nonmotor symptoms and principles of rehabilitation.

Conclusion: These protocols are expected to guide the clinical reasoning of nurses for comprehensive care of patients with Parkinson's disease and their families.

Keywords: Parkinson's disease, nursing role, specialist nurses, rehabilitation nurses, multidisciplinary teams

1. Introduction

Parkinson's disease (PD) affects approximately 1% of women and men worldwide, especially those over the age of 60 [1]. It is a multisystem and neurodegenerative disease with genetic and environmental factors that result in deficits in the production of neurotransmitters, including dopamine [2].

PD is diagnosed through a clinical evaluation of motor symptoms; the presence of nonmotor symptoms combined with the current lack of cure reflects the complexity of health care, which aims to control symptoms in order to maintain the quality of life of the patient and family [3–5].

Currently, health system remodelling is observed for the development of guidelines with multidisciplinary actions that address the complexity of care [6, 7].

Enabling health professionals with specific areas of knowledge allows standardization of behaviors that will minimize the challenges of interprofessional collaboration.

In this context, nursing care of patients with PD must focus on the biopsychosocial context and must be based on ethical, legal, operational, and theoretical assumptions of the profession for health promotion, prevention of complications, treatment, and rehabilitation [8].

Thus, the clinical reasoning of nurses should be based on the pathophysiology of the disease as well as the nursing process and should be structured in a standardized language for communication with other professionals on the team. Standardization of the nursing language enables communication and comparison of data between different contexts, countries, and languages, and maximizes dissemination of knowledge from clinical data [9, 10].

Among existing nursing terminologies is the International Classification for Nursing Practice (ICNP®), which was developed by the International Council of Nurses and is integrated into the family of international classifications of the World Health Organization [9]. This terminology allows development of terminological subsets of diagnoses, outcomes, and interventions targeted to specific areas of clinical nursing practice.

2. The role of nurses in Parkinson's disease

Research has shown increasing specialization among nurses who care for patients with PD [11–13]; thus, knowledge of the pathophysiology of this disease is arguably an important starting point for vocational training [14]. Based on this, we sought to hierarchically organize the major motor and nonmotor symptoms of PD using evidence gathered from the literature (**Figure 1**).

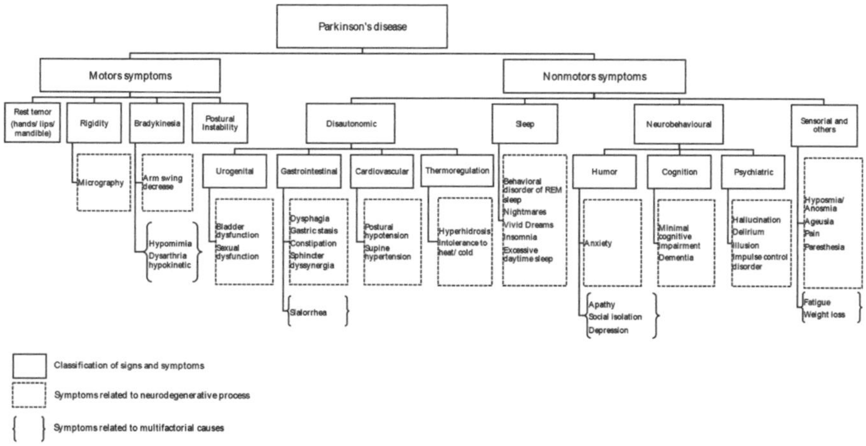

Figure 1. Classification of the main motor and nonmotor symptoms in Parkinson's disease.

The symptoms of PD are divided into motor and nonmotor; each of these classifications contains various other signs and symptoms related to both the neurodegenerative disease process itself as well as multifactorial causes. Thus, hierarchical organization of symptoms is not an easy task, and various descriptions have been proposed to facilitate understanding of the pathophysiology of the disease [15–18]; however, none of them have structured the symptoms into an organizational chart.

Our research on nursing diagnoses, outcomes, and interventions was based on this chart.

2.1. Nursing diagnoses/outcomes and interventions of ICNP® for patients with Parkinson's disease in rehabilitation

We analyzed 2123 nursing documentations from 352 medical records of patients with PD who participated in a rehabilitation program at a specialized centre in Rio de Janeiro, Brazil, from May 2009 to March 2014. From these documents, empirical evidence regarding nursing diagnoses, outcomes, and interventions was extracted. These dates were cross-mapped with ICNP® 2013 and validated by judges (nurses) to build a terminological subset of ICNP® for patients with PD in rehabilitation [19].

The diagnoses, outcomes, and interventions were divided into categories including motor symptoms, nonmotor symptoms, and principles of rehabilitation, as shown in **Figure 2**.

Greater variability was observed in nursing diagnoses, outcomes, and interventions related to nonmotor symptoms of Parkinson's disease; in general, it appears that nurses work in a comprehensive and communicative manner with other professionals on multidisciplinary teams.

Diagnoses and Outcomes ICNP® 2013 release	Interventions ICNP® 2013 release
Motor symptoms and Self Care and Safety	
Tremor Hypoactivity Impaired Ability To Communicate By Talking, Impaired Ability To Transfer, Impaired Bed Mobility, Impaired Mobility, Impaired Psychomotor Activity, Slurred Speech Self Care Deficit Impaired Ability To Bath, Impaired Ability To Dress, Impaired Ability to Feed Self, Impaired Ability To Groom, Impaired Ability To Perform Hygiene Impaired House Safety Risk For Fall, Risk for Fall Injury Impaired Walking Wheelchair Mobility Lack Of Knowledge Of Disease	Teaching the Patient to Self Care Teaching about Feeding Device Teaching Adaptation for Communication Teaching the Patient a to Applying Safety Device to Self Care Teaching the Family to Obtaining a Caregiver Teaching the Patient About House Safety Teaching The Family About Fall Prevention Teaching about Transfer Technique Referring To Physical Therapy Teaching the Patient About Rehabilitation Teaching the Group About Disease and About Rehabilitation Teaching About Health Seeking Behaviour Referring the Patient and Family to the Group to Teaching About Disease and Teaching About Rehabilitation
Non-motor Symptoms - Disautonomic - Urogenital	
Impaired Urinary System Process Enuresis, Stress Incontinence, Impaired Urine, Urge Incontinence, Urinary Incontinence Risk For Urine Infection, Urinary Tract Infection Impotence	Teaching Patient about the Urinary System Process, Evaluating Genitourinary Status, Assessing Bowel Status, Measuring Fluid Intake, Measuring Fluid Output, Assessing Urinary Retention Using Ultrasound, Teaching for Urination Controlling, Teaching Self Catheterisation, Referring to Interprofessional Team, Catheterising Bladder to Collecting Specimen of Urine, Collecting Specimen of Urine
Non-motor Symptoms - Disautonomic - Gastrointestinal	
Impaired Gastrointestinal System Process Constipation, Impaired Swallowing, Nausea, Perceived Constipation, Bowel Incontinence, Abnormal Salivation	Teaching the Group About Eating Pattern, Teaching the Patient About Eating Pattern, Collecting Specimen of Faeces, Teaching the Group About Fluid Intake, Teaching the Patient About Fluid Intake, Teaching the Group about Gastrointestinal System Process, Teaching the Patient about Gastrointestinal System Process
Non-motor Symptoms - Disautonomic - Cardiovascular	
Hypotension Peripheral Oedema	Measuring Blood Pressure, Teaching Measuring Blood Pressure, Teaching About Disease, Referring to Interprofessional Team
Non-motor Symptoms - Sleep Disorders	
Impaired Sleep Nightmare, Somnolence	Referring to Interprofessional Team Teaching About Sleep, Teaching About Disease
Non-motor Symptoms - Neuro Behavioral	
Impaired Mood Equilibrium Anxiety, Depression, Chronic Sadness, Impaired Adaptation, Impaired Coping Impaired Cognition Impaired Memory, Disorientation, Delirium, Hallucination, Agitation, Fear, Craving, Impaired Behaviour, Low Initiative	Facilitating the Family Ability to Participate in Care Planning Referring to Interprofessional Team Teaching Family Support Teaching About Disease
Non-motor Symptoms - Sensory	
Altered Perception Dizziness, Fatigue, Pain, Weakness Body Weight Problem	Referring to Interprofessional Team, Teaching About Managing Withdrawal Symptoms, Teaching the Patient About Disease, Teaching the Patient About Eating Pattern

Principles of Rehabilitation - Medication Regime	
Impaired Ability To Manage Medication Regime Lack Of Knowledge Of Medication Regime Medication Supply Deficit Negative Response to Medication	Assessing Risk for Negative Response to Medication, Referring for the Group to Teaching About Treatment Regime, Teaching About Medication Handling, Teaching the Group About Medication,, Teaching the Patient About Medication, Teaching the Group About Treatment Regime
Principles of Rehabilitation - Quality of life	
Caregiver Stress, Inadequate Routine, Impaired Socialisation, Impaired Quality of Life	Promoting Socialisation, Teaching the Adaptation of the Routine, Teaching the Patient to Contacting the Health Care Facility, Encouraging Positive Affirmations, Contracting for Adherence

Figure 2. The main Nursing Diagnoses/Outcomes and Interventions of Parkinson's disease mapped according to ICNP®.

2.1.1. Nursing diagnoses and outcomes related to motor symptoms, self-care, and safety

The motor symptoms of PD include resting tremor, muscle rigidity, bradykinesia, and postural instability. These symptoms were described in 1817 in a monograph by James Parkinson and are currently considered the cardinal signs for clinical diagnosis of the disease [20]. In the ICNP®, these symptoms are represented by the diagnoses and outcomes *tremor, hypoactivity,* and *risk for fall.*

2.1.1.1. Tremor

Resting tremor affects up to 75% of the patients with PD. It is characterized by involuntary tremors of the hands, lips, and jaw 4–6 Hz in intensity. They occur at rest but may worsen in stressful situations or while walking and stopping when actions are performed by the affected limb [21].

2.1.1.2. Hypoactivity

Muscle rigidity and bradykinesia are represented in the ICNP® by the term *hypoactivity*. This is a broad term that can be considered a syndrome that encompasses several specific terms corresponding to this diagnosis.

Muscle rigidity is characterized by disharmony of the flexor and extensor muscles, compromising joint mobility by making them rigid. Rigidity may lead to motor symptoms, among other problems, evidenced by reduced handwriting capacity, which is referred to as a micrograph in PD and is represented in the ICNP® by the term *impaired psychomotor activity*. Its prevalence in this population ranges from 10 to 63.2% [22].

Bradykinesia is defined as difficulty and slowness in initiating movement. It may affect the ability to perform simultaneous tasks and slow reaction times [14] and is associated with other disorders, such as decreased arm balance, hypomimia, and hypokinetic dysarthria, which are encompassed by the ICNP® terms *slurred speech* and *impaired ability to communicate by talking*.

Decreased arm balance occurs asymmetrically in the early stages of PD [3]. Hypomimia is defined as the reduction of voluntary orofacial movements that result in reduced facial expression in patients with PD. These symptoms may be related to bradykinesia [3], as well as other cognitive disorders that impair emotional recognition of facial expression [23].

Lack of motor control speech, called hypokinetic dysarthria, affects about 90% of patients with PD. It is characterized by deficits in vocalization related to the variation in the height and intensity during speech [24–26]. Its pathophysiological mechanisms have been studied, and there is empirical evidence that in addition to motor mechanisms associated with bradykinesia, cognitive mechanisms of self-perception, and self-monitoring of speech are involved [24, 25].

2.1.1.3. Risk for fall

Postural instability is related to the loss of postural reflexes, which occurs in the later stages of PD. Instability is measured by retropulsion or propulsion tests. Postural instability is defined as more than two steps backward or forward, or when there is an absence of postural response. This symptom is the most common cause of falls and contributes significantly to the risk of fractures [17].

2.1.1.4. Lack of knowledge of disease or self-care deficit

Knowledge about the disease and its symptoms promotes better patient and family management of limitations. The role of the family, both to encourage maximum independence in the patient's activities of daily living and to provide compensatory care for the deficits, is not an easy task. Thus, identification of these diagnoses is considered the starting point of the rehabilitation program.

2.1.2. Nursing diagnoses and outcomes related to nonmotor symptoms

The hierarchical organization of nonmotor symptoms includes disautonomic (urogenital, gastrointestinal, cardiovascular, and thermoregulation), sleep, neurobehavioral (mood, cognition, and psychiatric), sensory, and other subdivisions. In the ICNP®, these symptoms are represented by diagnoses and results, including impaired urinary system process, impotence, impaired gastrointestinal system process, hypotension, impaired sleep, impaired mood equilibrium, impaired cognition, and altered perception.

2.1.2.1. Impaired urinary system process

Bladder urogenital symptoms may be present in up to 96% of the patients with PD; they are characterized as storage symptoms (urgency, urge incontinence, increased daytime urinary frequency above eight micturitions, and two or more nocturnal micturitions) and emptying symptoms (hesitancy, decreased, or intermittent urine stream, sensation of incomplete emptying, and urinary retention) [27, 28].

2.1.2.2. Impotence

Sexual dysfunctions are the result of neurodegeneration and include difficulty with erection, loss of libido, and lack of orgasm. However, patients may also experience the opposite symptoms, mainly related to dopamine agonist therapy, which are characterized by obsessions or compulsions related to sex [15, 16].

2.1.2.3. *Impaired gastrointestinal system process*

In the ICNP® the diagnosis or outcome *impaired gastrointestinal system process* is also considered a broad term that may include specific diagnoses related to the same problem.

In PD, degenerative impairment of the vagus nerve, which is responsible for nervous control of the esophagus, stomach, and intestine via the parasympathetic and spinal cord system, causes dysfunction of the motility of the entire gastrointestinal tract, resulting in the following symptoms: oropharyngeal dysphagia (*impaired swallowing*), gastric stasis, constipation or slow motility (*constipation*), and sphincter dyssynergism and drooling (*abnormal salivation*) related to the decrease or absence of the swallowing reflex, which leads to the accumulation of saliva in the mouth [29, 30]. A review study also revealed that drooling may be related to both increased saliva production and slowed orofacial movements [31].

2.1.2.4. *Hypotension*

Orthostatic hypotension can result in dizziness during position changes (particularly to a standing position), fatigue, and even fainting and falls. This symptom may be subtle in early PD and does not necessarily worsen with disease progression [15, 16]. It affects about 40–60% of patients with PD, but only 20% may be symptomatic [32]. Supine hypertension, described in the organizational chart, is a sign recently debated among scientists who are in the early stages of studies on the pathophysiological mechanisms [33]. What we do know is that this symptom usually coexists with hypotension, both related to changes in the circadian rhythms of blood pressure [34].

2.1.2.5. *Impaired sleep*

Sleep disorders are very prevalent in patients with PD and have been studied extensively by scientists. Their pathophysiology is complex and results in overall impairment of the sleep–wake cycle [35, 36]. These disorders may negatively affect many biological functions and enhance associated symptoms such as cognitive, neuropsychiatric, and fatigue and affect quality of life of the patient/family [37].

2.1.2.6. *Impaired mood equilibrium*

Among neurobehavioral symptoms, mood disorders are present in 40–70% of patients with PD. The pathophysiological mechanisms of neurotransmitter regulation are demonstrably involved in the causes of depression (*depression*), apathy (*low initiative*), and social isolation (*impaired socialisation*) [16, 38, 39]. However, it is important to consider the impact of other symptoms, including motor symptoms, on the mood of patients with this disease [39].

2.1.2.7. Impaired cognition

The cognitive (minimum cognitive impairment and dementia) and neuropsychiatric (hallucination, delusion, illusion, and impulses control disorder) impairments associated with PD also have a complex pathophysiology; the manifestations vary in severity, tending to worsen with disease progression [39]. They deserve special attention from multidisciplinary health teams as they may endanger patient's health and overwhelm patient's families and caregivers [40].

2.1.2.8. Altered perception

Sensory symptoms directly related to the pathophysiology of PD include hyposmia and anosmia, ageusia, pain, and paresthesia [15, 16, 39, 41]. Fatigue has also been recently studied as an additional symptom. The prevalence of altered perception ranges from 33 to 58% and may be related to depression and apathy, sleep changes, cardiovascular dysfunction, motor symptoms, drug use, or insufficient blood flow in the frontal lobe [41].

2.1.2.9. Body weight problem

One review study described weight loss as a very common symptom in patients with PD, who have low body mass indexes compared with those of healthy controls matched by sex and age. The etiology has been described as multifactorial, related to motor symptoms, changes in eating habits, and medication use (especially levodopa) in addition to being potentially related to physiological changes in the neurodegenerative process [39].

2.1.3. Nursing diagnoses related to the principles of rehabilitation

Most of the symptoms of Parkinson's disease can be controlled by drugs, which make it necessary to assess patient adherence to treatment.

Drug treatment regimens for PD are complex since the variability in symptoms denotes the necessity of drug combination subdivided into smaller doses over 24 hours [42]. While the indication and prescription of drugs are obviously performed by physicians, nurses play an important role in treatment adherence.

There are several reasons why patients may not adhere to drug treatment, which are classified as intentional and unintentional [43].

2.1.3.1. Lack of knowledge of medication regime and negative response to medication

One of the unintentional reasons for compromised treatment adherence is a lack of patient's understanding on the importance of treatment. Patients often believe that drug therapy will cure their symptoms, not realizing that the therapy is aimed at reducing their severity in order to promote better quality of life. Moreover, the presence of motor fluctuations and complications of the therapy itself promotes disbelief regarding the effectiveness of treatment, which in turn contributes to nonadherence.

2.1.3.2. Medication supply deficit and impaired ability to manage medication regime

The factors associated with unintentional nonadherence are often a result of poor access to treatment because of the high cost of medications. Likewise, unintentional nonadherence may result from the patient's inability to self-manage their medications. This inability may result from cognitive deficits, education level, and cultural, religious, and behavioral factors.

Thus, accurate assessment of the causes of nonadherence to drug therapy in patients with PD underscores the importance of the nursing care plan, which therefore will complement multiprofessional health actions focused on the patient, promoting improvement of their quality of life through better control of their symptoms.

2.1.3.3. Impaired quality of life and socialisation, inadequate routine, and caregiver stress

The impact of the disease on routine activities, socialization, and quality of life of patients who are affected by the symptoms of PD may compromise their independence in performing the activities of daily life as well as their professional lives. In a ripple effect, these problems will results in individual, family, and social losses [13, 44, 45].

2.1.4. Nursing interventions related to nonmotor and motor symptoms and principles of rehabilitation

2.1.4.1. "Teaching" interventions

Among the main nursing interventions mapped, those related to educational practice and used by nurses as the main tool for health promotion were of particular importance.

Health education is considered a change of strategy in care models and is an alternative used to improve the quality of health and life of the population through increased understanding of health and disease [46].

Health promotion actions in neurological rehabilitation facilitate recovery and adaptation to the limitations imposed by disabilities on individual and contextualized bases. These actions mainly focus on functional, motor, psychosocial, and spiritual aspects [46].

Therefore, it is imperative for nurses to establish bonds with patients and their families when providing orientations in order to promote facilitation and implementation of learning. In this coparticipatory relationship, the focus is on personal autonomy for affirmation of the principles of citizenship and democracy, with the aim to improve health status [46].

2.1.4.2. "Referring" interventions

We highlight the interventions that reveal the important role played by interprofessional nurses, which are based on the best evidence to identify symptoms and collaborate with the team through discussion and referral of patients for evaluation. These interventions show that nurses are often the connection point with other members of the professional team in order to provide holistic care [47].

2.2. Nursing protocols for patients with Parkinson's disease

Accurate identification of nursing diagnoses is essential for clinical practice since it enables proper planning of care, implementation of interventions, and efficient evaluation of the results.

Therefore, it is necessary to use diagnostic support tools prepared in accordance with institutional settings and the complexity of patient's conditions. These tools should still be based on the best clinical evidence and recommendations described in the scientific literature.

This subchapter presents several nursing assessment protocols in the context of the activities of daily living, gastrointestinal and genitourinary function, sleep disorders, hypotension, and medication adherence.

Nursing assessment for daily life activities in patients with Parkinson's disease

Date: _____/_____/_______

Personal data
Name: ________________ Age: ___ Sex: ( ) Female ( ) Male Family/Caregiver:________________
Date of onset of symptoms of Parkinson's disease: ____
Concomitant diseases: _____________ Daily medications: ________________________________
Housing conditions and family support
( ) Own residence ( ) Rented residence ( ) Residence of relatives/friends ( ) Institutionalized
( ) House with a single level ( ) House with multiple levels ( ) Stairs with unilateral handrail ( ) Stairs with bilateral handrail ( ) Stairs without handrail ( ) No stairs ( ) Apartment with elevator ( ) Apartment with no elevator
Adaptation at residence? ( ) yes ( ) no Where?____
( ) Live alone ( ) Live with whom? ______________________ Family/caregiver support? ( ) Yes ( ) No
Routine
Describe your routine before the Parkinson's disease diagnosis:______________________________
____
Describe your current routine:____
____
Schwab and England activities of daily living [48]
100%-Completely independent. Able to do all chores without slowness, difficulty, or impairment. Essentially normal. Unaware of any difficulty.
90%-Completely independent. Able to do all chores with some degree of slowness, difficulty, and impairment. Might take twice as long. Beginning to be aware of difficulty.
80%-Completely independent in most chores. Takes twice as long. Conscious of difficulty and slowness.

70%-Not completely independent. More difficulty with some chores. Three to four times as long in some. Must spend a large part of the day with chores.

60%-Some dependency. Can do most chores but exceedingly slowly and with much effort. Errors; some impossible.

50%-More dependent. Help with half, slower, et cetera. Difficulty with everything.

40%-Very dependent. Can assist with all chores, but few alone.

30%-With effort, now and then does a few chores alone or begins alone. Much help needed.

20%-Nothing alone. Can be a slight help with some chores. Severe invalid.

10%-Total dependent, helpless. Complete invalid.

0%-Vegetative functions such as swallowing, bladder, and bowel functions are not functioning. Bed-ridden.

MDS-UPDRS Part II scale can be applied

Nursing diagnoses	Nursing interventions

Evaluation of patient's ability to perform activities of daily life is complex because it involves environmental aspects (usually related to the accessibility of the house), family support or caregivers, and commitment to the routine. The assessment should be based on standardized scales, such as the Unified Parkinson's Disease Rating Scale (UPDRS) Part II and the Schwab and England activities of daily living scales widely used in research and clinical practice [48–50].

Nursing assessment of bowel status in patients with Parkinson's disease

Date: ____/____/______

Personal data
Name: ____________ Age: ___ Sex: ( ) Female ( ) Male Family/Caregiver:______________
Onset date of symptoms of PD: ____
Concomitant diseases: ____
Daily medications:____
Digestive system function
Main complaint: ____
Onset of symptoms: ____ Presence of symptoms before PD: ( ) Yes ( ) No How many years? _____
Background surgical gastrointestinal tract: ( ) Yes ( ) No What: ___________________________
Regular monitoring by gastroenterologist: ( ) Yes ( ) No
Feel the urge for bowel movement? ( ) Several times/day ( ) Daily ( ) Every 1-2 days ( ) Every 1-_ days
Flatulence? ( ) Never ( ) Sometimes ( ) Often ( ) Always
Fecal Incontinence? ( ) Never ( ) Sometimes ( ) Often ( ) Always
When does fecal incontinence occur? (You can mark more than one answer)

( ) During a diarrheal episode ( ) Every time because of the urgency ( ) When coughing and rising ( ) Unexpectedly

Rome III Criteria [51]

Must include two or more of the following:

( ) Straining during at least 25% of defecations

( ) Lumpy or hard stools in at least 25% of defecations

( ) Sensation of incomplete evacuation for at least 25% of defecations

( ) Sensation of anorectal obstruction/blockage for at least 25% of defecations

( ) Manual maneuvers to facilitate at least 25% of defecations (e.g., digital evacuation)

( ) Fewer than three defecations per week

* Criteria fulfilled for the last three months with symptom onset at least six months prior to diagnosis

Bristol scale

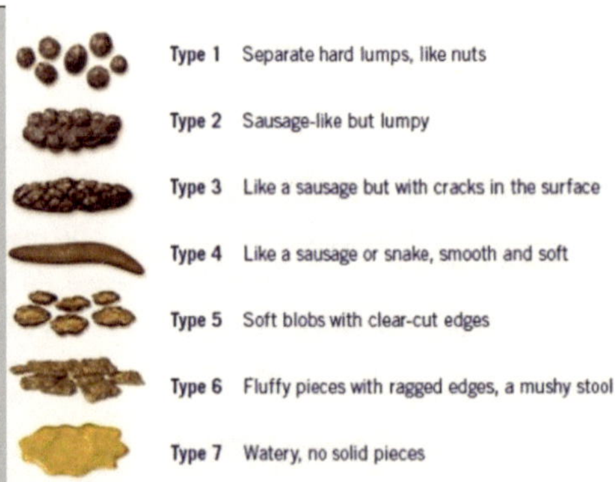

In most evacuations, what is the characteristic of the feces? ____________________

Devices for evacuation	Complications
( ) External device for evacuation ( ) Toilet	( ) Diverticulitis
( ) Diapers	( ) Hernia
( ) Have you ever undergone intestinal cleansing	( ) Volvulus
( ) Laxatives/or antigas medication Which?______	( ) Other: ____________________
How often do you use laxative or antigas medication? ( ) > 1×/month ( ) > 1×/week ( ) > 1×/day	

Mobility

Are you dependent on others for evacuation: ( ) Yes ( ) No

Transfer to lavatory seat: ( ) Independent ( ) Dependent

Locomotion: ( ) Without assistance and without support ( ) Locomotion assistance

Self-care

Dependant on others to eat and/or drink ( ) Yes ( ) No Why?__________ Daily water intake _____

Low tolerance for liquids? ( ) Yes ( ) No Do you have adipsia? ( ) Yes ( ) No

( ) Dysphagia for liquids ( ) Dysphagia for solids ( ) Need to change food consistency

Food routine:

Breakfast: ______________________________

Snack: ______________________________

Lunch: ______________________________

Snack: ______________________________

Dinner: ______________________________

Supper: ______________________________

Mental function

Dependant on others? ( ) Yes ( ) No Why?______________________________

Cognitive disorders? ( ) Yes ( ) No What: ______________________________

Behavioral disorders? ( ) Yes ( ) No What: ______________________________

Housing conditions

Easy access to the bathroom: ( ) Yes ( ) No

Modifications made to bathroom/home: ( ) Yes ( ) No What? ______________________________

Modifications to the bathroom/home are required: ( ) Yes ( ) No What? ______________________________

Community, social, and civic life

Impact on labour activities related to constipation ( ) Yes ( ) No ( ) Not applicable

Impact on leisure activities related to constipation ( ) Yes ( ) No

Impact on quality of life related to constipation ( ) Yes ( ) No

Have financial resources for modifications, medicines, and intestinal devices? ( ) Yes ( ) No

Physical examination

Inspection:

- Skin: ______________________________

- Contour: ( ) Plan ( ) Excavated ( ) Globular

- Symmetry: ______________________________

Abdominal auscultation (Intestinal noises): ( ) 2 to 5/min ( ) < 2 to 5/min ( ) > than 2 to 5/min

Percussion: ( ) Tympanic ( ) Hypertympanic ( )Massive Quadrant:______________________________

Abdominal palpation: ______________________________

Nursing diagnoses	Nursing interventions

Evaluation of intestinal symptoms in patients with PD focuses on constipation, which is the main problem. However, it is important to assess other symptoms such as fecal incontinence and related factors that enhance intestinal symptoms such as changes in mobility/accessibility, swallowing, and cognitive function, among others. The Rome III criteria and the Bristol Stool Scale are recommended tools for evaluation of constipation [51, 52].

Genitourinary nursing assessment in patients with Parkinson's disease

Date: ____/____/______

Personal data

Name: ____________ Age: __ Sex: ( ) Female ( ) Male Family/Caregiver:_________________

Date of onset of symptoms of Parkinson's disease: ______________________________________

Concomitant diseases: ____

Daily medications: ____

Genitourinary, reproductive, and bowel functions

Number of pregnancies and births: _______ ( ) Vaginal birth ( ) Caesarean ( ) Abortions: _______

Main complaint: ____

Onset of symptoms: ______________ Presence of symptoms before PD: ( ) Yes ( ) No

History of uro/gynaecology surgery: ( ) Yes ( ) No Which: _________________________

Regular monitoring by urologist/gynaecologist: ( ) Yes ( ) No

Sensation of bladder fullness ( ) Yes ( ) No

Bladder control ( ) Yes ( ) No Urinary Urgency ( ) Yes ( ) No Urinary Loss ( ) Yes ( ) No

Intestinal function: ( ) Regular ( ) Irregular Frequency:_____________________________

Do the bladder symptoms impact sexual capacity ( ) Yes ( ) No How? __________________

Storage symptoms

( ) Urinary Urgency ( ) Urge Incontinence

( ) Stress incontinence ( ) Enuresis

( ) Increased frequency of diurnal urinary

( ) Nocturia. How many times?_______

Voiding symptoms

( )Decreased urinary stream( )Hesitation

( )Urinary flow intermittent ( )Voiding Effort

( )Sensation of incomplete emptying ( )Dysuria

( )Dripping ( )Initial Dripping ( )Terminal Dripping

Urinary devices

( ) Toilet ( ) urinals bedpans

( ) Indwelling catheter

( ) Diapers

( ) Absorbent intimate feminine

( ) Catheterization intermittent bladder

( ) External condom collecting device

Complications of urinary tract

( ) Urethral fistula

( ) Cystocele

( ) Prostatic hyperplasia

( ) Urethral Stenosis

( )Hydronephrosis D/E

( ) Urethral diverticulum

( ) Lithiasis vescial

( ) Renal lithiasis

( ) Renal failure

( ) Lesion of penis

( ) Urinary tract infection

Self-care	
Daily water intake _________ Appropriate division of ingestion ( ) Yes ( ) No	
Liquid dysphagia ( ) Yes ( ) No Low tolerance for liquids ( ) Yes ( ) No	
Dependant on others for toileting ( ) Yes ( ) No	
Do you require instruction on how to use the urinary device? ( ) Yes ( ) No	
Mobility	
Dependant on others ( ) Yes ( ) No Why?_____________________________________	
Impairment: ( ) Bradykinesia ( ) Tremor ( ) Postural instability ( ) Motor complications	
Locomotion: ( ) Without Assistance and without support ( ) Locomotion with assistance Which?______	
Falls: ( ) Yes ( ) No ( ) Falls between bed- and bathroom: ( ) Yes ( ) No Risk of falls: ( ) Yes ( ) No Why? ____	
Mental function	
Cognitive/behavioral disorders: ( ) Yes ( ) No Which: ________________________	
Sleep	
Dependent on medication: ( ) Yes ( ) No Wakes from sleep by urinary desire: ( ) Yes ( ) No	
Sleep disorders: ( ) Yes ( ) No	
Housing conditions	
Live alone ( ) Yes ( ) No Accessible bathroom ( ) Yes ( ) No	
It is able to maintain a safe environment without help? ( ) Yes ( ) No	
Has made modification to the bathroom ( ) Yes ( ) No What? _________________________	
Needs to modify the bathroom/home ( ) Yes ( ) No What?________________________	
Community, social, and civic life	
Impact on labor activities related to genitourinary disorders ( ) Yes ( ) No ( ) Not applicable	
Impact on leisure activities related to genitourinary disorders ( ) Yes ( ) No	
Impact on quality of life related to genitourinary disorders ( ) Yes ( ) No	
Have financial resources for modifications, medicines, and urinary devices? ( ) Yes ( ) No	
Nursing diagnoses	**Nursing interventions**

Evaluation of bladder symptoms in patients with PD is complex because it involves investigation of urinary, gynecological/urological, cognitive/behavioral, and sleep symptoms, as well as mobility/accessibility and quality of life. Thus, nurse evaluations should focus on several aspects that may contribute to these changes in order to propose appropriate interventions. Some measurement scales may be used, including the Overactive Bladder questionnaire (OAB-q) [53], Questionnaire on Pelvic Organ Function [54], and the Scale for Outcomes in Parkinson's disease (SCOPA-AUT) [55].

Nursing assessment for sleep disorders in patients with Parkinson's disease

Date: ____/____/______

Personal data	
Name: ____________ Age: __ Sex: ( ) Female ( ) Male Family/Caregiver:______________	
Date of onset of symptoms of Parkinson's disease: ______________________________	
Concomitant diseases: ____	
Daily medications: ____	
Sleep assessment	
Complaint: _______________________ Onset of symptoms of sleep disorder: _________	
Use medication to sleep? ( ) yes ( ) no Impact on quality of life of the patient: ( ) yes ( ) no	
Has sleep routine? ( ) yes ( ) no Impact on quality of life of the family: ( ) yes ( ) no	
Sleep disorders related to motor symptoms	
Difficulty with movement in bed: ( ) Yes ( ) No	Morning dystonia: ( ) Yes ( ) No
Tremors that compromise the quality of sleep: ( ) Yes ( ) No	Restless leg syndrome: ( ) Yes ( ) No
Sleep disorders related to nonmotor symptoms	
Hallucinations: ( ) Yes ( ) No	Mental confusion: ( ) Yes ( ) No
Sleep apnoea/difficulty breathing: ( ) Yes ( ) No	Pain: ( ) Yes ( ) No
Nocturia: ( ) Yes ( ) No	
Specific symptoms of sleep disorders	
Initial insomnia: ( ) Yes ( ) No	Sleep-talking: ( ) Yes ( ) No
Terminal insomnia: ( ) Yes ( ) No	Nightmares: ( ) Yes ( ) No
Nonrestorative sleep: ( ) Yes ( ) No	Vivid dreams: ( ) Yes ( ) No
Specific symptoms of daytime sleep disorders	
Sleeping unexpectedly during the day: ( ) Yes ( ) No	Sleep while talking: ( ) Yes ( ) No
Sleeping while watching TV: ( ) Yes ( ) No	Sleep while sitting: ( ) Yes ( ) No
Difficulty staying awake during the day: ( ) Yes ( ) No	
Nursing diagnoses	**Nursing interventions**

Evaluations of symptoms that cause sleep disorders should be approached with care and cover various related aspects, including motor/nonmotor function and night/day sleep disorders. Measurement scales can be used for this assessment and may include those recommended by the Movement Disorders Society Task Force: the PD sleep scale (PDSS), Pittsburgh sleep quality index (PSQI), SCOPA-sleep (SCOPA), and the Epworth sleepiness scale (ESS) [56]. We also emphasize that the PDSS scale has been revised and the PDSS-2 version has been validated [57].

Nursing assessment for orthostatic hypotension in patients with Parkinson's disease

Date: _____/_____/_______

Personal data	
Name: ________________ Age: ___ Sex: ( ) Female ( ) Male Family/Caregiver:______________	
Date of onset of symptoms of Parkinson's disease: ______________________________________	
Concomitant diseases: ____	
Daily medications: ____	
Autonomic scale for outcomes in Parkinson's disease (SCOPA-AUT): Hypotension section	
In the past month, when standing up, have you had the feeling of either becoming light-headed, not seeing properly, or not thinking clearly?	
( ) Never ( ) Sometimes ( ) Regularly ( ) Often	
In the past month, did you become light-headed after standing for sometime?	
( ) Never ( ) Sometimes ( ) Regularly ( ) Often	
Have you fainted in the past six months?	
( ) Never ( ) Sometimes ( ) Regularly ( ) Often	
Composite Autonomic Symptom Scale (COMPASS 31): Hypotension section [59]	
1. In the past year, have you ever felt faint, dizzy, "goofy", or had difficulty thinking soon after standing up from a sitting or lying position? (1) Yes (2) No	
2. When standing up, how frequently do you get these feelings or symptoms?	
(1) Rarely (2) Occasionally (3) Frequently (4) Almost Always	
3. How would you rate the severity of these feelings or symptoms?	
(1) Mild (2) Moderate (3) Severe	
4. In the past year, have these feelings or symptoms that you have experienced:	
(1) Gotten much worse (2) Gotten somewhat worse (3) Stayed about the same	
(4) Gotten somewhat better (5) Gotten much better (6) Completely gone	
Physical Examination	
Blood pressure (BP) lying:_____X_____mmHg	Cardiac frequency (CF) lying:___hpm
BP in orthostasis:____X___mmHg (immediately)	CF in orthostasis:___hpm (immediately)
BP in orthostasis: ___X___mmHg (after 3min)	CF in orthostasis:___hpm (after 3min)
*Criteria for orthostatic hypotension: when a person moves from a supine to a sitting or a standing position occurs a decline of >20 mmHg in systolic blood pressure or a decline of >10 mmHg in diastolic blood pressure. The decrease must be present within 3 minutes after the postural change [60].	
Nursing diagnoses	**Nursing interventions**

Evaluation of orthostatic hypotension in patients with PD should be part of nursing protocol. Different measurement scales can be used, including those recommended by the Movement Disorders Society Task Force [58]: SCOPA-AUT and the Composite Autonomic Symptom Scale (COMPASS) [59]. Nursing care can be based on "Clinical Practice Guidelines: Patient Self-Management of BP Instability in Multiple System Atrophy, Parkinson's Disease and Other Neurological Disorders" [60].

Nursing assessment for medication adherence in patients with Parkinson's disease

Date: _____/_____/_______

Personal Data		
Name: _______________ Age: ___ Sex: ( ) Female ( ) Male Family/Caregiver:________________		
Date of onset of symptoms of Parkinson's disease: ____		
Daily medication		
Number of pills/time of ingestion	Number of pills/time of ingestion	Medication action/Side effects
		Time-action:______________________ ( ) dyskinesia ( ) wearing-off ( ) ON/OFF ( ) nausea/vomiting ( ) No side effect ( ) Other: ( ) take the pills with food/protein
Morisky Medication Adherence Scale: High adherence (8 points), medium (6 to < 8 points) and low adherence (<6 points) [61]		
1) Do you sometimes forget to take your pills for PD?		(0) Yes (1) No
2) People sometimes miss taking their medications for reasons other than forgetting. Thinking over the past two weeks, were there any days when you did not take your medicine?		(0) Yes (1) No
3) Have you ever cut back or stopped taking your medicine without telling your doctor because you felt worse when you took it?		(0) Yes (1) No
4) When you travel or leave home, do you sometimes forget to bring along your medicine?		(0) Yes (1) No
5) Did you take all your medicine yesterday?		(0) Yes (1) No
6) When you feel like your symptoms are under control, do you sometimes stop taking your medicine?		(0) Yes (1) No
7) Taking medicine every day is a real inconvenience for some people. Do you ever feel hassled about sticking to your treatment plan?		(0) Yes (1) No
8) How often do you have difficulty remembering to take all your medicine?		( )Never/rarely ( )Once in a while ( )Sometimes ( )Usually ( )All the time
Self-care		

Dependent on others for management of medications? ( ) yes ( ) no
( )Dysphagia for liquids ( )Dysphagia for solids: capsules/tablets ( )Change the consistency of medications
Mental function
Cognitive disorders: ( ) Yes ( ) No What: ___
Neuropsychiatric disorders: ( ) No ( ) Visual hallucinations ( ) Auditory hallucinations ( ) Impulsivity
( ) Hypersexuality ( ) Anxiety
Housing conditions
Live alone ( ) Yes ( ) No Easy access to where medications are stored ( ) Yes ( ) No
Community, social, and civic life
Impact on labor activities related to drug use? ( ) Yes ( ) No ( ) Not applicable
Impact on leisure activities related to drug use? ( ) Yes ( ) No
Impact on quality of life related to drug use? ( ) Yes ( ) No
Have financial resources to purchase medicines? ( ) Yes ( ) No
Support and relationships
Requires support of family/caregiver for management of medicines? ( ) Yes ( ) No
Resources to remember to take medication (box organizer, alarms, cellular)? ( )Yes ( ) No
Have financial resources to purchase medicines? ( ) Yes ( ) No
Acquires the medications by the public health system? ( ) Yes ( ) No
Suffers consequences of insufficient supply of medicines? ( ) Yes ( ) No ( ) Public services ( ) Private service
Nursing diagnoses Nursing interventions

Evaluation of medication adherence should consider aspects related to medication (expected, adverse, and side effects; action time; costs; etc.), other symptoms of PD (dysphagia, cognitive/neuropsychiatric disorders), impact on the quality of life, and family support/caregiver for management of treatment. The scale most commonly used in research and clinical practice is the Morisky Medical Adherence Scale (MMAS) [62–64].

3. Conclusion

The important role of nurses in the multidisciplinary care of patients with PD is obvious, and training of increasing numbers of professionals to meet the growing demand is an absolutely plausible goal.

Health actions based on comprehensive care centered on patients and their families, based on ethical, legal, operational, and theoretical premises of the profession and grounded in the concepts of prevention, promotion, treatment, and rehabilitation, provide quality and scientific rigor for patient care. These actions may help to improve the quality of life of individuals with neurodegenerative diseases that are multisystem, incurable, and often disabling.

Development of an organizational chart of the motor and nonmotor symptoms of PD and a survey of the main diagnoses/outcomes and nursing interventions based on a standardized language can direct clinical reasoning of professionals who care for these patients. Moreover, these tools may enable the development and/or improvement of clinical protocols that underlie the systematization of nursing care.

Author details

Michelle Hyczy de Siqueira Tosin[1*] and Beatriz Guitton Renaud Baptista de Oliveira[2]

*Address all correspondence to: michellehyczy@gmail.com

1 Sarah Network of Rehabilitation Hospitals, Rio de Janeiro, RJ, Brazil

2 School of Nursing, Federal Fluminense University, Niterói, RJ, Brazil

References

[1] Martinez-Martin P, Jeukens-Visser M, Lyons KE, Rodriguez-Blazquez C, Selai C, Siderowf A, et al. Health-related quality-of-life scales in Parkinson's disease: critique and recommendations. Mov Disord. 2011;26(13):2371–80.

[2] Nalls MA, McLean CY, Rick J, Eberly S, Hutten SJ, Gwinn K, et al. Diagnosis of Parkinson's disease on the basis of clinical and genetic classification: a population-based modelling study. Lancet Neurol. 2015;14(10):1002–9.

[3] Postuma RB, Berg D, Stern M, Poewe W, Olanow CW, Oertel W, et al. MDS clinical diagnostic criteria for Parkinson's disease. Mov Disord. 2015;30(12):1591–601.

[4] Martinez-Martin P, Rodriguez-Blazquez C, Paz S, Forjaz MJ, Frades-Payo B, Cubo E, et al. Parkinson symptoms and health related quality of life as predictors of costs: a longitudinal observational study with linear mixed model analysis. PLoS One. 2015;10(12):e0145310.

[5] Skelly R, Lindop F, Johnson C. Multidisciplinary care of patients with Parkinson's disease. Prog Neurol Psychiatry. 2012;16(2):10–4.

[6] Cohen EV, Hagestuen R, Gonzalez-Ramos G, Cohen HW, Bassich C, Book E, et al. Interprofessional education increases knowledge, promotes team building, and changes practice in the care of Parkinson's disease. Parkinsonism Relat Disord. 2016;22:21–7.

[7] Noorden RV. Interdisciplinary research by the numbers. Nature. 2015;525:306–7.

[8] Tosin MH, Campos DM, Blanco L, Santana RF, Oliveira BG. Mapping nursing language terms of Parkinson's disease. Rev Esc Enferm USP. 2015;49(3):409–16.

[9] Kim TY, Hardiker N, Coenen A. Inter-terminology mapping of nursing problems. J Biomed Inform. 2014;49:213–20.

[10] Tosin MH, Mecone CA, Oliveira BG. International Classification for Nursing Practice —ICNP(R): application to the Brazilian reality. Rev Bras Enferm. 2015;68(4):730–1.

[11] Cotton P, Heisters D. How to care for people with Parkinson's disease. Nurs Times. 2012;108(16):12–3.

[12] Campos DbM, Tosin MHdS, Blanco L, Santana RF, Oliveira BGRBd. Nursing diagnoses for urinary disorders in patients with Parkinson's disease. Acta Paul Enferm. 2015;28(2): 190–5.

[13] Beaudet L, Ducharme F. Living with moderate-stage Parkinson disease: intervention needs and preferences of elderly couples. J Neurosci Nurs. 2013;45(2):88–95.

[14] Gopalakrishna A, Alexander SA. Understanding Parkinson disease: a complex and multifaceted illness. J Neurosci Nurs. 2015;47(6):320–6.

[15] Chen W, Xu ZM, Wang G, Chen SD. Non-motor symptoms of Parkinson's disease in China: a review of the literature. Parkinsonism Relat Disord. 2012;18(5):446–52.

[16] Hou J-GG, Lai EC. Nonmotor symptoms of Parkinson's disease. Int J Gerontol. 2007;1(2):53.

[17] Jankovic J. Parkinson's disease: clinical features and diagnosis. J Neurol Neurosurg Psychiatry. 2008;79(4):368–76.

[18] Vernon GM. Parkinson disease and the nurse practitioner: diagnostic and management challenges. J Nurse Pract. 2009;5(3):195–206.

[19] Tosin, MHS. Subconjunto terminológico da CIPE® para pacientes com doença de Parkinson em reabilitação. 2016. 193 f. Dissertação (Mestrado Profissional em Enfermagem Assistencial) - Escola de Enfermagem Aurora de Afonso Costa, Niterói, 2016 URL: http://www.repositorio.uff.br/jspui/handle/1/1775

[20] Kurtis MM, Rodriguez-Blazquez C, Martinez-Martin P, Group E. Relationship between sleep disorders and other non-motor symptoms in Parkinson's disease. Parkinsonism Relat Disord. 2013;19(12):1152–5.

[21] Behari M, Bhattacharyya KB, Borgohain R, Das SK, Ghosh B, Kishore A, et al. Parkinson's disease. Ann Indian Acad Neurol. 2011;14(Suppl 1):S2–6.

[22] Letanneux A, Danna J, Velay JL, Viallet F, Pinto S. From micrographia to Parkinson's disease dysgraphia. Mov Disord. 2014;29(12):1467–75.

[23] Ricciardi L, Bologna M, Morgante F, Ricciardi D, Morabito B, Volpe D, et al. Reduced facial expressiveness in Parkinson's disease: A pure motor disorder? J Neurol Sci. 2015;358(1–2):125–30.

[24] New AB, Robin DA, Parkinson AL, Eickhoff CR, Reetz K, Hoffstaedter F, et al. The intrinsic resting state voice network in Parkinson's disease. Hum Brain Mapp. 2015;36(5):1951–62.

[25] Kwan LC, Whitehill TL. Perception of speech by individuals with Parkinson's disease: a review. Parkinsons Dis. 2011;2011:389767.

[26] Ramig LO, Fox C, Sapir S. Speech treatment for Parkinson's disease. Expert Rev Neurother 2008;8(2):299–311.

[27] Uchiyama T, Sakakibara R, Yamamoto T, Ito T, Yamaguchi C, Awa Y, et al. Urinary dysfunction in early and untreated Parkinson's disease. J Neurol Neurosurg Psychiatry. 2011;82(12):1382–6.

[28] Xue Peng WT, Zong Huantao and Zhang Yong. Urodynamic analysis and treatment of male Parkinson's disease. Chin Med J. 2014;127(5):878–81.

[29] Jost WH. Gastrointestinal dysfunction in Parkinson's Disease. J Neurol Sci. 2010;289(1–2):69–73.

[30] Sung H-Y, Park J-W, Kim J-S. The frequency and severity of gastrointestinal symptoms in patients with early Parkinson's disease. Mov Disord. 2014;7(1):7–12.

[31] Zlotnik Y, Balash Y, Korczyn AD, Giladi N, Gurevich T. Disorders of the oral cavity in Parkinson's disease and parkinsonian syndromes. Parkinsons Dis. 2015;2015:379482.

[32] Isaacson SH, Skettini J. Neurogenic orthostatic hypotension in Parkinson's disease: evaluation, management, and emerging role of droxidopa. Vasc Health Risk Manag. 2014;10:169–76.

[33] Mazza A, Ravenni R, Antonini A, Casiglia E, Rubello D, Pauletto P. Arterial hypertension, a tricky side of Parkinson's disease: physiopathology and therapeutic features. Neurol Sci. 2013;34(5):621–7.

[34] Berganzo K, Díez-Arrola B, Tijero B, Somme J, Lezcano E, Llorens V, et al. Nocturnal hypertension and dysautonomia in patients with Parkinson's disease: are they related? J Neurol. 2013;260(7):1752–6.

[35] Postuma RB, Adler CH, Dugger BN, Hentz JG, Shill HA, Driver-Dunckley E, et al. REM sleep behavior disorder and neuropathology in Parkinson's disease. Mov Disord. 2015;30(10):1413–7.

[36] Boeve BF. Idiopathic REM sleep behaviour disorder in the development of Parkinson's disease. Lancet Neurol. 2013;12(5):469–82.

[37] Maass A, Reichmann H. Sleep and non-motor symptoms in Parkinson's disease. J Neural Transm. 2013;120(4):565–9.

[38] Robert G, Le Jeune F, Lozachmeur C, Drapier S, Dondaine T, Peron J, et al. Apathy in patients with Parkinson disease without dementia or depression: a PET study. Neurology. 2012;79(11):1155–60.

[39] Munhoz RP, Moro A, Silveira-Moriyama L, Teive HA. Non-motor signs in Parkinson's disease: a review. Arq Neuropsiquiatr. 2015;73(5):454–62.

[40] Martinez-Martin P, Rodriguez-Blazquez C, Forjaz MJ, Frades-Payo B, Agüera-Ortiz L, Weintraub D, et al. Neuropsychiatric symptoms and caregiver's burden in Parkinson's disease. Parkinsonism Relat Disord. 2015;21(6):629–34.

[41] Berardelli A, Conte A, Fabbrini G, Bologna M, Latorre A, Rocchi L, et al. Pathophysiology of pain and fatigue in Parkinson's disease. Parkinsonism Relat Disord. 2012;18:S226–S8.

[42] Connolly BS, Lang AE. Pharmacological treatment of Parkinson disease: a review. JAMA. 2014;311(16):1670–83.

[43] Shin JY, Habermann B, Pretzer-Aboff I. Challenges and strategies of medication adherence in Parkinson's disease: a qualitative study. Geriatr Nurs. 2015;36(3):192–6.

[44] Starhof C, Anker N, Henriksen T, Lassen CF. Dependency and transfer incomes in idiopathic Parkinson's disease. Dan Med J. 2014;61(10):1–5.

[45] Young-Mason J. The fine art of caring: people with Parkinson disease and their care partners. Clin Nurse Spec. 2015;29(2):121–2.

[46] Silva KnLd, Sena RRnd, Grillo MJC, Horta NldCs, Prado PMC. Nursing education and the challenges for health promotion. Rev Bras Enferm. 2009;62(1):86–91.

[47] Vaughn S, Mauk KL, Jacelon CS, Larsen PD, Rye J, Wintersgill W, et al. The competency model for professional rehabilitation nursing. Rehabil Nurs. 2015;0:1–12.

[48] Rehabilitation Measures Database [Internet]. Available from: http://www. rehabmeasures.org/Lists/RehabMeasures/DispForm.aspx?ID=1012. [Accessed: 2016-03-13].

[49] Lawrence BJ, Gasson N, Kane R, Bucks RS, Loftus AM. Activities of daily living, depression, and quality of life in Parkinson's disease. PLoS One. 2014;9(7):e102294.

[50] Martinez-Martin P, Prieto L, Forjaz MJo. Longitudinal metric properties of disability rating scales for Parkinson's disease. Value Health. 2006;9(6):386–93.

[51] Guidelines WGOG. Constipation: a global perspective; 2010.

[52] Evatt ML, Chaudhuri KR, Chou KL, Cubo E, Hinson V, Kompoliti K, et al. Dysautonomia rating scales in Parkinson's disease: sialorrhea, dysphagia, and constipation—critique and recommendations by movement disorders task force on rating scales for Parkinson's disease. Mov Disord. 2009;24(5):635–46.

[53] Iacovelli E, Gilio F, Meco G, Fattapposta F, Vanacore N, Brusa L, et al. Bladder symptoms assessed with overactive bladder questionnaire in Parkinson's disease. Mov Disord. 2010;25(9):1203–9.

[54] Sakakibara R, Shinotoh H, Uchiyama T, Sakuma M, Kashiwado M, Yoshiyama M, et al. Questionnaire-based assessment of pelvic organ dysfunction in Parkinson's disease. Auton Neurosci. 2001(92):76–85.

[55] Visser M, Marinus J, Stiggelbout AM, Van Hilten JJ. Assessment of autonomic dysfunction in Parkinson's disease: the SCOPA-AUT. Mov Disord. 2004;19(11):1306–12.

[56] Hogl B, Arnulf I, Comella C, Ferreira J, Iranzo A, Tilley B, et al. Scales to assess sleep impairment in Parkinson's disease: critique and recommendations. Mov Disord. 2010;25(16):2704–16.

[57] Trenkwalder C, Kohnen R, Hogl B, Metta V, Sixel-Doring F, Frauscher B, et al. Parkinson's disease sleep scale—validation of the revised version PDSS-2. Mov Disord. 2011;26(4):644–52.

[58] Pavy-Le Traon A, Amarenco G, Duerr S, Kaufmann H, Lahrmann H, Shaftman SR, et al. The movement disorders task force review of dysautonomia rating scales in Parkinson's disease with regard to symptoms of orthostatic hypotension. Mov Disord. 2011;26(11):1985–92.

[59] Sletten DM, Suarez GA, Low PA, Mandrekar J, Singer W. COMPASS 31: a refined and abbreviated Composite Autonomic Symptom Score. Mayo Clin Proc. 2012;87(12):1196–201.

[60] Viscomi P, Jeffrey J. Development of clinical practice guidelines or patient management of blood pressure in stability in multiple system atrophy, Parkinson's disease, and other neurological disorders. Can J Neurosci Nurs. 2010;32(2):6–19.

[61] Morisky Medication Adherence Scales: MMAS-4 and MMAS-8 [Internet]. https://www.mainequalitycounts.org/image_upload/5_Morisky_Medication_Adherence.pdf. [Accessed: 2016-03-13].

[62] Fabbrini G, Abbruzzese G, Barone P, Antonini A, Tinazzi M, Castegnaro G, et al. Adherence to anti-Parkinson drug therapy in the "REASON" sample of Italian patients with Parkinson's disease: the linguistic validation of the Italian version of the "Morisky Medical Adherence Scale-8 items." Neurol Sci. 2013;34(11):2015–22.

[63] Lakshminarayana R, Wang D, Burn D, Chaudhuri KR, Cummins G, Galtrey C, et al. Smartphone- and Internet-assisted self-management and adherence tools to manage Parkinson's disease (SMART-PD): study protocol for a randomised controlled trial. Trials. 2014;7(15).

[64] Santos-García D, Prieto-Formoso M, Fuente-Fernández Rdl. Levodopa dosage determines adherence to long-acting dopamine agonists in Parkinson's disease. Neurol Sci. 2012;318(1–2):90–3.